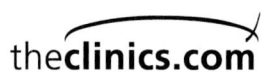

A. Simon Turner, BVSc, MS
CONSULTING EDITOR

VETERINARY CLINICS OF NORTH AMERICA

Equine Practice

Evidence-Based Veterinary Medicine

GUEST EDITOR
David W. Ramey, DVM

August 2007 • Volume 23 • Number 2

SAUNDERS

An Imprint of Elsevier, Inc.
PHILADELPHIA   LONDON   TORONTO   MONTREAL   SYDNEY   TOKYO

W.B. SAUNDERS COMPANY
A Division of Elsevier Inc.

Elsevier, Inc., 1600 John F. Kennedy Blvd., Suite 1800, Philadelphia, PA 19103-2899

http://www.vetequine.theclinics.com

VETERINARY CLINICS OF NORTH AMERICA: Volume 23, Number 2
EQUINE PRACTICE ISSN 0749-0739
August 2007 ISBN-13: 978-1-4160-5133-6
Editor: John Vassallo; j.vassallo@elsevier.com ISBN-10: 1-4160-5133-3

Copyright © 2007 by Elsevier Inc. All rights reserved. No part of this publication may be reproduced or transmitted in any form or by any means, electronic or mechanical, including photocopy, recording, or any information retrieval system, without written permission from the Publisher.

Single photocopies of single articles may be made for personal use as allowed by national copyright laws. Permission of the publisher and payment of a fee is required for all other photocopying, including multiple or systematic copying, copying for advertising or promotional purposes, resale, and all forms of document delivery. Special rates are available for educational institutions that wish to make photocopies for non-profit educational classroom use. Permission may be sought directly from Elsevier's Global Rights Department in Oxford, UK: phone 215-239-3804 or +44 (0)1865 843830, fax +44 (0)1865 853333, email healthpermissions@elsevier.com. Requests may also be completed online via the Elsevier homepage (http://www.elsevier.com/permissions). In the USA, users may clear permissions and make payments through the Copyright Clearance Center, Inc., 222 Rosewood Drive, Danvers, MA 01923, USA; phone: (978) 750-8400, fax: (978) 750-4744, and in the UK through the Copyright Licensing Agency Rapid Clearance Service (CLARCS), 90 Tottenham Court Road, London WIP 0LP, UK; phone: (+44) 171 436 5931; fax: (+44) 171 436 3986. Other countries may have a local reprographic rights agency for payments.

The ideas and opinions expressed in *Veterinary Clinics of North America: Equine Practice* do not necessarily reflect those of the Publisher. The Publisher does not assume any responsibility for any injury and/or damage to persons or property arising out of or related to any use of the material contained in this periodical. The reader is advised to check the appropriate medical literature and the product information currently provided by the manufacturer of each drug to be administered to verify the dosage, the method and duration of administration, or contraindications. It is the responsibility of the treating physician or other health care professional, relying on independent experience and knowledge of the patient, to determine drug dosages and the best treatment for the patient. Mention of any product in this issue should not be construed as endorsement by the contributors, editors, or the Publisher of the product or manufacturers' claims.

Veterinary Clinics of North America: Equine Practice (ISSN 0749-0739) is published in April, August, and December by Elsevier Inc., 360 Park Avenue South, New York, NY 10010-1710. Business and Editorial Offices: 1600 John F. Kennedy Blvd., Suite 1800, Philadelphia, PA 19103-2899. Customer Service office: 6277 Sea Harbor Drive, Orlando, FL 32887-4800. Subscription prices are $165.00 per year for US individuals, $265.00 per year for US institutions, $83.00 per year for US students and residents, $193.00 per year for Canadian individuals, $324.00 per year for Canadian institutions, $209.00 per year for international individuals, $324.00 per year for international institutions and $105.00 per year for Canadian and foreign students/residents. To receive student/resident rate, orders must be accompanied by name of affiliated institution, date of term, and the *signature* of program/residency coordinator on institution letterhead. Orders will be billed at individual rate until proof of status is received. Foreign air speed delivery is included in all *Clinics* subscription prices. All prices are subject to change without notice. **POSTMASTER:** Send address changes to *Veterinary Clinics of North America: Equine Practice*, Elsevier Periodicals Customer Service, 6277 Sea Harbor Drive, Orlando, FL 32887-4800, USA; phone: 1-800-654-2452 [toll free number for US customers], or 1-407-345-4000 [customers outside US]; fax: 1-407-363-1354; e-mail: usjcs@elsevier.com.

Reprints. For copies of 100 or more, of articles in this publication, please contact the Commercial Reprints Department, Elsevier Inc., 360 Park Avenue South, New York, New York 10010-1710. Tel. (212) 633-3813, Fax: (212) 462-1935 email: reprints@elsevier.com.

Veterinary Clinics of North America: Equine Practice is covered in *Index Medicus, Excerpta Medica, Current Contents/Agriculture, Biology and Environmental Sciences,* and *ISI.*

Printed in the United States of America.

EVIDENCE-BASED VETERINARY MEDICINE

CONSULTING EDITOR

A. SIMON TURNER, BVSc, MS, Diplomate, American College of Veterinary Surgeons; Professor, Department of Clinical Sciences, College of Veterinary Medicine and Biomedical Sciences, Colorado State University, Fort Collins, Colorado

GUEST EDITOR

DAVID W. RAMEY, DVM, Ramey Equine, Calabasas, California

CONTRIBUTORS

NURIA BARQUERO, DVM, MSc, MRCVS, Centre for Preventive Medicine, Animal Health Trust, Kentford, Newmarket, Suffolk, United Kingdom

WARREN L. BEARD, DVM, MS, Diplomate, American College of Veterinary Surgeons; Professor of Equine Surgery, Department of Clinical Sciences, College of Veterinary Medicine, Kansas State University, Manhattan, Kansas

DANIELA BEDENICE, Dr med vet, Diplomate, American College of Veterinary Internal Medicine; Diplomate, American College of Veterinary Emergency and Critical Care; Department of Clinical Sciences, Cummings School of Veterinary Medicine, Tufts University, North Grafton, Massachusetts

JOSEPH J. BERTONE, DVM, MS, Diplomate, American College of Veterinary Internal Medicine; Professor, Equine Medicine, Western University of Health Sciences, College of Veterinary Medicine, Pomona, California

STEVEN P. BRINSKO, DVM, MS, PhD, Diplomate, American College of Theriogenologists; Associate Professor of Theriogenology, Department of Large Animal Clinical Sciences, College of Veterinary Medicine and Biomedical Sciences, Texas A&M University, College Station, Texas

JAMES L. CARMALT, MA, VetMB, MVetSc, MRCVS, Diplomate, American Board of Veterinary Practitioners; Diplomate, American College of Veterinary Surgeons; Registered Specialist in Equine Surgery, Scone Veterinary Hospital, Scone, Australia

STEPHANIE S. CASTON, DVM, LA, Diplomate, American College of Veterinary Surgeons; Clinician, Equine Surgery, Department of Veterinary Clinical Sciences, College of Veterinary Medicine, Iowa State University, Ames, Iowa

MICHAEL S. DAVIS, DVM, PhD, Associate Professor, Department of Physiological Sciences, Oklahoma State University Center for Veterinary Health Sciences, Stillwater, Oklahoma

EHUD ELIASHAR, BSc, DVM, MRCVS, Diplomate, European College of Veterinary Surgeons; Lecturer in Equine Surgery, Department of Veterinary Clinical Sciences, The Royal Veterinary College, North Mymms, Hatfield, United Kingdom

JAMES R. GILKERSON, BVSc, PhD, Senior Lecturer in Veterinary Microbiology, Equine Infectious Disease Laboratory, Veterinary Pre-Clinical Centre, Faculty of Veterinary Science, University of Melbourne, Victoria, Australia

MARK A. HOLMES, MA, VetMB, PhD, MRCVS, Senior Lecturer in Preventive Veterinary Medicine, Department of Veterinary Medicine, University of Cambridge, Cambridge, United Kingdom

PHILIP J. JOHNSON, BVSc (Hons), MS, MRCVS, Diplomate, American College of Veterinary Internal Medicine; Diplomate, European College of Equine Internal Medicine; Professor of Equine Internal Medicine, Department of Veterinary Medicine and Surgery, Veterinary Medical Teaching Hospital at Clydesdale Hall, College of Veterinary Medicine, University of Missouri, Columbia, Missouri

KEVIN G. KEEGAN, DVM, MS, Diplomate, American College of Veterinary Surgeons; Director, E. Paige Laurie Endowed Program in Equine Lameness; and Associate Professor, Department of Veterinary Medicine and Surgery, College of Veterinary Medicine, University of Missouri, Columbia, Missouri

RICARDO LOINAZ, VMD, Urb. Tintillo Gardens, Guaynabo, Puerto Rico

TIM S. MAIR, PhD, MRCVS, Diplomate, Equine Internal Medicine; Diplomate, Equine Soft Tissue Surgery; Bell Equine Veterinary Clinic, Mereworth, Maidstone, Kent, United Kingdom

NAT T. MESSER IV, DVM, Diplomate, American Board of Veterinary Practitioners (Equine Practice); Associate Professor of Equine Medicine, Department of Veterinary Medicine and Surgery, Veterinary Medical Teaching Hospital at Clydesdale Hall, College of Veterinary Medicine, University of Missouri, Columbia, Missouri

J. RICHARD NEWTON, BVSc, MSc, PhD, FRCVS, Diplomate, London School of Hygiene and Tropical Medicine; Diplomate, European College of Veterinary Public Health; Centre for Preventive Medicine, Animal Health Trust, Kentford, Newmarket, Suffolk, United Kingdom

ROSE NOLEN-WALSTON, DVM, Diplomate, American College of Veterinary Internal Medicine; Assistant Professor of Medicine, School of Veterinary Medicine, University of Pennsylvania, Kennett Square, Pennsylvania

JULIA PAXSON, PhD, DVM, Resident, Cummings School of Veterinary Medicine, Tufts University, North Grafton, Massachusetts

SARAH L. RALSTON, VMD, PhD, Diplomate, American College of Veterinary Nutrition; Department of Animal Science, School of Environmental and Biological Sciences, Rutgers, The State University of New Jersey, New Brunswick, New Jersey

DAVID W. RAMEY, DVM, Ramey Equine, Calabasas, California

ERIC L. REINERTSON, DVM, MS, Associate Professor, Equine Surgery, Department of Veterinary Clinical Sciences, College of Veterinary Medicine, Iowa State University, Ames, Iowa

DEAN W. RICHARDSON, DVM, Diplomate, American College of Veterinary Surgeons; Charles W. Raker Professor of Surgery, University of Pennsylvania School of Veterinary Medicine, New Bolton Center, Kennett Square, Pennsylvania

CERI E. SHERLOCK, MRCVS, Bell Equine Veterinary Clinic, Mereworth, Maidstone, Kent, United Kingdom; University of Georgia, College of Veterinary Medicine, Athens, Georgia

LUISA J. SMITH, MRCVS, Bell Equine Veterinary Clinic, Mereworth, Maidstone, Kent; Royal Veterinary College, Hawkshead Campus, North Mymms, Hatfield, Hertfordshire, United Kingdom

CHRISTINE A. UHLINGER, VMD, MPH, Brandywine Equine Clinic, Apex, North Carolina

JÉRÔME VAN BIERVLIET, DVM, Diplomate, American College of Veterinary Internal Medicine; Neuronal Cell Biology and Gene Transfer Laboratory, Department for Molecular and Developmental Genetics; Neuronal Cell Biology and Gene Transfer Laboratory, Center for Human Genetics, Leuven, Belgium

SARAH WAXMAN, BS, Veterinary Student, College of Veterinary Medicine, Kansas State University, Manhattan, Kansas

KATHERINE K. WILLIAMSON, DVM, Research Associate, Department of Physiological Sciences, Oklahoma State University Center for Veterinary Health Sciences, Stillwater, Oklahoma

EVIDENCE-BASED VETERINARY MEDICINE

CONTENTS

Preface   xv
David W. Ramey

An Introduction to Evidence-Based Veterinary Medicine   191
Mark A. Holmes and David W. Ramey

> Evidence-based veterinary medicine is not impossible to practice, nor does it restrict its followers from using their best clinical judgment in individual case management. Based on the experiences in the various fields of human medicine, veterinarians should expect that the base of evidence for veterinary treatments is likely to expand rapidly, with positive expectations for improved treatment results. They would be well served by learning and applying evidence-based approaches to veterinary care, for the benefit of all who participate in the veterinarian-client-patient interaction.

Evidence-Based Drug Use in Equine Medicine
and Surgery   201
Joseph J. Bertone

> The nature of the equine industry and equine veterinary medicine often requires veterinarians to prescribe drugs with little evidence for a drug's formulation safety or efficacy, or even assurance of the chemistry of the drug used. This means that equine veterinarians must remain skeptics and understand the limitations in their ability to attribute safety and efficacy to a particular drug or treatment. An evidence-based approach to pharmacology demands rigorous testing and an unbiased analysis of results.

Evidence-Based Respiratory Medicine in Horses   215
Katherine K. Williamson and Michael S. Davis

> It is clear from a review of the current scientific literature that an evidence-based approach to medical treatment of equine respiratory disease can be applied, at least in the instance of common

lower respiratory diseases. In particular, there is clear evidence for efficacious treatments for recurrent airway obstruction and exercise-induced pulmonary hemorrhage, and with the recognition of this evidence, these treatments should be the first to be considered by a practitioner when treating these conditions. The purpose of this article is not only to identify the existence of relevant high-quality studies for incorporation into an evidence-based veterinary medicine approach to patient care, but to highlight the features of those studies that should be considered when evaluating their value in individual situations.

Evidence-Based Equine Upper Respiratory Surgery 229
Warren L. Beard and Sarah Waxman

The purpose of this article is to review the veterinary literature for various surgical procedures of the equine upper respiratory tract in an effort to evaluate the evidence supporting various therapies. This article focuses on the therapeutic benefit from more widely occurring conditions, such as laryngeal hemiplegia, dorsal displacement of the soft palate, arytenoid chondritis, and epiglottic entrapment.

Evidence-Based Gastrointestinal Medicine in Horses: It's Not About Your Gut Instincts 243
Rose Nolen-Walston, Julia Paxson, and David W. Ramey

The use of an evidence-based approach allows veterinary clinicians to assess questions that are clinically relevant to the diagnosis and treatment of equine gastrointestinal tract disease. This approach involves formulating a clinical question, searching the literature, and answering the question with the best available evidence, with the results summarized as a clinical "bottom line." This article is organized to reinforce the principle that the cornerstone of evidence-based medicine is the clinical question. Specific questions are further categorized as to topic, with epidemiologic risk factors, diagnostic process, clinical examination, differential diagnosis, diagnostic tests, treatment, harm, prognosis, and prevention as general themes. The topics covered in this article are by no means exhaustive but give an example of how the veterinary literature can be used to answer clinically important questions in an evidence-based manner.

Evidence-Based Gastrointestinal Surgery in Horses 267
Tim S. Mair, Luisa J. Smith, and Ceri E. Sherlock

Colic surgery is now performed at many equine hospitals around the world. Despite the tremendous improvements in survival rates over the past 30 years, the morbidity and mortality rates remain relatively high. This fact, coupled with the high cost of treatment, makes it important to apply evidence-based medicine principles to establish the best possible treatment plans and surgical techniques whereby the outcomes can be optimized. Factors affecting survival rates and rates of major complications (incisional complications and postoperative ileus) are discussed. Preoperative assessment and postoperative care are not considered in this review.

Evidence-Based Medicine in Equine Critical Care 293
Daniela Bedenice

One of the fundamental skills required for practicing evidence-based medicine is the development of a well-built clinical question, which specifies the patient group or problem, intervention, and outcome of interest. For this purpose, various "levels of evidence" have been developed in the human literature, which rank the validity of evidence. Our established conclusions and advice are thus supported by specific "grades of recommendations," which are intended to give an indication of the "strength" of a clinical recommendation. This article was compiled with these principles in mind.

An Evidence-Based Approach to Clinical Questions in the Practice of Equine Neurology 317
Jérôme Van Biervliet

The practice of equine neurology has special challenges posed by the size of the animal being examined. Many diagnostic procedures routinely used in small animal practice are unsafe when applied to the equine patient or unavailable to the equine practitioner. Therefore, astute observation is the mainstay of making a neuroanatomic diagnosis, and detailed evidence on the deficits present may be difficult to obtain. Because clinical observation can sometimes be ambiguous and somewhat subjective, it is even more important to approach equine neurology from an evidence-based point of view. Here, such an approach is outlined for the diagnosis of cervical vertebral compressive myelopathy (CVCM), one of the most common noninfectious causes of equine neurologic disease. This article is an attempt to summarize all aspects of making a diagnosis of CVCM on the basis of signalment, clinical examination, ancillary diagnostic tests, and pathologic examination. Each of these considerations has inherent limitations regarding diagnostic accuracy, which are discussed.

Evidence-Based Literature Pertaining to Thyroid Dysfunction and Cushing's Syndrome in the Horse 329
Nat T. Messer IV and Philip J. Johnson

The evidence-based literature pertaining to thyroid dysfunction and Cushing's syndrome is discussed in this article. Summaries of and recommendations for the treatment of these conditions are made. There is a need for reliable diagnostic tests for these conditions in horses.

Evidence-Based Equine Nutrition 365
Sarah L. Ralston

> One of the most difficult problems in equine nutrition research is often the lack of objective and clinically relevant end points. Nevertheless, this article attempts to present the best evidence (or lack thereof) for some of the most common clinical questions pertaining to such topics as the evaluation of glucose and insulin tolerance and factors that may confound results, dietary management of horses prone to laminitis and rhabdomyolysis, nutritional prevention of gastric ulcers and developmental orthopedic disease, the efficacy of commonly used herbal products, and feeding geriatric horses.

Common Procedures in Broodmare Practice: What Is the Evidence? 385
Steven P. Brinsko

> Many procedures performed as part of routine broodmare practice are based on sound clinical judgment and experience or scientific evidence; however, others are based on perceived problems and needs to address them. This article presents four procedures commonly used in broodmare practice, for which there is questionable evidence to substantiate their use.

Evidence-Based Lameness Detection and Quantification 403
Kevin G. Keegan

> Kinematic and kinetic gait analysis potentially offers veterinarians an objective method of determining equine limb lameness. Subjective analyses have been shown to be somewhat flawed, and there does not seem to be a high degree of intraobserver agreement when evaluating individual horses. In addition, recognition of the compensatory effects of primary lameness may be helpful for the practicing equine veterinarian.

An Evidence-Based Assessment of the Biomechanical Effects of the Common Shoeing and Farriery Techniques 425
Ehud Eliashar

> The first aim of this article is to review the progress made in the field of distal limb biomechanics. By understanding limb biomechanics, it is then possible to review the rationale behind a few

of the more common techniques that veterinarians routinely use when treating their patients and to evaluate the evidence in support of them.

An Evidence-Based Approach to Selected Joint Therapies in Horses   443
Dean W. Richardson and Ricardo Loinaz

There is an enormous volume of published material about most of the agents used to treat or prevent arthritis in horses. Unfortunately, most of the claims made by nearly all purveyors of arthritis medications in such media are largely unsubstantiated. In addition, the quality of the available information is highly inconsistent, making evidence-based recommendations difficult. This article concentrates on injectable polysulfated glycosaminoglycan, injectable hyaluronan, and the common oral "nutraceuticals".

Evidence-Based Musculoskeletal Surgery in Horses   461
Stephanie S. Caston and Eric L. Reinertson

Musculoskeletal disorders comprise a large portion of the conditions treated by equine veterinarians. Surgical intervention is the treatment of choice in many cases. The body of literature describing and exploring surgical correction of musculoskeletal disorders in horses is steadily growing but still lacking. At this juncture, we can use what information we have with the understanding that as the quality of research advances, we should apply stricter standards to the evidence we use to answer our clinical questions.

Evidence-Based Immunization in Horses   481
Nuria Barquero, James R. Gilkerson, and J. Richard Newton

Evidence of vaccine efficacy is essential for practitioners when giving advice to clients about the relative merits of different vaccines or when trying to evaluate the economic benefits of instituting a vaccine program. In equine veterinary medicine, this sort of data, which are necessary to make informed decisions about vaccine use and effectiveness, are often not available. Veterinarians need to consider the epidemiology of the disease in question, the type of vaccine that they are administering to the animal, the immunologic constraints of the vaccine technology, and the available evidence of efficacy when they are evaluating which vaccine to use or whether to vaccinate at all.

Evidence-Based Parasitology in Horses   509
Christine A. Uhlinger

This article focuses on what has been established concerning the interaction of equine parasites and their hosts, highlighting those issues for which convincing data are still lacking. There is a compelling need for the participation of the veterinarian in the design of appropriate anthelmintic treatments and prevention strategies.

Evidence-Based Equine Dentistry: Preventive Medicine 519
James L. Carmalt

Dental problems are some of the most common reasons for a horse to be presented to an equine veterinarian. Despite the importance of anecdotal evidence as a starting point, the science of equine dentistry (especially prophylactic dentistry) has remained poorly supported by evidence-based approaches to diagnosis and treatment. In the 21st century, veterinarians have an ethical responsibility to promote and use the results of evidence-based research and not propagate statements attesting to the purported benefits of intervention without supporting research. Consider also that society is becoming more litigious and therefore is basing treatment plans and advice on published research, which protects the profession from legal challenges concerning our professional conduct. This article reviews the current published evidence concerning the role of equine dentistry in feed digestibility and performance.

Index 525

FORTHCOMING ISSUES

December 2007
   Urinary Tract Disorders
   Harold C. Schott II, DVM, PhD, *Guest Editor*

April 2008
   Orthopedic Challenges in Performance Horses
   Antonio Cruz, DVM, MVM, MSc,
   Guest Editor

August 2008
   Clinical Pathology
   Bruce W. Parry, BVSc, PhD, *Guest Editor*

RECENT ISSUES

April 2007
   Trauma and Emergency Care
   Eileen K. Sullivan, DVM, MS, *Guest Editor*

December 2006
   Advances in Reproduction
   Elaine M. Carnevale, DVM, PhD,
   Guest Editor

August 2006
   Advances in Diagnosis and Management of Infection
   Louise L. Southwood, BVSc, PhD,
   Guest Editor

The Clinics are now available online!

Access your subscription at:
www.theclinics.com

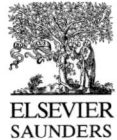

VETERINARY CLINICS
Equine Practice

Preface

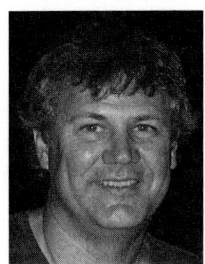

David W. Ramey, DVM
Guest Editor

For nearly as long as there are records of domesticated horses, there are records of people who took care of them. Over the centuries, these people made earnest efforts to treat diseases of unknown origin with treatments of uncertain efficacy. In many cases and in many cultures, these efforts were recorded and passed down by word of mouth, and occasionally, on the written page. Still, until the 18th century, the essential basis for clinical decision making was primarily a certainty of knowledge (preferably in accordance with the wisdom of the Ancients). This essential basis persists today.

Critical assessments of the effectiveness of therapeutic interventions first became a subject for discussion in 18th century British medicine and surgery. For example, James Lind's 1753 account [1] of his comparison of different treatments for scurvy describes how he tried to make sure that the sailors who took part in his trial were clinically "as similar as I could have them," "lay together in one place," and had "one diet common to all" [2]. Still, it was not until 1948 that a patient allocation schedule based on random number tables was used in a British Medical Research Council trial of streptomycin for pulmonary tuberculosis [3].

In human medicine in the mid-1990's, a movement began that tried to gather reliable information, by using the best current available evidence obtained from rigorously conducted clinical trials, in an effort to improve the clinical decisions made during the care of individual patients. The momentum from the movement has been overwhelming. Now there are workshops on how to practice and teach what is formally known as "Evidence-Based Medicine"(EBM), undergraduate and postgraduate training programs for

0749-0739/07/$ - see front matter © 2007 Elsevier Inc. All rights reserved.
doi:10.1016/j.cveq.2007.04.006

vetequine.theclinics.com

EBM; there are even centers (in the UK, "centres") for EBM. The Cochrane Collaboration [4] and Bandolier [5], among others, are providing systematic reviews of the effects of health care; new evidence-based practice journals are being launched, and it has become a common topic in the lay media.

Even so, enthusiasm for EBM has not been universal. EBM has also spawned some negative reaction, with criticism ranging from EBM being "old hat" (otherwise stated, "Isn't that what we've always done?"), to being a dangerous innovation, which is perpetrated by arrogant inhabitants of ivory towers to suppress the clinical "freedom" of the practitioners in the field.

In spite of such criticisms, and following the lead of human medicine, a movement (in veterinary medicine) toward EBM appears to be forming. A book on the topic was published in 2003 [6], and the Society for Evidence-Based Veterinary Medicine was formed in 2006, at Mississippi State University [7]. The evidentiary cat appears to be out of the clinical bag.

I got into practice to help horses. As a practicing clinician for over 20 years, I have often been bewildered by the array of therapeutic choices presented to me at conferences, in advertisements, and at stall-side conferences with my clients. It has always seemed to me that veterinary practice should be more than providing a poker table full of therapeutic "options," then letting the chips fall where they may. I have come to believe that an evidence-based approach to medicine offers veterinarians a clear-cut path to help make more rational clinical decisions—decisions that directly benefit horses and the people who own them, and it allows veterinarians to more efficiently and economically practice high quality medicine.

Apparently, a number of esteemed colleagues agree with me. That a sole practitioner, such as myself, was able to put together an issue of a major publication such as this, would have been unthinkable without the assistance of people much more knowledgeable than I. In assembling this issue, I have been overwhelmed by the enthusiasm and dedication of the researchers, clinicians, and practitioners who have blazed the way in exploring a novel approach to the assessment of information in equine practice. Of course, it would be impossible to make a text of this relatively short length comprehensive, so the authors have taken the approach of asking answerable clinical questions for which there may be answers based on available evidence. I believe that this approach is as valuable for practicing clinicians in private practice as it is to instructors and researchers in educational institutions. It's one that will also be seen monthly, in a regular column in the *Equine Veterinary Education* journal published in the United Kingdom. And, of course, ultimately, if an evidence-based approach is of benefit to horses, then everyone involved in the veterinarian–client–patient transaction will be the better for it.

I thank Dr. Simon Turner, an unforgettable teacher during my years at Colorado State University in the early 1980's, and who is also an enthusiastic supporter of the concept of this issue of *Veterinary Clinics of North*

America: Equine Practice. I also thank John Vassallo and the editorial staff at Elsevier for their patience, help, support, and enthusiasm. Finally, I offer my most heartfelt thanks and love to my irrepressible wife, Oryla, and to my eager and enthusiastic boys, Jackson and Aidan, for helping me to keep it all in perspective.

David W. Ramey, DVM
Ramey Equine
P.O. Box 9114, Calabasas, CA 91372, USA

E-mail address: ponydoc@pacbell.net

References

[1] Troehler U. To improve the evidence of medicine: the 18th century British origins of a critical approach. Edinburgh: Royal College of Physicians; 2000.
[2] Lind J. A treatise of the scurvy. In three parts. Containing an inquiry into the nature, causes and cure, of that disease. Together with a critical and chronological view of what has been published on the subject. Edinburgh: Printed by Sands, Murray and Cochran for A Kincaid and A Donaldson; 1753.
[3] Medical Research Council. Streptomycin treatment of pulmonary tuberculosis: a Medical Research Council investigation. BMJ 1948;2:769–82.
[4] The Cochrane collaboration. Available at: http://www.cochrane.org. Accessed May 18, 2007.
[5] Bandolier. Evidence based thinking about health care. Available at: http://www.jr2.ox.ac.uk/bandolier. Accessed May 18, 2007.
[6] Holmes M, Cockroft P. Handbook of evidence-based veterinary medicine. Blackwell Publishing 2003.
[7] Evidence Based Veterinary Medicine Association. Available at: http://www.ebvma.org. Accessed May 18, 2007.

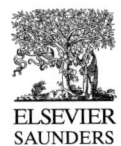

VETERINARY CLINICS
Equine Practice

An Introduction to Evidence-Based Veterinary Medicine

Mark A. Holmes, MA, VetMB, PhD, MRCVS[a],*,
David W. Ramey, DVM[b]

[a]*Department of Veterinary Medicine, University of Cambridge, Madingley Road, Cambridge CB3 0ES, UK*
[b]*Ramey Equine, P.O. Box 9114, Calabasas, CA 91372, USA*

When politicians, or skeptical surgeons, start using the term *evidence-based* ... or start referring to the "evidence base," alarm bells start ringing in the minds of the cynical. It cannot have escaped any veterinarian who looks at the scientific literature, even briefly, that the concept of evidence-based medicine has become established as a new medical dogma embraced by scientific zealots and health management organization (HMO) managers (who may use a lack of evidence to justify not having to pay for procedures). Before you discard this issue of *Veterinary Clinics of North America: Equine Practice*, however, you should at least give some thought to the following account of how invalid health information is potentially lethal.

As a recent medical graduate in the mid-1960s, Dr. Iain Chalmers, now Sir Iain Chalmers and better known as a distinguished health services researcher, bought a copy of Dr. Benjamin Spock's famous book, *Baby and Child Care*. In his copy, he marked a passage that read: "There are two disadvantages to a baby's sleeping on his back. If he vomits, he's more likely to choke on the vomitus. Also he tends to keep his head turned toward the same side ... I think it is preferable to accustom a baby to sleeping on his stomach from the start." Persuaded by these suggestions, Dr. Chalmers passed on and acted on this apparently rational and authoritative advice, no doubt like millions of Dr. Spock's other readers.

Sadly, collation of the results of many simple observational studies contradicted this advice, ultimately culminating in a recommendation issued by the American Academy of Pediatrics in 1992 that infants be placed on their backs to reduce the risk of sudden infant death syndrome (SIDS). Before

---

* Corresponding author.
E-mail address: mah1@cam.ac.uk (M.A. Holmes).

this advice, more than 70% of US infants were placed on their fronts to sleep. By the year 2000, however, approximately 80% of infants slept on their backs and the incidence of SIDS had decreased by more than 40% (from 1.4 deaths per 1000 births to 0.8 deaths per 1000 births; Fig. 1) [1]. In a letter to the *British Medical Journal*, Dr. Chalmers [2] later wrote: "We now know that the advice promulgated so successfully in Spock's book led to thousands, if not tens of thousands, of avoidable cot deaths." This example should provide a sobering warning to those of us who disseminate or use health information based on "common sense," without also ensuring, to the best of our ability, that evidence from reliable empiric research has shown that our prescriptions and proscriptions are more likely to help than to harm our patients.

Although this example supports the use of good-quality clinical research and effective communication, it also illustrates the fundamental scientific principles that underpin the practice of veterinary medicine as applied by an individual practitioner caring for an individual patient. Of course, there are important skill sets other than an ability to appraise the scientific literature critically that contribute to our performance as veterinarians. A good clinician needs good powers of observation, empathy with patients and clients, manual dexterity, and a host of other skills. Apart from these, however, a good clinician needs to accept that his or her clinical decisions

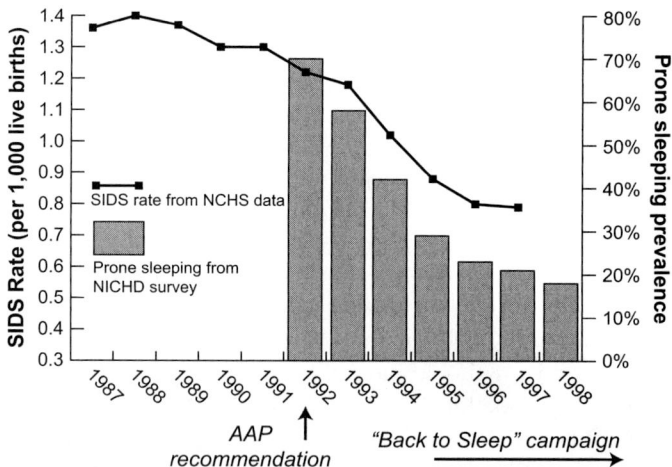

Fig. 1. SIDS rate in the United States from National Center for Health Statistics (NCHS) data and prone-positioning rate from National Institute for Child Health and Human Development (NICHD) surveys over the years 1987 to 1998. The recommendation of the American Academy of Pediatrics (AAP) against prone sleeping was made in 1992, and the "Back to Sleep" campaign was begun in 1994. (*From* American Academy of Pediatrics. Task Force on Infant Sleep Position and Sudden Infant Death Syndrome. Changing concepts of sudden infant death syndrome: implications for infant sleeping environment and sleep position. Pediatrics 2000;105:651; with permission.)

might be wrong and to constantly ask the question: "Can I obtain better information that can increase the likelihood that my clinical decisions will be good ones?"

The natural world is riven with uncertainty; indeed, it would not function without it. Human beings are poorly equipped to deal with it; consequently, our judgments are influenced by hope, fear, and desire. We take pleasure in paying magicians to mislead us, and we play games of chance, such as roulette and lotteries, even though we know that our risk of losing is ultimately a certainty. Even when it comes to our cardinal sense ("I'll believe it when I see it"), we still cannot trust the evidence it provides (Fig. 2).

Individual clinicians acquire proficiency and judgment through clinical experience and clinical practice. Good clinicians routinely overestimate the value of their own experience, however, and may thereby misinterpret or skew results. Researchers and clinicians often end up selectively recalling events or overestimating successes, whereas ignoring, downplaying, or rationalizing failures. Existing literature on experimenter bias shows that even the most honest and best trained individuals anticipate the results that they hope to see when they try to make judgments after the outcome of complex events. Certainly, noticing interesting correlations between therapy and response is a good starting point for a more systematic investigation; however, such ad hoc correlations should never be the end point in the search for effective new therapies. Unfortunately, over time, reliance on educated guesses and uncontrolled observations may lead to an overconfidence that ultimately blurs the line between opinion and evidence. The knowledge that chance and our human frailties mislead us means we must develop and use skills that enable us to make objective judgments on the strength of the evidence that we use for making clinical decisions.

Of course, every good practitioner already has a philosophy encompassing the desire to achieve best practice, which manifests itself in our attempts

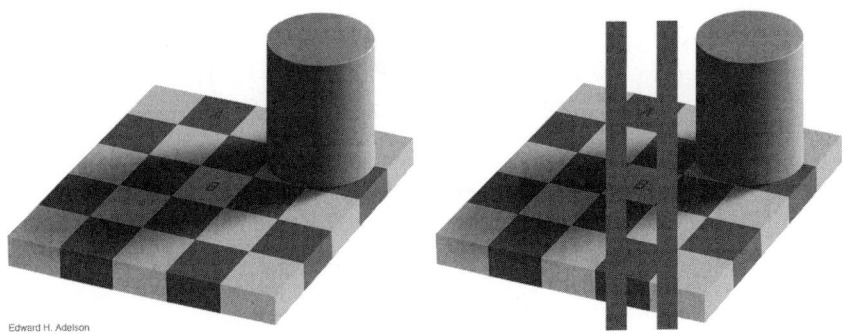

Fig. 2. An impressive optical illusion. Based on the image on the left, it is almost impossible to believe that the squares marked A and B are identical shades of gray. Looking at the image on the right, however, on which two thick lines of the same gray have been superimposed, it becomes clear that this is true. (*Courtesy of* Edward H. Adelson, Cambridge, MA).

to keep up with the literature in our specialty interest. Evidence-based medicine evolved as a result of the failure of research results to reach patients and out of our perennial problem of too much to read and too little time to read it.

What is evidence-based veterinary medicine?

Simply stated, evidence-based veterinary medicine (EBVM) is the conscientious, explicit, and judicious use of the current best evidence in making decisions about the care of individual patients [3,4]. The practice of EBVM integrates individual clinical expertise with the best available external clinical evidence from systematic research. EBVM is not a blind reliance on clinical research; rather, it attempts to incorporate the best information obtained from clinical research and the best clinical judgment of the practitioner (Fig. 3).

The main difference in emphasis of EBM from traditional approaches to learning is a move away from an emphasis on textbooks, lecture notes, and narrative reviews toward the use of primary clinical research. It is a change from our attempts to accumulate all the knowledge just in case we need it to an approach that enables us to find the information when we need it.

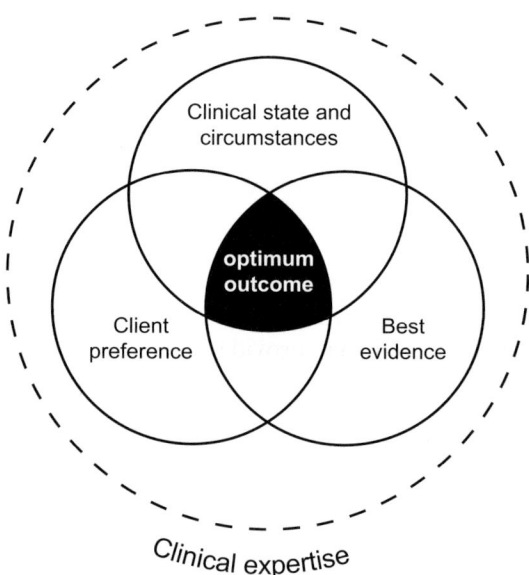

Fig. 3. Decision making in EBVM. The decision-making process in EBVM is represented in this Venn diagram. The optimal outcome depends on the clinical situation, best evidence, and wishes of the client (and patient). Veterinary clinical expertise is required for all aspects of the decision-making process.

It would be laughable to suggest that an evidence-based practitioner would immediately start searching the literature every time he or she was asked to give an influenza vaccination or treat a case of laminitis. Conversely, stop for a moment, and think about how you choose the diagnostic tests, vaccines, and treatment strategies you use. As a rational and conscientious veterinarian, you do not make an arbitrary decision. Instead, you use the best evidence at hand, probably influenced by a recent review article or notes from a recent equine meeting.

This practice could be extended broadly. A practice of adopting EBVM would examine common procedures on a regular basis to establish that practice policy was backed up by the current best evidence. This goal could be achieved by agreeing that one veterinarian, or a group of veterinarians, should search and appraise the primary literature and then circulate a summary for discussion.

How do we perform evidence-based veterinary medicine?

As has already been stated, to perform EBVM, we combine clinical judgment and the individual circumstances of our patient with the best evidence from clinical research (see Fig. 3). The unfamiliar part of the process is finding, appraising, and evaluating the evidence. For example, an evidence-based equine veterinarian faced with a nonroutine clinical decision searches the literature databases, such as PubMed and CAB abstracts, to find the scientific evidence to inform that decision.

The process of EBVM consists of turning our information need into an answerable clinical question, performing a literature search, formally appraising the articles we find, and then applying the information acquired to our situation.

Such a process requires some time, effort, and education. It is beyond the scope of this introduction to provide detailed information on the process and skills required to appraise the literature and apply the evidence to patients. There are many excellent books and sources of information on evidence-based medicine [3–10] that provide detail beyond the scope of this introduction.

Levels of evidence

To practice EBVM, veterinarians must become familiar with the types of evidence that are available and recognize the strengths and weaknesses inherent in each of them. In that regard, attempts have been made to rank evidence based on its relative strength.

Level one evidence is obtained from systematic reviews, with homogeneity (that is, the treated conditions are the same) of randomized controlled trials (RCTs), individual RCTs with narrow confidence intervals, or "all or none" case series (all patients died or got diseased before the diagnosis became available, but some now survive, or some patients died or got diseased before the diagnosis became available, but none now do).

Level two evidence comes from systematic reviews, with homogeneity, of cohort studies (two groups [cohorts] of patients, with one receiving the exposure of interest and one not, and following these cohorts forward for the outcome of interest), individual cohort studies, or "outcomes" research (studies a cohort of patients with the same diagnosis and relates their clinical and health outcomes to the care that they received).

Level three evidence comes from systematic reviews, with homogeneity, of case-control studies (identifying patients who have the outcome of interest [cases] and control patients without the same outcome and looking back to see if they had the exposure of interest) or from individual case-control studies.

Level four evidence comes from case series and poor-quality cohort and case-control studies. Unfortunately, poor-quality studies seem to have been the rule rather than the exception in veterinary medicine. Poor-quality studies may fail to define comparison groups clearly, fail to measure exposures and outcomes in the same (preferably blinded) objective way in exposed and nonexposed individuals, fail to identify or control known confounders appropriately, or fail to carry out a sufficiently long and complete follow-up. So, for example, even if a study on horses with navicular disease is blinded and randomized, it may not be a particularly good study if the treated horses are only followed for a few weeks.

Level five evidence comes from clinical practice based on expert opinion without explicit critical appraisal or based on physiology, on bench research, or solely on pathophysiologic principles. This sort of information is extremely common in veterinary medicine, particularly at conferences. Although it is perhaps the most persuasive evidence (after all, why would a paid conference speaker get up and lie), it is almost certainly the weakest type of evidence available unless it is buttressed by good supporting information.

Is medicine evidence based?

It is sometimes claimed that strict standards of evidence hold some forms of veterinary practice to a "higher standard" than others and that little of medicine is actually evidence based. For example, it has been claimed that only 20% or less of standard "Western" medicine in human beings is evidence based, and this claim has been repeated widely by health professionals and others [11]. This statement is simply not true, however. In fact, a growing body of evidence demonstrates that the practice of evidence-based medicine is widespread and is becoming more so [12].

Regardless of its prevalence, perhaps a more salient question is: "Does practicing evidence-based medicine make any difference for patients?" In human medicine, it is clear that patients who receive treatments based on the best available evidence benefit. For example, myocardial infarction survivors prescribed aspirin [13] or beta-blockers [14] have a lower mortality rate than those who are not prescribed those drugs. When clinicians use more warfarin and stroke unit referrals, mortality attributable to stroke declines by greater than 20% [15]. For a negative example, patients undergoing carotid surgery despite failing to meet evidence-based operative criteria, when compared with surgical patients who meet those criteria, are more than three times as likely to experience a major stroke or death in the next month [16].

In veterinary medicine, no studies on EBVM seem to have been conducted; however, it seems clear that EBVM does benefit human patients, and there is no reason to believe that it would not benefit veterinary patients. Furthermore, the lack of such studies in veterinary medicine does not mean that more therapies lacking in evidence should be incorporated. Even if veterinary medicine is 100% non-evidence based, this does not argue for failing to look for good evidence to support veterinary treatments.

Practice-based clinical research

The best place to perform clinical research that is of greatest relevance to most equine clinicians is in equine practices. Ideally, the practice of EBVM should identify the questions to which field practitioners need answers. The acquisition of appraisal skills by practitioners provides excellent initial training for performing research. Practitioners often bemoan the fact that experience accumulated over many years of veterinary work is lost to the profession. Equine surgeons in practice may develop new surgical techniques and often report their difficulties in getting results published.

Although it may be of value to have these techniques described, it is virtually impossible to evaluate the relative merits of a new technique, or the actual value of accumulated years of experience using a particular technique, in the absence of some form of comparison. Although a case series in which all the horses are operated on using a technique demonstrating 100% success with almost no adverse effects illustrates the surgeon's skill and ability, it fails to provide strong evidence that another surgeon is likely to have the same success. Conversely, should the surgeon compare results from two techniques on two groups of horses and demonstrate an advantage, it does provide evidence on the benefits of adopting this surgical technique.

Good clinical research asks a focused question that almost inevitably involves some form of comparison. It would be naive in the extreme to expect randomized, blind, controlled trials in equine surgery; however, a prospective cohort study or trial always provides better evidence than a case study or an anecdote. A recent development in the United Kingdom has been the establishment of a Clinical Research Outreach Program at the University of Cambridge to provide training and support for all veterinary practitioners [17].

The way forward

There are two main thrusts in the development of EBVM. The first follows the acceptance that the "best evidence" may not be reaching individual patients and that we can ameliorate this by acquiring (or improving) skills in locating sources of information, in appraising the evidence, and in incorporating the evidence into our clinical practice. The second developing area is the presentation and delivery of the results of research in forms that help clinicians to obtain the evidence.

Traditionally, scientific papers place a great emphasis on communication of results and methodology to fellow researchers. Although epidemiologists and statisticians may have little difficulty in understanding subtle variations in statistical tests, even academic clinicians reviewing such papers may find it difficult to interpret the magnitude or certainty of the results reported. The use of confidence intervals to describe the variability of results and the use of absolute differences (absolute risk reduction or increase) make it far easier to judge the clinical significance of a finding, as opposed to relative risk or odds ratios. When the favorable results from two therapies are compared, the inverse of the absolute risk provides a measure known as the number needed to treat (NNT). An NNT value of 20 (ie, there was a 5% advantage in using the better treatment) indicates that if the better therapy was applied to 20 patients, there would be 1 extra patient with a favorable outcome than if the less good treatment was used. This makes it much easier for a clinician to evaluate the advantages and disadvantages (eg, extra cost) of changing to the better therapeutic option.

A further advance that has been widely applied in human medicine is the use of secondary research. In veterinary medicine, we are familiar with the narrative review, in which a respected colleague "reviews" the literature to provide an overview of current expert opinion. In contrast, systematic reviews perform a formal systematic appraisal of the scientific literature to provide an overall "result." In the systematic reviews on the literature looking at SIDS described at the beginning of this article, the many different studies on SIDS were combined using special statistical techniques to provide a statistically validated combined result using a process known as meta-analysis. Centers for secondary research, such as the Cochrane Collaboration, [18] have contributed greatly to human medical understanding in areas in which there are often studies with what seem to be conflicting or inconclusive results. Unfortunately, systematic reviews are not often performed in veterinary medicine because the literature base is too small (examples of a veterinary systematic review and a meta-analysis can be found in 2 articles on atopic dermatitis in dogs by Olivry and Mueller [19] and Steffan and colleagues [20]).

Another development, however, the use of clinically appraised topics (CATs), might be of considerable value in veterinary medicine. CATs are miniature systematic reviews that address a simple clinical question (eg, likelihood of death attributable to anesthesia in a 2-year-old Thoroughbred colt undergoing routine orthopedic surgery). The author would search the literature, find the best evidence to answer that question, and summarize the results in a "clinical bottom line." CATs are ephemeral in nature (ie, they become obsolete as soon as new data are produced); thus, they tend to be published on the Internet. A good example is the human critical care CAT Web site, BestBETS [21]. The publication of veterinary CATs may well provide better training for diplomate candidates of the many veterinary specialist colleges and boards than the publication of case reports, which are often produced as a qualification requirement; they would certainly be of greater use to many general practitioners.

Summary

EBVM is not impossible to practice, nor does it restrict its followers from using their best clinical judgment in individual case management. Based on the experiences in the various fields of human medicine, veterinarians should expect that the base of evidence for veterinary treatments is likely to expand rapidly, with positive expectations for improved treatment results. They would be well served by learning and applying evidence-based approaches to veterinary care, for the benefit of all who participate in the veterinarian-client-patient interaction.

References

[1] American Academy of Pediatrics Task Force on Infant Positioning and SIDS. Positioning and SIDS: changing concepts of sudden infant death syndrome: implications for infant sleeping environment and sleep position. Pediatrics 1992;89:1120–6.
[2] Chalmers I. Invalid health information is potentially lethal [letter]. BMJ 2001;322:998.
[3] Sackett DL, Strauss SE, Richardson WS, et al. Evidence-based medicine: how to practice and teach EBM. Edinburgh (UK): Churchill-Livingstone; 2000.
[4] Cockroft PD, Holmes MA. Handbook of evidence-based veterinary medicine. Ames (IA): Blackwells Scientific; 2003.
[5] Dahoo IR, Waltner-Toews D. Interpreting clinical research: part I. General considerations. Compendium Of Continuing Education 1985;7,9:S474–7.
[6] Dahoo IR, Waltner-Toews D. Interpreting clinical research: part II. Descriptive and experimental studies. Compendium Of Continuing Education 1985;7,9:S513–9.
[7] Dahoo IR, Waltner-Toews D. Interpreting clinical research: part III. Observational studies and interpretation of results. Compendium Of Continuing Education 1985;7,9:S605–13.
[8] Holmes MA, Cockroft PD. Evidence-based veterinary medicine 1. Why is it important and what skills are needed? In Pract 2004;26:28–33.

[9] Cockcroft PD, Holmes MA. Evidence-based veterinary medicine 2. Identifying information needs and finding the evidence. In Pract 2004;26:96–102.
[10] Holmes MA, Cockcroft PD. Evidence-based veterinary medicine 3. Appraising the evidence. In Pract 2004;26:154–64.
[11] Smith R. Where is the wisdom ... the poverty of medical evidence. BMJ 1991;303:798–9.
[12] Imrie R, Ramey DW. The evidence for evidence-based medicine. Complement Therap Med 2000;8:123–6.
[13] Krumholz HM, Radford MJ, Ellerbeek FF, et al. Aspirin for secondary prevention after acute myocardial infarction in the elderly; prescribed use and outcomes. Ann Intern Med 1996;124:292–8.
[14] Krumholz HM, Radford MJ, Wang Y, et al. National use and effectiveness of beta-blockers for the treatment of elderly patients after acute myocardial infarction. National Cooperative Cardiovascular Project. JAMA 1998;280:623–9.
[15] Mitchell JG, Ballard DJ, Whisnant JP, et al. What role do neurologists play in determining the costs and outcomes of stroke patients? Stroke 1996;27:1937–43.
[16] Wong JH, Findlay JM, Suarez-Almazor ME. Regional performance of carotid endarterectomy appropriateness, outcomes and risk factors for complications. Stroke 1997;28:891–8.
[17] The Cambridge Clinical Research Outreach Programme. Cambridge (UK). Available at: http://www.vet.cam.ac.uk/cidc/training/outreach.html. Accessed October 13, 2006.
[18] The Cochrane Collaboration. Available at: http://www.cochrane.org/index.htm. Accessed October 13, 2006.
[19] Olivry T, Mueller RS. Evidence-based dermatology: a systematic review of the pharmacotherapy of canine atopic dermatitis. Vet Dermatol 2003;14:121–46.
[20] Steffan J, Favrot C, Mueller R. A systematic review and meta-analysis of the efficacy and safety of cyclosporin for the treatment of atopic dermatitis in dogs. Vet Dermatol 2006; 17:3–16.
[21] BestBETs: best evidence topics. Available at: http://www.bestbets.org/. Accessed October 13, 2006.

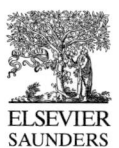

VETERINARY
CLINICS
Equine Practice

Evidence-Based Drug Use in Equine Medicine and Surgery

Joseph J. Bertone, DVM, MS

Equine Medicine, Western University of Health Sciences, College of Veterinary Medicine, 309 East 2nd Street, Pomona, CA 91766, USA

The nature of the equine industry and equine veterinary medicine often requires veterinarians to prescribe drugs with little evidence for a drug's formulation safety or efficacy, or even assurance of the chemistry of the drug used. Relative to the volume of information available in other health professions, equine veterinarians often fly by the seat of their pants in terms of drug use as well as with many other treatments and procedures. (They are not alone here, because some areas of veterinary medicine, for example, exotic and zoo animal medicine, are arguably even less evidence based). This situation does not also mean that it is impossible to make good clinical decisions, however. It only means that equine veterinarians must remain skeptics and understand the limitations in their ability to attribute safety and efficacy to a particular drug or treatment. An evidence-based approach to pharmacology demands rigorous testing and an unbiased analysis of results.

What is a drug, and how has potion mixing been preserved in veterinary medicine?

A drug is defined, for the purposes of this article, as well as legally (at least in part) as the entire formulation, which includes the active ingredient, excipients (eg, water, preservatives), packaging, and directions for use and storage. Legally, the US Food and Drug Administration (FDA) adds the advertising and other literature as part of the drug, (those additions are not discussed here). For the purposes of veterinary medicine, it is much more appropriate to define a drug as everything in the package than it is to define a drug as only the active ingredient. The formulation and

E-mail address: jbertone@westernu.edu

packaging and handling instructions determine the pharmacokinetics, safety, efficacy, and stability of the product.

Unfortunately, veterinary literature tends to overemphasize the active molecule alone and de-emphasizes the formulation. The near absence of pharmaceutics training in veterinary education (there are notable exceptions) leaves veterinary medicine unprepared to understand this issue and its importance. This educational void also opens the veterinary profession to pirates and profiteers who take advantage of that ignorance. Pharmaceutics, the science of drug formulation, is critical because of the comparative nature of our discipline. Arguably, veterinary journals and proceedings would serve veterinarians better if they allowed the use of drug names (eg, Dormosedan [detomidine hydrochloride], Sedivet [romifidine hydrochloride], Ketaset [ketamine hydrochloride], Buscopan [N-butylscopolammonium bromide, Naxel [ceftiofur sodium]) in studies investigating the use of those drugs. That would give proper credit to the drug formulation being evaluated in a study.

The focus on the active ingredient alone in the veterinary literature does a disservice to the profession. Drugs are not just the active ingredients alone, and their pharmacokinetics and pharmacodynamics, shelf-life, and almost every other feature depend on the formulation, which includes such things as the conjugate or salt of the active ingredient used. Thus, it is generally a particular formulation, as opposed to a particular active ingredient, that satisfies research requirements to show that the formulation is stable and actually in the product that is ultimately used by the practitioner.

Three studies looking at digoxin pharmacokinetics in horses highlight this issue. Each set of investigators administered three different formulations of digoxin orally to normal horses. In reality, these were three different drugs, and many pharmacokinetic differences were evident. As examples, the calculated dose (μg/kg/h) and mean half-time ($T_{1/2}$ hours), respectively, from each study were 44 and 16.9 [1], 35 and 23.1 [2], and 17.4 and 28.8, depending on the formulation [3]. Those are dramatic differences for a drug with such a small window of safety and efficacy.

Differing effects of active ingredient salts or conjugates are also obvious and evident. Excede (ceftiofur crystalline free acid) is associated with severe life-threatening diarrhea and colitis in horses, whereas Naxel is much safer. Other examples include the varied clinical uses associated with the drugs SoluMedrol (methylprednisolone sodium succinate) versus DepoMedro (methylprednisolone acetate) or differences in the uses, dosages, safety, and efficacy of potassium, sodium, benzathine, and procaine penicillins [4].

Although veterinary medicine often stresses the active ingredient in lectures, notes, continuing education, and scientific literature, that view of a drug incorrectly assumes that the only issue of any importance is the active ingredient. That approach assumes that active ingredients are absorbed, distributed, metabolized, and excreted independent of the other substances (excipients) in the bottle, pill, or tube. That assumption is clearly incorrect, and that opinion needs to change. Not even all generic formulations meet the specifications of the pioneer compounds.

Evidence-based pharmacology

Pharmacology is the study of how chemical substances interact with living systems. If substances have medicinal properties, they are considered pharmaceutic agents. The science is believed to have been invented in Baghdad by Arab physicians during the Golden Age of Islam, and pharmacopoeias were authored in Arabic as early as the seventh century [5].

Evidence-based medicine (EBM) is the process of systematically finding, appraising, and using contemporaneous research findings as the basis for clinical decisions. This requires self-directed and lifelong learning techniques. The use of EBM as a technique follows four general steps that include formulation of a clear clinical question from a patient's problem, a literature search for the best available evidence, evaluation of the evidence for its validity and usefulness, and implementation of useful findings in clinical practice [6]. As pertains to pharmacology, however, this process clearly requires knowledge of what drug (ie, everything in the bottle) is being administered. Evidence-based pharmacology depends on the evidence supporting the repeatability of a response in association with the administration of a drug, which then allows confidence in attributing that response to the drug.

Many governments regulate the manufacture, sale, and administration of medications to protect the consumer and prevent abuse. In the United States, the main body regulating pharmaceutic agents is the FDA, which enforces standards set by the US Pharmacopoeia. Given that few FDA-approved drugs are specifically formulated for horses relative to the number of drugs used in horses, however, and the various ways in which they are used, federal regulation often has little influence on equine veterinary practice other than as pertains to controlled substances. Accordingly, from an evidence-based perspective, the main question becomes, "What does it take to attribute effectiveness and safety to a chemical mixture, known as a drug?"

What is being given?

Assurances of drug quality, purity, and strength are essential to attributing effectiveness and safety. Assuming that such qualities are assured, most veterinarians use drugs believing in the accuracy of the package label and use the label concentration to calculate a dosage. Such an assumption presumes strong government oversight and protection, however. Unfortunately, this presumption is only appropriate in the case of FDA-approved pioneer, generic, and registered formulations. Essentially, these are the only medicaments in which the essential qualities necessary for acceptable medical use are regulated and, more importantly, enforced.

Another category of drugs includes drug-listed formulations, which are regulated for manufacturing and safety but for which efficacy has not been demonstrated (eg, calcium borogluconate, Normosol [balanced polyionic fluid], other vitamins, and replacement fluids). All the FDA-approved and -registered drugs are listed in the "Green Book" [7].

Although there are many good compounding pharmacies, there is always some lack of assuredness with compounded products compared with FDA-approved or -registered formulations. This is because, in most cases, the pharmacist has only the label on the container of raw materials as well as any excipients to use as assurance of purity, quality, and strength of the enclosed chemical. There may be unexpected interactions within a formulation, and the stability of a compounded product is rarely evaluated. Hence, even when appropriately indicated, there is a short shelf-life on compounded products, which is often just the length of the prescription period.

Compounding and poor formulation errors do occur [8,9]. In fact, it was a tragic compounding error that was the final impetus for enactment of the Food, Drug, and Cosmetic Act as we know it. The government was essentially inactive, in terms of drugs, throughout the early part of the past century. Well into the 1930s, pharmaceutical companies still manufactured many 19th and early 20th century drugs that were sold in bulk to pharmacists, who then compounded them into physicians' prescriptions. In 1937, Massengill Company produced a liquid sulfanilamide drug for oral administration. The company used diethylene glycol for the suspension and ultimately sold this syrup, which was called Elixir Sulfanilamide. The drug was on the market for 2 months; during that time, it was associated with fulminant renal failure and deaths of 106 people, including many children [10].

The United States Congress passed the Food, Drug, and Cosmetic Act of 1938, which banned drugs that were dangerous and required drug labels to include directions for use and appropriate warnings for other drugs. The act also required new drugs to be tested for safety before being granted federal government approval and created a new category of drugs that could be dispensed to a patient only at the request of a physician (before the act was passed, patients could purchase any drug, except narcotics, from pharmacists). The FDA (the regulatory division established in 1927 from the former Bureau of Chemistry) was given responsibility for implementing these laws. Manufacturing, purity, quality, and strength standards followed. It was not until the 1940s that the Federal Trade Commission required drug manufacturers to substantiate claims made about their products.

The nature of equine medicine and future equine pharmaceutic development requires, and is likely to continue to require, compounding pharmacies. The needs of the equine industry are not a priority for the pharmaceutic industry, with the exception of some classes of drugs in wide use (eg, parasiticides, anti-inflammatories). In large, part, this is attributable to the relative small size of the equine market, and the resultant lesser ability of that market to generate profit as compared with small animal medicine, as well as to the exuberant, arguably nonvalue, added regulatory burdens that require a large market to recoup costs. Here, compounding pharmacies attempt to fill a void. Although some compounding pharmacies are ethical and quality driven, others still continue to make and sell products with known formulation issues [11]. Compounded drugs are reasonable to use when there is no FDA-approved drug to use for the same purpose; however, it is unethical to use a compounded drug because the profit margin is more advantageous [12].

Some human formulations used in equine medicine are devices and not approved as drugs. For example, a bottled formulation intended to be applied to wounds is most likely approved as a human device, because topical wound dressings are most often regulated as devices (FDA, Center for Devices and Radiological Health). The required quality assurance standards for devices are far less rigorous than the assurance regulations for products marketed as drugs. When human devices are used by veterinarians as drugs, practitioners must know that the devices do not bear the same level of regulatory assurance of strength, purity, and stability as FDA-approved drugs. In addition, the Animal Medical Drug Use Clarification Act (AMDUCA), which allows the extralabel use of drugs by veterinarians, does not allow for extralabel use of a device, and adverse reactions may lead to malpractice legal issues with these products because they can be excluded from coverage by the Professional Liability Insurance Trust.

To increase the complexity, substances that do not even have human device approval but are marketed as veterinary devices are being injected into horse's veins, soft tissues, and joints with no manufacturing oversight. The Center for Veterinary Medicine (CVM) at the FDA regulates veterinary devices but chooses to provide no manufacturing, safety, or efficacy enforcement. In fact, the CVM has provided little enforcement of claims made by these sponsors that clearly label the product as an adulterated drug

Can a horse absorb the drug, or are systemic effective concentrations durable to have a significant effect?

Bioavailability is a serious issue for many drugs given to horses, because orally, intramuscularly, and intravenously (rapid clearance issues) administered drugs are so variably handled in this species [13–15]. With the oral route, questions include "Does the drug get absorbed from the gastrointestinal tract?" or "Does it get past the liver?" Even when administered intramuscularly or intravenously, a drug's plasma concentration or duration of action may not be sufficient enough to have an effect.

Oral isoxsuprine in horses is an example of a drug that is poorly bioavailable. Evidence indicates that when given orally, isoxsuprine concentrations are nearly immeasurable; thus, the drug does not attain levels sufficient for an effect [14]. When the drug is given intravenously, its duration of effect is less than 14 minutes [14] and no localized effect is evident [16]. In addition, no analgesic effect has been shown in masked studies [17]. Yet, in spite of this evidence, the product is still widely used. Similarly, no studies to date have identified albuterol concentrations in plasma when the drug is given orally at any concentration (there are positive urine test cases for both drugs, but this merely reflects urine concentration rather than free and active concentrations in blood). Some drugs, even when administered by the intravenous or intramuscular route, are poorly bioavailable because of rapid clearance rates. For example, benzathine penicillin cannot be given at a rate to horses to achieve the minimum inhibitory concentration (MIC) for *Streptococcus* spp [15].

There is no treatment effect if a disease does not exist

Extrapolations from other species plague rational drug use in horses. For example, there are no adequate and well-controlled studies that provide evidence to suggest that horses with low plasma thyroxin levels are overweight or have associated reproductive challenges, insulin resistance, laminitis, poor hair coats, or any other clinical signs. Many of these signs can be loosely related to hypothyroidism in other species but have not been associated with any certainty in relation to hypothyroidism in horses. When a test result from a screening panel suggests low plasma concentration, based on a reference range built from a small number of animals (common practice), there is no need whatsoever to provide the horse with supplemental thyroxin and a clinical change (eg, pregnancy) cannot necessarily be attributed to the treatment.

The use of reference ranges alone to identify a questionably mild anemic horse and then to supplement iron in the form of various tonics is also without foundation. Indeed, there is nearly no place for iron supplements in horses, regardless of the level of anemia. Almost all equine diets are replete with iron, and iron deficiency is absolutely rare in horses and only occurs under special restrictive situations [18,19]. If a horse is truly anemic, iron deficiency is not the cause.

Supplemental progesterone in mares in the first trimester of pregnancy lacks an evidence base. There is no evidence that pregnancy loss in the first trimester is associated with failure of the corpus luteum to produce adequate quantities of progesterone. In the one study that measured serial plasma progesterone concentration in early pregnancy, almost all mares lost their pregnancies well before plasma progesterone decreased to lower than 2 ng/mL or less [20]. Nevertheless, progesterone supplementation is common practice in early pregnancy in mares.

Accurate diagnosis is required for treatment efficacy to be established

To be assured that a drug is responsible for clinical improvement, the disease should be accurately diagnosed and identified. Many horses with vague gait abnormalities have been labeled as having neurologic deficits caused by equine protozoal myelitis (EPM) based on the results of a Western blot test plagued with false-positive results, even from cerebrospinal fluid (CSF) samples [21]; hence, these horses were treated for EPM. Clinical improvement in such cases cannot be reliably attributed to treatment, because the presence of disease was never reliably determined.

Certainly, it is possible to treat a disease effectively, even if the disease is undiagnosed. An example here might be the treatment of a horse with fever of unknown origin with systemic antibiotics when the horse has occult pleuropneumonia (pleuropneumonia with a low-volume pleural exudate and no other respiratory signs) and the drug is chosen on a best guess of *Streptococcus* spp. Treatment is effective, but the disease is not specifically diagnosed. Conversely, not all horses with fever of unknown origin require antibiotic therapy, and it is unwarranted to attribute resolution of the fever to antibiotic administration in every case.

If the disease exists, is the treatment appropriate?

It is perhaps obvious that successful therapy requires that the right drug be given; by the correct route of administration; and at the right dose, frequency, and interval for the correct treatment based on your best information. If, for example, an animal with a mild case of strangles improves with the administration of gentamicin administered intramuscularly, it is likely that the animal improved on its own, because the drug has a low likelihood of having a positive effect on gram-positive cocci at pharmacologic doses. Similarly, attributing or taking credit for a positive response of a horse that was acutely febrile, depressed, and had a fine watery nasal discharge to administration of procaine penicillin (10 mL) simply because the dose of penicillin is inadequate and the drug has no efficacy on the influenza virus that likely caused the problem.

Is the expected clinical effect from a drug obvious? Not every effect requires a randomized controlled trial for confirmation. Some effects can be identified with great accuracy. For example, if an anesthetic or euthanasia drug is administered, an effect is immediately obvious and it would be reasonable to attribute efficacy to the drug. If a severely painful animal responds to administration of Sedivet, the response is most likely attributable to the drug's analgesic properties, especially when the clinical signs of pain return after the drug effect has dissipated. When Dobutrex (dobutamine) is administered at the correct dosage and a quantitative measure of blood pressure with a direct arterial line is in place, a clear effect can be identified.

The ability to assess the efficacy of a drug used in more subtle cases, such as mild subtle lameness, poor hair coat, behavioral issues, and hoof quality, or in diseases that often spontaneously resolve is far more difficult, especially when a drug has been administered chronically. Biologic systems are in constant change, and change is expected.

Further confounding the ability to assess efficacy are such factors as chronicity as well as incidence and prevalence of disease. The efficacy of drugs administered as prophylaxis for rare diseases is difficult to assess. Concomitant therapies also confound assessments of treatment success. For example, supplements that guarantee a better hair coat when started before the show season, which are given while the grooms learn to use fine soft brushes and toweling, are sure to be coincident with a better hair coat eventually but may not be the only cause for the horse's shine.

When the disease is rare and uncommon, drugs used as preventives are unlikely to have any assurance of efficacy without study. Laminitis prevention, claimed as a rationale for the administration of endotoxin or *Salmonella* vaccines, cannot be said to have reliable efficacy at least in part because of the rarity of the condition in the population as a whole.

Conflict of interest and publication bias

Conflict of interest is defined as "a conflict between the private interests and official responsibilities of a person in a position of trust" [22]. Conflicts of interest potentially occur when an investigator has a financial relation (often research funding and sometimes more) with a sponsor whose product is being studied by the investigator. There is nothing intrinsically wrong with conflicts of interest; indeed, they are ubiquitous, because in veterinary and human medicine, so many trials are funded by the manufacturer of the product being studied. The problem is less conflict of interest itself but that the conflict of interest is a risk factor for conscious or subconscious scientific misconduct. Several authors have identified a significant association between industry funding and the outcome of studies. In fact, the industry-desired result was far more prevalent in the industry-supported research and far less likely to be the result of a study in research not funded by industry [23–26]. In veterinary medicine, there are barely enough studies on any one drug to make such an analysis. In addition, the reluctance to publish negative results, a form of publication bias, adds to this issue [27]. Accordingly, if a product does not work, veterinarians may have a difficult time in learning about it.

Herbs

The pharmacologic water has been most recently made muddy by the wide availability of various plant preparations, with numerous, largely unsupported, claims of effectiveness. Some plants do contain pharmacoactive substances, and a significant percentage of modern pharmaceutic agents have been derived from plants. These products are largely unregulated, however. Even if effective, the effects of weather and the growing environment mean that the content of the active ingredient is always in question from batch to batch. Using such substances is essentially a form of therapeutic roulette [28].

Tool for thought

There are many variables to account for when assuring the efficacy and safety of a drug. Although not a rigid guide, Table 1 can be employed in the consideration of procedure and evidence when using drugs in horses. Generally, the table can be applied on a case-by-case basis. To use the table, an item is chosen under each heading that applies to a particular drug use

Table 1
Evidence calculator for safety and efficacy of drug use in horses

Drug formulation	Score
FDA approved for horses	10
FDA approved for nonequine mammalian species	8
Compounded product, not pirate of approved drug[a]	6
Human devices used as drugs[a]	2
Veterinary device used as a drug[a]	0
Unregulated herbs[a]	0
Unregulated homeopathic preparations[a]	0
Dose	
Approved dose	10
Dose effective in laboratory studies	6
No clinical or laboratory studies on dose	0
Route of administration	
Intended route	10
Oral route when intended is intravenous or intramuscular	2
Evidence for efficacy	
Label claim	10
Nonregulatory clinical trial in horse	8
Laboratory study, intact horse	6
Pharmacokinetic study in horse	5
Pharmacokinetic in nonhorse mammal	0
Anecdote alone	2
Laboratory study, intact nonhorse mammal	0
Laboratory study, in vitro horse cells	1
Laboratory study, in vitro nonhorse cells	0
No evidence for efficacy	0
Evidence for safety	
FDA approved for horses at the dose and for the label use	10
Anecdote	4
No evidence	0
Total score	

Abbreviation: FDA, US Food and Drug Administration.

[a] In practice, but there is no allowance under the Food, Drug, and Cosmetic Act (http://www.fda.gov/opacom/laws/fdcact/fdctoc.htm) or the Animal Medical Drug Use Clarification Act of 1994 (http://www.fda.gov/cvm/amducatoc.htm) that allows for extralabel use of drugs in veterinary medicine.

(drug formulation, dose, route of administration, evidence for efficacy, and evidence for safety). An associated score can then be noted and summed. In the veterinary field, a reasonable score is 40 or higher, although special circumstances may make that target figure variable. For example, when there is a labeled dose and spectrum of an antibiotic (determined when it was approved) but there are changes in the bacterial population, the necessary dose or frequency of administration of the drug may increase. Of course, such dosing changes may also alter the safety profile of the drug.

Clinical examples

0

Oral albuterol, ciprofloxacin, and isoxsuprine are good examples of 0's. Not only are the formulations not assured; there is also no evidence of bioavailability to effective concentrations. Albuterol and isoxsuprine urine analysis positive test results do occur, but none is evident in blood when administered by means of the oral route. Ciprofloxacin is measurable in blood, but its bioavailability is marginal at best [13].

Near 0

An oral glucosamine combination has recently been shown to have a positive effect on gait in older horses [29]. The evidence for the product is still ranked as a near 0, however, because the formulation varies with sources. However, this score could change if manufacturing is regulated for quality, strength, and purity, and if the new product is re-evaluated for efficacy and safety in adequate and well controlled trials.

Score of 20 to 50

Not all FDA-approved drugs have science-based studies associated with their FDA approvals. For example, Naxcel was approved for treatment of equine respiratory infections associated with *Streptococcus zooepidemicus* [30]. It is approved in horses (10 points). The FDA-approval studies were designed to meet an interpretation of the regulatory requirements that was dubious at best, however, rather than being science based. That is, Naxcel was arguably only shown to be as effective as the label dose of an approved ampicillin product that, even at the time of the study, was known to be labeled with an ineffective dose (6.6 mg/kg administered twice daily). Even now, tissue penetration studies have shown that the labeled dose of ampicillin is woefully inadequate (an adequate dose has now been clearly identified in the area of 15 mg/kg administered once daily) [31]. In fact, the Freedom of Information summary indicates that, "at Day 7 post-treatment, 11 (73%) of the ceftiofur patients and 7 (50%) of the horses treated with ampicillin had completely recovered/cured" [30].

Nevertheless, further studies have shown that Naxcel does have a scientific basis for use with gram-positive infection. Naxcel for use in gram negative infections is a more complex issue, because the dosing interval is more frequent so as to maintain concentrations in the MIC range for most gram-negative organisms. Hence, the safety of the drug is less assured with that use. The interpretation of a recent study of Naxcel administered by means of regional limb perfusion as support for that route [32] is questionable for a time-dependent drug. In that study, 2 g (essentially 4.4 mg/kg) was administered by means of regional limb perfusion in one dose. The study discussion implied that higher local concentrations would be associated with greater efficacy. Cephalosporins are categorized as having have type II activity, however. This means that they depend on time greater than MIC, with minimal persistent effects. Conversely, aminoglycosides, described originally for use in regional limb perfusion, show type III activity in that they are concentration dependent and have prolonged persistent effects [33–35]. In addition, the effective break point (>1 µg/mL) of ceftiofur concentrations found in the horses treated with Naxcel and regional limb perfusion are actually no more likely to be effective or of a greater duration than if the drug were administered at a rate of 2.2 mg/kg (total of 4.4 mg/kg over 24 hours) every 12 hours [36].

Full 50 points

Buscopan is an FDA-approved drug (NADA 141-228) whose approval was based on a masked, adequate, and well-controlled study of 200 horses with uncomplicated colic (not requiring surgery or extensive medical management). There is no other study of abdominal pain medications in horses that is within this class of evidence. Colic is easily diagnosed, and the response to time or treatment is clear. In the masked study, a saline placebo was the control. The saline-administered control horses had a positive colic score response in 5 minutes. The Buscopan-treated horses had a response that was significantly greater, in terms of reduced colic score, than did the saline placebo-treated horses at all posttreatment points (5–30 minutes), however.

In contrast, Banamine (flunixin meglumine), a commonly used first-line colic drug, is supported by a much weaker base of evidence. In the only clinical trial published on its pain-relieving effect, which was not masked, 38% of 118 horses showed improvement in 15 minutes and 68% showed improvement within 1 hour [37]. In comparing these two studies, the colic scores of horses treated with Banamine were similar to those of horses treated with placebo in the FDA approval study for Buscopan in managing uncomplicated colic. Hence, Banamine did not outperform the saline placebo. In the FDA approval study, pretreatment with flunixin meglumine did not affect the results of treatment with Buscopan or the placebo.

Summary

Veterinarians should be skeptical of any attribution of efficacy and safety for a pharmacologic product under the following conditions:

1. There is no assurance of what is being given.
2. There are no data to support whether or not the drug can be absorbed to an effective concentration or duration.
3. The expected response is subtle and not clinically obvious (eg, death, anesthesia, complete analgesia, sedation).
4. The treatment is chronic or long-term recovery is needed.

References

[1] Brumbaugh GW, Thomas WP, Enos LR, et al. A pharmacokinetic study of digoxin in the horse. J Vet Pharmacol Ther 1983;6(3):163–72.
[2] Button C, Gross DR, Johnston JT, et al. Digoxin pharmacokinetics, bioavailability, efficacy, and dosage regimens in the horse. Am J Vet Res 1980;41(9):1388–95.
[3] Pedersoli WM, Ravis WR, Belmonte AA, et al. Pharmacokinetics of a single, orally administered dose of digoxin in horses. Am J Vet Res 1981;42(8):1412–4.
[4] Dowling P. Antimicrobial therapy. In: Bertone JJ, Horspool LJI, editors. Equine clinical pharmacology. London: Elsevier Science; 2004. p. 13–47.
[5] Khairallah AA. Outline of Arabic contributions to medicine. Beirut (Lebanon): 1946.
[6] Guyatt GH, Rennie D. Users' guides to the medical literature: editorial. JAMA 1993;270: 2096–7.
[7] US Food and Drug Administration. Available at: http://www.fda.gov/cvm/Green_Book/elecgbook.html.
[8] Romano MJ, Dinh A. 1000-fold overdose of clonidine caused by a compounding error in a 5-year-old child with attention-deficit/hyperactivity disorder. Pediatrics 2001;108(2):471–2.
[9] Jones TF, Feler CA, Simmons BP, et al. Neurologic complications including paralysis after a medication error involving implanted intrathecal catheters. Am J Med 2002;112(1):31–6.
[10] Wax PM. Elixirs, diluents, and the passage of the 1938 Federal Food, Drug, and Cosmetic Act. Annals of Internal Medicine 1995;122(6):456–61.
[11] Merritt AM, Sanchez LC, Burrow JA, et al. Effect of GastroGard and three compounded oral omeprazole preparations on 24 h intragastric pH in gastrically cannulated mature horses. Equine Vet J 2003;35(7):691–5.
[12] Rollins BA, Bertone JJ. The ethical debate: drug piracy. DVM Magazine 2003;21–4.
[13] Dowling PM, Wilson RC, Tyler JW, et al. Pharmacokinetics of ciprofloxacin in ponies. J Vet Pharmacol Ther 1995;18(1):7–12.
[14] Matthews NS, Gleed RD, Short CE, et al. Cardiovascular and pharmacokinetic effects of isoxsuprine in the horse. Am J Vet Res 1986;47(10):2130–3.
[15] Sullins KE, Messer NT, Nelson L. Serum concentration of penicillin in the horse after repeated intramuscular injections of procaine penicillin G alone or in combination with benzathine penicillin and/or phenylbutazone. Am J Vet Res 1984;45(5):1003–7.
[16] Ingle-Fehr JE, Baxter GM. The effect of oral isoxsuprine and pentoxifylline on digital and laminar blood flow in healthy horses. Vet Surg 1999;28(3):154–60.
[17] Lizarraga I, Castillo F, Valderrama ME. An analgesic evaluation of isoxsuprine in horses. J Vet Med A Physiol Pathol Clin Med 2004;51(7–8):370–4.
[18] Fleming KA, Barton MH, Latimer KS. Iron deficiency anemia in a neonatal foal. J Vet Intern Med 2006;20(6):1495–8.
[19] Brommer H, van Oldruitenborgh-Oosterbaan MM. Iron deficiency in stabled Dutch Warmblood foals. J Vet Intern Med 2001;15(5):482–5.

[20] Irvine CH, Sutton P, Turner JE, et al. Changes in plasma progesterone concentrations from days 17 to 42 of gestation in mares maintaining or losing pregnancy. Equine vet J 1990;22(2): 104–6.
[21] Daft BM, Barr BC, Gardner IA, et al. Sensitivity and specificity of Western blot testing of cerebrospinal fluid and serum for diagnosis of equine protozoal myeloencephalitis in horses with and without neurologic abnormalities. J Am Vet Med Assoc 2002;221(7):1007–13.
[22] Council on Scientific Affairs and Council on Ethical and Judicial Affairs. Conflicts of interest in medical center/industry research relationships. JAMA 1990;263:2790–3.
[23] Davidson RA. Source of funding and outcome of clinical trials. J Gen Intern Med 1986;1: 155–8.
[24] Stelfox HT, Chua G, O'Rourke K, et al. Conflict of interest in the debate over calcium-channel antagonists. N Engl J Med 1998;338:101–6.
[25] Friedberg M, Saffran B, Stinson TJ, et al. Evaluation of conflict of interest in economic analyses of new drugs used in oncology. JAMA 1999;282:1453–7.
[26] Cho MK, Bero LA. The quality of drug studies published in symposium proceedings. Ann Intern Med 1996;124:485–9.
[27] Chalmers I. Underreporting research is scientific misconduct. JAMA 1990;263:1405–8.
[28] Ramey DW. A skeptical view of herbal medicine. In: Wynn S, Fougere B, editors. Veterinary herbal medicine. St. Louis (MO): Mosby, Inc; 2007. p. 121–35.
[29] Forsyth RK, Brigden CV, Northrop AJ. Double blind investigation of the effects of oral supplementation of combined glucosamine hydrochloride (GHCL) and chondroitin sulphate (CS) on stride characteristics of veteran horses. Equine Vet J Suppl 2006;(36):622–5.
[30] US Food and Drug Administration. Freedom of information summary. NADA 140-338. Available at: http://www.fda.gov/cvm/FOI/1496.htm. Accessed June 8, 2007.
[31] van den Hoven R, Hierweck B, Dobretsberger M, et al. Intramuscular dosing strategy for ampicillin sodium in horses, based on its distribution into tissue chambers before and after induction of inflammation. J Vet Pharmacol Ther 2003;26(6):405–11.
[32] Pille F, De Baere S, Ceelen L, et al. Synovial fluid and plasma concentrations of ceftiofur after regional intravenous perfusion in the horse. Vet Surg 2005;34(6):610–7.
[33] Rodvold KA. Pharmacodynamics of antiinfective therapy: taking what we know to the patient's bedside. Pharmacotherapy 2001;21(11 Pt 2):319S–30S.
[34] Nicolau DP. Optimizing outcomes with antimicrobial therapy through pharmacodynamic profiling. J Infect Chemother 2003;9(4):292–6.
[35] Scheuch BC, Van Hoogmoed LM, Wilson WD, et al. Comparison of intraosseous or intravenous infusion for delivery of amikacin sulfate to the tibiotarsal joint of horses. Am J Vet Res 2002;63(3):374–80.
[36] Jaglan PS, Roof RD, Yein FS, et al. Concentration of ceftiofur metabolites in the plasma and lungs of horses following intramuscular treatment. J Vet Pharmacol Ther 1994;17(1):24–30.
[37] Vernimb GD, Hennessey PW. Clinical studies on flunixin meglumine in the treatment of equine colic. J Equine Medicine Surg 1977;1:111–6.

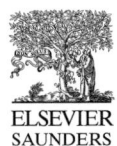

Evidence-Based Respiratory Medicine in Horses

Katherine K. Williamson, DVM,
Michael S. Davis, DVM, PhD*

Department of Physiological Sciences, Oklahoma State University Center for Veterinary Health Sciences, 264 McElroy Hall, Stillwater, OK 74078, USA

The application of evidence-based veterinary medicine (EBVM) to the medical treatment of respiratory diseases reveals a wide spectrum of evidence for a particular treatment. Some common conditions, particularly those of the upper airways (nares, pharynx, and larynx), are notable in the striking paucity of published reports of rigorous clinical trials. At the opposite end of the spectrum, there exists a relative abundance of high-quality published studies evaluating treatments for various lower airway inflammatory conditions in horses. This abundance, however, does not necessarily make the job of the practitioner easier when it comes to applying the principles of EBVM to these diseases, because the application of EBVM requires the careful evaluation of these studies and the concurrent application of the practitioner's clinical judgment as to whether they apply to the patient in question. The purpose of this article is not only to identify the existence of relevant high-quality studies for incorporation into an EBVM approach to patient care but to highlight the features of those studies that should be considered when evaluating their value in individual situations.

Lower airway conditions

Recurrent airway obstruction

Recurrent airway obstruction (RAO, historically also described as chronic obstructive pulmonary disease [COPD] and more casually referred to as "heaves") has the greatest body of literature that can be used directly

---

* Corresponding author.
E-mail address: michael.davis@okstate.edu (M.S. Davis).

or indirectly in an EBVM approach to treating lower respiratory disease in horses. Many of the published studies incorporate rigorous experimental designs, such as blinding, randomization, placebo, or positive treatment controls, which substantially increase the value of the report from an EBVM perspective. In assessing the relevant clinical value, however, it is necessary for the practitioner to consider not just experimental design but the test population (client-owned versus research herd), mechanism of disease induction (naturally occurring versus experimentally induced), and, perhaps most importantly, the end point measured (eg, clinical signs, pulmonary mechanical properties, gas exchange, indices of airway inflammation). A therapy that effectively reduces peripheral airway neutrophilia in a university-owned horse with signs of RAO elicited by controlled exposure to moldy hay may not extrapolate perfectly to the typical client-owned horse with naturally occurring disease that is presented for clinical signs of dyspnea and coughing. (For the sake of simplicity of discussion in this article, all studies addressing treatments for heaves, COPD, and RAO are cited as being relevant to RAO.)

The most relevant parameter for a private practitioner evaluating the efficacy of therapy for RAO is clinical signs of dyspnea. Unfortunately, this parameter is unavoidably subjective, and therefore probably less precise than objective measurements, such as pulmonary resistance, arterial oxygen tension, or neutrophil concentration in bronchoalveolar lavage fluid (BALF). Objective measurements are thus preferred by researchers seeking to minimize the numbers of subjects (and attendant costs) required to demonstrate a desirable biologic effect of a therapy. A subjective clinical scoring system that assigned numeric values to the severity of clinical signs of dyspnea (nasal flaring and abdominal lift) had a statistically significant relation to most measurements of pulmonary mechanical properties and breathing strategy; however, perhaps unfortunately, this relation was driven primarily by concordance in the most severely affected animals [1]. The relation was less reliable in horses with a lower clinical score. For example, a decrease in two grades of clinical severity corresponded to a 12% drop in pulmonary resistance when resistance and clinical score were highest, but a 24% decrease in pulmonary resistance was required to decrease the clinical score by two grades when the subjects were only moderately affected. The authors interpreted this to indicate that in mildly affected horses, even a statistically significant improvement in pulmonary mechanical properties may not be reflected by an improvement in clinical score.

It is important that practitioners recognize that improvements in pulmonary function may not be apparent clinically. This is true when evaluating published literature that relies on pulmonary mechanical properties as the key end point for evaluating efficacy as well as when a practitioner creates expectations for the client when recommending a specific treatment for RAO. Nevertheless, despite these caveats, changes in pulmonary mechanical properties are probably the objective evidence that is most closely related to clinical signs of disease. Therefore, in this article, the strength of evidence for the efficacy of a particular treatment for RAO is evaluated only from the standpoint of changes in pulmonary mechanical properties, especially when clinical signs of disease are not reported.

RAO can be considered an environmentally induced disease of airway inflammation that results in bronchoconstriction. Addressing one or more of these three features forms the backbone of treatment. A host of oral, systemic, and aerosolized bronchodilators have been evaluated in the scientific literature, and most show efficacy in improving pulmonary mechanical properties, and in some cases, clinical signs of disease. The efficacy of aerosolized β_2 agonists has been reported in the peer-reviewed literature, and the quality of this evidence is quite good.

Aerosolized drugs must be delivered through an administration device, and the specific device may substantially affect the delivery of the drug (and, by inference, its efficacy). The reported efficacy of drugs delivered through systems that are not available to the practitioner, such as fenoterol delivered through a custom-made face mask [2] and pirbuterol [3] and albuterol [4] delivered through the Torpex (Boehringer Ingelheim Vetmedica, Inc.) delivery device (no longer available), must therefore be viewed with caution. In the case of albuterol, however, improvement in pulmonary mechanics in horses with RAO has also been reported using a metered-dose inhaler and the Equine Aeromask (Trudell Medical International, London, Ontario, Canada) [5]. Improvement in pulmonary mechanical properties and clinical severity score has been reported for salmeterol (a long-acting β_2 agonist) administered from a metered-dose inhaler through an Equine Aeromask [6]. Both studies employed randomized crossover designs with untreated controls using university-owned horses and experimentally induced signs of disease, and thus do not meet the most rigorous standards for application to the true target population of patients. These studies are substantially stronger than studies without controls, however. Salmeterol may be superior to albuterol for relief of bronchoconstriction because of its longer duration of action, but it is also important to note that although there was a statistically significant reduction in pulmonary mechanical properties for 6 hours after a single dose, the significant improvement in clinical severity score lasted only 2 hours. Nevertheless, the evidence for efficacy of aerosolized β_2 agonists to provide transient improvement in the clinical signs and pulmonary function of horses with RAO is strong.

Anticholinergic drugs have also been evaluated for use in relieving airway obstruction and clinical signs of RAO. Intravenous atropine decreases airway resistance in horses [7] and ponies with RAO [8] and is frequently used as a positive control in research studies as well as a diagnostic tool to determine the potential for bronchodilation in clinical subjects. Concern regarding the adverse gastrointestinal effects of repeated systemic dosing of anticholinergic drugs limits their therapeutic use for RAO, however. Nebulized ipratropium bromide solution (a derivative of atropine) has been shown to result in prolonged (4–6 hours) improvement in pulmonary mechanical properties in horses with RAO [9], and the same drug caused a reduction in pulmonary resistance for at least 1 hour when administered as a dry powder aerosol [10]. Although neither study reported measurements of clinical disease severity, the reduction in pulmonary resistance in both studies was substantial (50%), and thus likely associated with an improvement in clinical condition.

Clenbuterol hydrochloride is a β_2 agonist approved for use in the treatment of RAO. High-quality evidence for the efficacy of this drug in horses is surprisingly lacking in the peer-reviewed literature, however. At a dose of 0.4 mg per horse administered by mouth twice daily, clenbuterol failed to improve the clinical signs of disease in horses diagnosed with RAO [11] compared with placebo-treated control animals. Clenbuterol administered at an increasing dose (starting at 0.8 µg/kg and increasing by 0.8 µg/kg every 3 days until an effect was observed) resulted in improvement of clinical signs of RAO, but this study did not include a control group of untreated or placebo-treated horses [12]. The lack of a control group is an important point for interpreting this study, because the clinical signs of heaves can wax and wane and horses can seem to improve spontaneously. Thus, the overall evidence for the efficacy of oral clenbuterol for the treatment of RAO in horses is modest at best, despite being approved for use in horses for this indication by the US Food and Drug Administration.

Another (and not necessarily separate) therapeutic option for reducing pulmonary resistance in horses with RAO is to decrease the amount of intraluminal debris that is obstructing the airway. Accordingly, and despite its classification as a bronchodilator, clenbuterol may be more efficacious as a drug used to increase the clearance of intraluminal exudates. Intravenous clenbuterol at the lowest recommended dose (0.8 µg/kg) acutely increases the rate of mucociliary clearance in horses with RAO [13]. Unfortunately, there was no concurrent measurement of clinical score in this study, and extrapolation using studies discussed in the preceding paragraph would suggest that the efficacy of clenbuterol in improving clinical score remains open for debate, regardless of the mechanism by which it might improve the clinical score. Nevertheless, it is worthwhile to note that improvement in clinical score based only on increased rate of mucociliary clearance is not likely to be rapid; thus, it is possible that the previous studies evaluating the effect of clenbuterol on clinical score may not have been long enough to detect a benefit from decreased intraluminal mucus. Another report that investigated the use of rapid intravenous administration of isotonic saline to reduce the viscosity of intra-airway secretions, and thus improve clearance, actually caused acute worsening of pulmonary mechanical properties in horses with heaves [14]. In summary, at this time, there is minimal evidence of a clinical benefit of increased mucociliary clearance in horses with RAO.

Other treatments that have been reported in the peer-reviewed literature for treatment of RAO through improvement of pulmonary mechanical properties include acupuncture and herbal preparations. A controlled study of a single acupuncture treatment by a professional acupuncturist that included numerous controls (handling with no acupuncture and acupuncture by an untrained veterinarian) found no benefit from acupuncture that was not also observed by simple handling of the subject [15]. A study of a herbal preparation of thyme and cowslip found approximately a 38% reduction in pulmonary resistance after 1 month of treatment, but, interestingly, no improvements in clinical severity score [16]. This study contained only five horses and did not include a control group, substantially diminishing its value in EBVM. A second study investigating a herbal preparation containing yellow gentian, garden sorrel, common elder, and verbena included five treated horses and four control (untreated) horses in a crossover study and found a significant effect of treatment on maximum transpulmonary pressure (an indicator of effort associated with breathing) but no significant effect of treatment on pulmonary resistance or clinical score [17]. At the present time, there is no reliable evidence for a beneficial effect of acupuncture or herbal remedies for the improvement of the clinical condition of horses with RAO.

RAO is widely considered to be an inflammatory disease resulting in adverse changes in pulmonary mechanical properties; thus, it is logical to presume that reducing the inflammation would have a beneficial effect on pulmonary mechanical properties and clinical condition. There are many peer-reviewed publications that describe the effect of anti-inflammatory drugs on various aspects of RAO, but not all are particularly persuasive from an EBVM point of view. Dexamethasone, whether administered intravenously at a dose of 0.04 mg/kg once daily [18,19], intravenously at a dose of 0.1 mg/kg once daily [20–22], or orally at a dose of 0.164 mg/kg once daily [22], resulted in improvement in pulmonary resistance, although the specific time course of the statistical improvement seems to have depended on the time of measurement after treatment and the statistical power of the study. Most of these studies included concurrent untreated controls or used the treated horses as their own controls by demonstrating stability of clinical disease for 1 to 2 weeks before treatment with dexamethasone. Dexamethasone isonicotinate, conversely, seems to be less efficacious at the doses tested, with one investigator [23] failing to demonstrate a statistically significant improvement in pulmonary mechanical properties after a single intramuscular dose of 0.06 mg/kg and another [21] reporting modest results with intramuscular dosing at 0.04 mg/kg every 3 days. Interestingly, only two studies concurrently measured and reported pulmonary mechanical properties and clinical severity scores. In one study, dexamethasone resulted in statistically significant clinical improvement starting 2 days after initial treatment and lasting throughout the treatment period [20]. In the second study, no improvement in clinical score was detected after a single treatment with dexamethasone isonicotinate [23]. Taken collectively, however, the evidence for efficacy of dexamethasone for the improvement of clinical signs of RAO is quite good.

The efficacy of aerosolized corticosteroids for the treatment of RAO is also widely reported in the peer-reviewed literature. Beclomethasone dipropionate, delivered at a rate of 500 μg twice daily for 10 days using a handheld delivery device similar to the now-defunct Torpex device, effectively improved the clinical score of horses with RAO after 10 days of treatment but, interestingly, did not have a statistically significant effect on pulmonary resistance [23]. Similarly, rapid improvement (within 3 days) was demonstrated in clinical score with a dose of 1320 μg administered twice daily using a similar delivery system, with significant improvement in pulmonary resistance detected after 10 days of treatment [20]. Unfortunately, as is the case with aerosolized bronchodilators, the value of these reports to the practitioner is somewhat diminished by the current lack of availability of the unique delivery system used in the studies. Beclomethasone dipropionate aerosol delivered from a metered-dose inhaler using an Equine Aeromask at a rate of 3750 μg administered twice daily for 15 days has been reported effective [24], however, with improvement in clinical signs detected after 4 days of treatment and improvement in pulmonary resistance detected after 7 days of treatment.

Aerosolized fluticasone propionate has also been investigated for the treatment of RAO, producing strong evidence for efficacy. In a double-blind, randomized, placebo- or prednisone-controlled study conducted on privately owned horses, in which at least some of the treatments were administered by the owners instead of the investigators, fluticasone delivered from a metered-dose inhaler through an Equine Aeromask at an initial rate of 1980 μg administered twice daily resulted in improvement in clinical score and pulmonary resistance values after 4 weeks of treatment [25]. The design of this study is, in the opinion of the authors, the most valuable in terms of clinical application of the principles of evidence-based medicine and provides the strongest evidence for the use of aerosolized fluticasone as a treatment for RAO.

Other anti-inflammatory drugs have less compelling evidence for efficacy. Oral prednisone has been widely used as a therapeutic agent for RAO, but critical evidence for its efficacy is weak. Highly variable but generally poor bioavailability of oral prednisone in RAO-affected horses has been reported [26]. Bioactivity depends on conversion of prednisone to prednisolone, and this process was also lacking. In the same study, the lack of concurrent depression of endogenous cortisol was viewed as further evidence of a lack of endogenous glucocorticoid activity of orally administered prednisone. Thus, perhaps not surprisingly, oral prednisone failed to improve pulmonary function at a dose of 2.2 mg/kg administered by mouth once daily for 10 days [21]. Improvement in clinical score was noted in one study [25] using a roughly equivalent dose (500 mg administered once daily), but similar to the study of Robinson and colleagues [21], no improvement in pulmonary mechanical properties was measured.

Other drugs have also been evaluated. Pentoxifylline administered orally at a dose of 16 g/d per horse resulted in a 43% reduction in pulmonary resistance after 15 days, but no measurement of clinical score was provided [27]. Given the tendency for dissociation between improvement in pulmonary mechanics and improvement in clinical score when evaluating anti-inflammatory treatments (in contrast to bronchodilators), the assumption that this magnitude of improvement would have resulted in an improved clinical score must be made with caution. Furthermore, the authors noted considerable variability in the pharmacokinetics of pentoxifylline when administered orally, making its reliability even more uncertain. Nutritional antioxidant supplementation has been advocated but has only been evaluated in horses with RAO in remission [28], and is therefore of uncertain value in clinically affected horses.

RAO is a disease triggered by environmental factors. Thus, it is certainly logical to treat the disease by correcting the environmental conditions that elicit the clinical disease. Removing horses from dusty barns and feeding low-dust forage have been mainstays of treatment whenever it is possible to implement these measures. The efficacy of removing horses from a dusty environment to allow the disease to go into remission is indirectly demonstrated by the dozens of mechanistic research studies in which university-owned herds of RAO-affected horses are maintained in remission between studies by being released into pasture. Not all horsemen have this option available; thus, there is considerable interest in stable management practices that might reduce the clinical signs of RAO in susceptible horses. Studies have indicated that bedding horses on shredded paper [29], wood shavings [30], cardboard [31], or good-quality straw [30] may allow RAO-susceptible horses to remain asymptomatic. In all these studies, however, some form of low-dust forage was concurrently provided in place of hay. The possible effect of this second variable is important, because studies of the aeroallergen exposure of horses strongly suggest that forage is the major source of particles that are inhaled by a horse [32]. Indeed, in one study, clinical exacerbation of RAO was achieved by using the same good-quality straw bedding but by replacing the low-dust forage with regular hay [30]. Fresh grass silage [30,31] or forage processed into cubes [29] also seems to be efficacious in preventing exacerbation of RAO in stabled horses. Although the quality of any individual study, from an EBVM standpoint, may not be high (ie, no blinding or randomization of treatments), the consistent and dramatic clinical response to a change in a single variable provides good evidence that the change was responsible for the response, and this response has been repeatedly demonstrated in independent studies.

Exercise-induced pulmonary hemorrhage

Exercise-induced pulmonary hemorrhage (EIPH) is a frequent target of therapy in equine veterinary medicine, but the critical evaluation of the strength of evidence for a purported efficacious treatment is complicated by the wide variety of end points used to evaluate treatment. EIPH is most often diagnosed by endoscopic visualization of blood in the trachea of a horse after exercise. The relative abundance of blood is typically scored using an ordinal scoring system to approximate the severity of the condition, and in most cases, this approach has been shown to have an acceptable degree of reproducibility [33,34]. This approach has significant value in the clinical application of EBVM because it (or some version of it) is the approach used in most situations in which EIPH and the response thereof to treatment are evaluated. In addition, the severity of EIPH in laboratory settings has been quantified through the enumeration of erythrocytes in BALF [35–37]. Unfortunately, the precision of this approach relative to the semiquantitative approach of endoscopic scoring is currently unknown [38]. As a final complication, none of these measures unequivocally reflect the true owner or agent complaint regarding a horse with EIPH—poor athletic performance. Unfortunately, methods of defining this end point are quite imprecise, although there have been admirable efforts to conduct studies with sufficient numbers to overcome this difficulty statistically.

Furosemide is the most common pharmacologic treatment for EIPH, and there is considerable evidence for its efficacy, as first demonstrated in the reduction of the severity of EIPH in approximately 64% of treated horses in a placebo-controlled study conducted using racehorses performing routine strenuous workouts [33]. The substitution of workouts for racing in this study highlights the difficulty of conducting EBVM-relevant studies on this condition, because the regulated nature of racing effectively precludes the use of random prospective assignment to treatment groups or the use of placebos. The possible relevance of this point is highlighted by the subsequent report in which the efficacy of furosemide was minimal under actual racing conditions [39]. Furosemide also has been shown to reduce the severity of EIPH (as defined by postexercise BALF erythrocyte concentrations) under laboratory conditions by two placebo-controlled, randomized, crossover studies [36,37].

The effect of furosemide on athletic performance has also been the subject of considerable study, and the consensus seems to be that administration of furosemide before an athletic event can improve performance in that event [40–43]. Although it is possible that the mechanism of action of furosemide relative to athletic performance may not rest entirely in its ability to attenuate EIPH (furosemide causes significant acute weight loss, and may therefore make the horse more energy efficient [44,45]), a recent study clearly defined a connection between racing performance and EIPH [46], providing a degree of legitimacy for this treatment that had been presumed but not proven.

Adhesive nasal strips that stabilize the external nares have been shown to reduce EIPH under laboratory conditions. Two similar studies from different laboratories [36,37] reported similar results, in that application of the nasal strip reduced the concentration of erythrocytes in postexercise BALF compared with no treatment. Both studies also concurrently evaluated pre-exercise treatment with furosemide, with slightly different conclusions.

One study found no difference between nasal strips and furosemide individually or when combined [37]; however, another study found that the combination of furosemide and the nasal strip was more efficacious than the nasal strip alone [36]. No benefit of the nasal strip on the endoscopic appearance of EIPH was found in a third study [47]; however, the quantification of EIPH was limited to a simple binomial grading scale (ie, whether fresh blood was present in the airways) rather than to the more commonly used subjective grading scale; thus, this study did not possess sufficient sensitivity to detect changes in the magnitude of EIPH. Finally, none of these studies have been conducted under actual racing conditions (as have the studies examining the efficacy of furosemide); thus, although there seems to be potential benefit in the use of nasal strips for lessening the severity of EIPH, the quality of evidence is less than that for furosemide.

Many other treatments, such as water-saturated vapor [48], cromolyn sodium [49], and hesperidin-citrus bioflavonoids [39], have been advocated and tested for EIPH, with disappointing results. In all cases, these studies were conducted using endoscopic scoring as the measurement of EIPH and a reasonable number of experimental subjects (comparable to the number initially needed to demonstrate an effect of furosemide on EIPH [33]). There is little basis for use of these treatments for EIPH in the realm of EBVM.

Upper airway diseases

There is less rigorous evidence of the efficacy of medical treatments of upper airway conditions in the horse compared with medical treatments for lower airway conditions. Many of the upper airway conditions, such as laryngeal hemiplegia, arytenoids chondritis, epiglottic entrapment, and dorsal displacement of the soft palate, are generally treated surgically and are discussed elsewhere in this issue. Other conditions, such as bacterial or viral infections of the upper airway structures, may be treated medically. There is a near-complete lack of reports that can be used in an EBVM approach, however. The potential reasons for this lack of research include the self-limiting nature of many of the diseases, the lack of experimental models to facilitate laboratory study of the diseases, and the anticipated reluctance of private horse owners to participate in a study in which their horse may receive a placebo treatment. The authors recognize the difficulty of conducting placebo-controlled studies on populations of horses that would almost certainly include client-owned animals, but such an approach is necessary when evaluating treatments for diseases for which spontaneous recovery is common.

Guttural pouches

Guttural pouch mycosis is an infrequent but serious disease in horses. Treatment of horses with guttural pouch mycosis consists of medical treatment (typically with antifungal drugs applied directly to the lesions in the guttural pouch [50,51]) or surgical ligation of the internal carotid artery [50,52,53]. There are numerous reports of multiple cases and treatment outcomes, but there are no studies that evaluate treatment in a comparative fashion. One can make the assumption that not treating a horse with guttural pouch mycosis universally results in that horse succumbing to the disease and can apply this hypothetic "control group" to these case studies. With that approach to evaluating these reports, treatment with medical or surgical management seems to be quite efficacious. It is impossible, based on the published evidence, to determine the relative value of a particular treatment as opposed to another, even within a single study, however, because all the published studies are retrospective and, in all instances, the assignment of treatment strategy was not random. Thus, although a practitioner probably is correct in concluding that any of the treatments that have been associated with a positive outcome are efficacious to some degree, there is little objective evidence to rank one treatment as being superior to another.

Summary

It is clear from a review of the current scientific literature that an evidence-based approach to medical treatment of equine respiratory disease can be applied, at least in the instance of common lower respiratory diseases. In particular, there is clear evidence for efficacious treatments for RAO and EIPH, and with the recognition of this evidence, these treatments should be the first to be considered by a practitioner when treating these conditions. As would be reasonably expected, there is less critical evidence for specific treatment efficacy for less common diseases, but the principles of EBVM can still be applied in those situations by the recognition of the lack of strong evidence for a particular treatment. In those situations, the practitioner should continue to rely more on his or her own experience and rational inferences drawn from the pathophysiology of the condition and the mechanisms of action of a particular therapy.

References

[1] Robinson NE, Olszewski MA, Boehler D, et al. Relationship between clinical signs and lung function in horses with recurrent airway obstruction (heaves) during a bronchodilator trial. Equine Vet J 2000;32:393–400.

[2] Tesarowski DB, Viel L, McDonell WN, et al. The rapid and effective administration of a beta 2-agonist to horses with heaves using a compact inhalation device and metered-dose inhalers. Can Vet J 1994;35:170–3.

[3] Derksen FJ, Olszewski M, Robinson NE, et al. Use of a hand-held, metered-dose aerosol delivery device to administer pirbuterol acetate to horses with 'heaves.' Equine Vet J 1996; 28:306–10.

[4] Derksen FJ, Olszewski MA, Robinson NE, et al. Aerosolized albuterol sulfate used as a bronchodilator in horses with recurrent airway obstruction. Am J Vet Res 1999;60: 689–93.

[5] Mazan MR, Hoffman AM, Kuehn H, et al. Effect of aerosolized albuterol sulfate on resting energy expenditure determined by use of open-flow indirect calorimetry in horses with recurrent airway obstruction. Am J Vet Res 2003;64:235–42.

[6] Henrikson SL, Rush BR. Efficacy of salmeterol xinafoate in horses with recurrent airway obstruction. J Am Vet Med Assoc 2001;218:1961–5.

[7] Murphy JR, McPherson EA, Dixon PM. Chronic obstructive pulmonary disease (COPD): effects of bronchodilator drugs on normal and affected horses. Equine Vet J 1980;12:10–4.

[8] Broadstone RV, Scott JS, Derksen FJ, et al. Effects of atropine in ponies with recurrent airway obstruction. J Appl Physiol 1988;65:2720–5.

[9] Robinson NE, Derksen FJ, Berney C, et al. The airway response of horses with recurrent airway obstruction (heaves) to aerosol administration of ipratropium bromide. Equine Vet J 1993;25:299–303.

[10] Duvivier DH, Votion D, Vandenput S, et al. Airway response of horses with COPD to dry powder inhalation of ipratropium bromide. Vet J 1997;154:149–53.

[11] Traub-Dargatz JL, McKinnon AO, Thrall MA, et al. Evaluation of clinical signs of disease, bronchoalveolar and tracheal wash analysis, and arterial blood gas tensions in 13 horses with chronic obstructive pulmonary disease treated with prednisone, methyl sulfonmethane, and clenbuterol hydrochloride. Am J Vet Res 1992;53:1908–16.

[12] Erichsen DF, Aviad AD, Schultz RH, et al. Clinical efficacy and safety of clenbuterol HCl when administered to effect in horses with chronic obstructive pulmonary disease (COPD). Equine Vet J 1994;26:331–6.

[13] Turgut K, Sasse HH. Influence of clenbuterol on mucociliary transport in healthy horses and horses with chronic obstructive pulmonary disease. Vet Rec 1989;125:526–30.

[14] Jean D, Vrins A, Lavoie JP. Respiratory and metabolic effects of massive administration of isotonic saline solution in heaves-affected and control horses. Equine Vet J 2004;36: 628–33.

[15] Wilson DV, Berney CE, Peroni DL, et al. The effects of a single acupuncture treatment in horses with severe recurrent airway obstruction. Equine Vet J 2004;36:489–94.

[16] van den HR, Zappe H, Zitterl-Eglseer K, et al. Study of the effect of Bronchipret on the lung function of five Austrian saddle horses suffering recurrent airway obstruction (heaves). Vet Rec 2003;152:555–7.

[17] Anour R, Leinker S, van den HR. Improvement of the lung function of horses with heaves by treatment with a botanical preparation for 14 days. Vet Rec 2005;157:733–6.

[18] Lavoie JP, Leguillette R, Pasloske K, et al. Comparison of effects of dexamethasone and the leukotriene D4 receptor antagonist L-708,738 on lung function and airway cytologic findings in horses with recurrent airway obstruction. Am J Vet Res 2002;63:579–85.

[19] Picandet V, Leguillette R, Lavoie JP. Comparison of efficacy and tolerability of isoflupredone and dexamethasone in the treatment of horses affected with recurrent airway obstruction ('heaves'). Equine Vet J 2003;35:419–24.

[20] Rush BR, Raub ES, Rhoads WS, et al. Pulmonary function in horses with recurrent airway obstruction after aerosol and parenteral administration of beclomethasone dipropionate and dexamethasone, respectively. Am J Vet Res 1998;59:1039–43.

[21] Robinson NE, Jackson C, Jefcoat A, et al. Efficacy of three corticosteroids for the treatment of heaves. Equine Vet J 2002;34:17–22.

[22] Cornelisse CJ, Robinson NE, Berney CE, et al. Efficacy of oral and intravenous dexamethasone in horses with recurrent airway obstruction. Equine Vet J 2004;36:426–30.

[23] Couetil LL, Art T, de Moffarts B, et al. Effect of beclomethasone dipropionate and dexamethasone isonicotinate on lung function, bronchoalveolar lavage fluid cytology, and transcription factor expression in airways of horses with recurrent airway obstruction. J Vet Intern Med 2006;20:399–406.

[24] Ammann VJ, Vrins AA, Lavoie JP. Effects of inhaled beclomethasone dipropionate on respiratory function in horses with chronic obstructive pulmonary disease (COPD). Equine Vet J 1998;30:152–7.
[25] Couetil LL, Chilcoat CD, DeNicola DB, et al. Randomized, controlled study of inhaled fluticasone propionate, oral administration of prednisone, and environmental management of horses with recurrent airway obstruction. Am J Vet Res 2005;66:1665–74.
[26] Peroni DL, Stanley S, Kollias-Baker C, et al. Prednisone per os is likely to have limited efficacy in horses. Equine Vet J 2002;34:283–7.
[27] Leguillette R, Desevaux C, Lavoie JP. Effects of pentoxifylline on pulmonary function and results of cytologic examination of bronchoalveolar lavage fluid in horses with recurrent airway obstruction. Am J Vet Res 2002;63:459–63.
[28] Kirschvink N, Fievez L, Bougnet V, et al. Effect of nutritional antioxidant supplementation on systemic and pulmonary antioxidant status, airway inflammation and lung function in heaves-affected horses. Equine Vet J 2002;34:705–12.
[29] Thomson JR, McPherson EA. Effects of environmental control on pulmonary function of horses affected with chronic obstructive pulmonary disease. Equine Vet J 1984;16:35–8.
[30] Vandenput S, Duvivier DH, Votion D, et al. Environmental control to maintain stabled COPD horses in clinical remission: effects on pulmonary function. Equine Vet J 1998;30: 93–6.
[31] Kirschvink N, Di Silvestro F, Sbai I, et al. The use of cardboard bedding material as part of an environmental control regime for heaves-affected horses: in vitro assessment of airborne dust and aeroallergen concentration and in vivo effects on lung function. Vet J 2002;163: 319–25.
[32] Woods PS, Robinson NE, Swanson MC, et al. Airborne dust and aeroallergen concentration in a horse stable under two different management systems. Equine Vet J 1993;25:208–13.
[33] Pascoe JR, McCabe AE, Franti CE, et al. Efficacy of furosemide in the treatment of exercise-induced pulmonary hemorrhage in Thoroughbred racehorses. Am J Vet Res 1985;46: 2000–3.
[34] Hinchcliff KW, Jackson MA, Brown JA, et al. Tracheobronchoscopic assessment of exercise-induced pulmonary hemorrhage in horses. Am J Vet Res 2005;66:596–8.
[35] Meyer TS, Fedde MR, Gaughan EM, et al. Quantification of exercise-induced pulmonary haemorrhage with bronchoalveolar lavage. Equine Vet J 1998;30:284–8.
[36] Geor RJ, Ommundson L, Fenton G, et al. Effects of an external nasal strip and furosemide on pulmonary haemorrhage in Thoroughbreds following high-intensity exercise. Equine Vet J 2001;33:577–84.
[37] Kindig CA, McDonough P, Fenton G, et al. Efficacy of nasal strip and furosemide in mitigating EIPH in Thoroughbred horses. J Appl Physiol 2001;91:1396–400.
[38] Hinchcliff KW. Counting red cells—is it an answer to EIPH? Equine Vet J 2000;32:362–3.
[39] Sweeney CR, Soma LR. Exercise-induced pulmonary hemorrhage in Thoroughbred horses: response to furosemide or hesperidin-citrus bioflavonoids. J Am Vet Med Assoc 1984;185: 195–7.
[40] Soma LR, Laster L, Oppenlander F, et al. Effects of furosemide on the racing times of horses with exercise-induced pulmonary hemorrhage. Am J Vet Res 1985;46:763–8.
[41] Sweeney CR, Soma LR, Maxson AD, et al. Effects of furosemide on the racing times of Thoroughbreds. Am J Vet Res 1990;51:772–8.
[42] Gross DK, Morley PS, Hinchcliff KW, et al. Effect of furosemide on performance of Thoroughbreds racing in the United States and Canada. J Am Vet Med Assoc 1999;215:670–5.
[43] Soma LR, Birks EK, Uboh CE, et al. The effects of furosemide on racing times of Standardbred pacers. Equine Vet J 2000;32:334–40.
[44] Hinchcliff KW, McKeever KH. Fluid administration attenuates the haemodynamic effect of furosemide in running horses. Equine Vet J 1998;30:246–50.
[45] Hinchcliff KW, McKeever KH, Muir WW III, et al. Effect of furosemide and weight carriage on energetic responses of horses to incremental exertion. Am J Vet Res 1993;54:1500–4.

[46] Hinchcliff KW, Jackson MA, Morley PS, et al. Association between exercise-induced pulmonary hemorrhage and performance in Thoroughbred racehorses. J Am Vet Med Assoc 2005; 227:768–74.
[47] Goetz TE, Manohar M, Hassan AS, et al. Nasal strips do not affect pulmonary gas exchange, anaerobic metabolism, or EIPH in exercising Thoroughbreds. J Appl Physiol 2001;90: 2378–85.
[48] Sweeney CR, Hall J, Fisher JR, et al. Efficacy of water vapor-saturated air in the treatment of exercise-induced pulmonary hemorrhage in Thoroughbred racehorses. Am J Vet Res 1988; 49:1705–7.
[49] Hillidge CJ, Whitlock TW, Lane TJ. Failure of inhaled disodium cromoglycate aerosol to prevent exercise-induced pulmonary hemorrhage in racing Quarter Horses. J Vet Pharmacol Ther 1987;10:257–60.
[50] Church S, Wyn-Jones G, Parks AH, et al. Treatment of guttural pouch mycosis. Equine Vet J 1986;18:362–5.
[51] Davis EW, Legendre AM. Successful treatment of guttural pouch mycosis with itraconazole and topical enilconazole in a horse. J Vet Intern Med 1994;8:304–5.
[52] Greet TR. Outcome of treatment in 35 cases of guttural pouch mycosis. Equine Vet J 1987; 19:483–7.
[53] Speirs VC, Harrison IW, van Veenendaal JC, et al. Is specific antifungal therapy necessary for the treatment of guttural pouch mycosis in horses? Equine Vet J 1995;27:151–2.

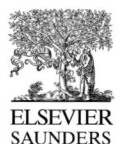

Evidence-Based Equine Upper Respiratory Surgery

Warren L. Beard, DVM, MS[a],*, Sarah Waxman, BS[b]

[a]*Department of Clinical Sciences, College of Veterinary Medicine, Kansas State University, 1800 Denison Avenue, Manhattan, KS 66506, USA*
[b]*College of Veterinary Medicine, Kansas State University, Manhattan, KS, USA*

The purpose of this article is to review the veterinary literature for various surgical procedures of the equine upper respiratory tract in an effort to evaluate the evidence supporting various therapies. The list of conditions to be covered is not, and need not be, all-inclusive. Indeed, the treatment of many conditions should be intuitive, and the benefit of intervention self-evident, such as drainage of pulmonary abscesses or excision of a neoplastic mass. Therapeutic benefit from such procedures is obvious and need not necessarily be supported by randomized controlled trials. This article instead focuses on the therapeutic benefit from more widely occurring conditions, such as laryngeal hemiplegia (LH), dorsal displacement of the soft palate (DDSP), arytenoid chondritis (AC), and epiglottic entrapment (EE).

An evidence-based approach to surgery can be challenging, and equine practice itself presents its own unique challenges. Some conditions do not necessarily lend themselves to experimental models. For example, some intermittent conditions, such as DDSP and EE, are only present during exercise, and the circumstances that induce the abnormality are not easily reproducible at rest. The diagnosis in such instances is often speculative, based on a compatible history, and often leads to differing inclusion criteria. As a result, studies may not be directly comparable. In addition, the effect of treatment and the prognosis for future performance can be difficult to determine, because horses often have multiple problems.

There are also variables between groups of horses to consider. Athletic horses perform widely varying tasks for a living, and the demands placed on the horses can dramatically affect the surgical outcome. For example, hunters and jumpers that exercise for short durations at submaximal intensity can be expected to have a lower requirement for air flow than a racehorse

* Corresponding author.
E-mail address: wbeard@ksu.edu (W.L. Beard).

galloping at speeds in excess of 14 m/s. Studies comparing results in these different disciplines confirm this.

Many of the surgical procedures for the upper respiratory tract are technically demanding. There can be tremendous variation in results between surgeons depending on training, level of expertise, and the frequency with which the surgeon performs the procedure. Many of the surgical procedures are exceedingly difficult to perform, and it is unreasonable to expect that an untrained individual would achieve results similar to a specialist who performs the procedure on a regular basis. As a result, retrospective studies that compile results from many surgeons tend to have more pessimistic results than studies in which one or a small number of surgeons perform all the procedures.

Many conditions do not occur with enough frequency to perform clinical trials on par with the large studies that are commonplace in human medicine. Owners keep these animals to perform in their chosen equestrian discipline; the goal is to win. This presents its own set of problems for clinical research in equine respiratory surgery. Owners may be unwilling to accept a sham treatment if they recognize a performance-limiting problem with their horse. Thus, placebo-controlled trials are nonexistent in equine surgery. Similarly, studies that compare a new treatment with the previous standard therapy are infrequent, because clients may be reluctant to participate in them. Clients are astute enough to recognize that the new treatment is being investigated because of shortcomings in the standard therapy; there is always the impression that newer equates to better. Unfortunately, such obstacles to collection of evidence are accompanied by even less noble reasons for the active promotion of unvalidated new procedures, including a disregard of scientific methodology, vanity, and financial incentive.

The result has been a succession of studies of new procedures that differ in equine populations, inclusion criteria, measure of success, and control population. The appearance of these procedures generally precedes their appearance in the peer-reviewed literature. Nevertheless, these therapies may be actively promoted in Web pages, lay publications, and non–peer-reviewed publications. This makes it difficult for the practitioner to assess the importance of many new procedures by any method other than to see how the technique fares with the passage of time.

The evidence-based medicine approach is relatively new in human and veterinary medicine. Most of the studies cited in this article were written long before the practice of evidence-based medicine was established. All the studies cited here were written by established researchers and clinicians doing what they were supposed to be doing: engaging in state-of-the-art practice, developing and testing new techniques, and reporting their findings in peer-reviewed literature. In light of present knowledge, it is easy to critique their methodology retrospectively; however, one must remember that many of these studies were in fact "landmark" articles that shaped the direction of future study. There has been a noticeable improvement in the quality of the studies over time as newer studies strive to avoid the weaknesses of prior publications.

This review is intended solely to evaluate the evidence in the literature; it is not intended to be a critique of the authors. The authors of this article took the liberty of mining the various publications for results and performed calculations that may not have been presented in the original studies. This was done to provide meaningful comparisons between studies and was performed without favoritism to any of the studies. Original technique descriptions, small case series, or reports that use methodologies dramatically different from current practice were ignored in favor of larger retrospective or prospective studies so as to present the best current evidence.

Laryngeal hemiplegia

LH is caused by paralysis of the recurrent laryngeal nerve, the effect of which can be mimicked by transaction of the nerve. This is significant, because there is a research model for this condition that closely replicates the naturally occurring disease and allows investigation of the various surgical procedures to treat LH under controlled conditions.

The goals of treatment of LH are to restore air flow and eliminate respiratory noise, although these two outcomes are somewhat interrelated. The prosthetic laryngoplasty, as described by Marks and colleagues [1] in 1970, has been the mainstay for restoring the normal airway mechanics by means of abduction and stabilization of the arytenoid cartilage. Two other procedures are occasionally used to restore normal airway mechanics; arytenoidectomy to remove the paralyzed cartilage and laryngeal reinnervation. Noise reduction may be accomplished by a ventriculectomy performed through a ventral laryngotomy, transendoscopically with a laser, or by means of a ventriculocordectomy.

Prosthetic laryngoplasty

Four experimental studies on LH induced by transection of the recurrent laryngeal nerve have evaluated the effects of LH on respiratory and blood gas variables in instrumented horses before neurectomy, after neurectomy, and after a prosthetic laryngoplasty [2–5]. LH caused decreases in respiratory frequency, minute ventilation, Pa_{O_2}, and pH and increases in upper airway impedance, negative inspiratory pressure, and Pa_{CO_2}. In all cases, prosthetic laryngoplasty restored the variables to preneurectomy values or significantly improved the variables compared with presurgical values [2–5]. Obviously, not all studies measured the same variables, but there was complete agreement between the studies that looked at the same variables. Furthermore, there have been no subsequent studies to contradict these findings. Taken together, these studies provide strong evidence that a prosthetic laryngoplasty can be successful in eliminating or attenuating the effects of induced

LH on respiratory and blood gas variables. Unfortunately, the clinical relevance of these studies is diminished by the fact that the effects of a prosthetic laryngoplasty were measured at treadmill speeds of 4.3 [2], 7.2 [3], 8.3 [4], and 10 [5] m/s; all of which are substantially less than the speed achieved by racehorses Fig. 1.

The outcome for clinical cases undergoing a prosthetic laryngoplasty is much less clear. Interpretation of results is confounded by all the customary factors that plague retrospective studies. Differences in surgeons, techniques, case selection, breed and use of horse, follow-up interval, and criteria for success make it difficult to compare among studies. Analysis is also complicated, because horses often have more than one respiratory condition. Racing data are especially difficult to analyze, because there is a high loss of horses to follow-up. In addition, grouping of horses into the four permutations of raced and unraced before and after surgery leaves small groups and unconvincing statistical analysis. For these reasons, all the authors in clinical studies have used subjective owner satisfaction as the criterion for success. The more recent literature strives to use more objective outcome criteria by employing racing data. Results from five retrospective studies are tabulated in Table 1. These results are based on owner assessment of outcome and do not account for horses lost to follow-up.

From these data, several generalizations can be made. The prognosis for successful racing performance, based on subjective owner or trainer assessment, ranges from 48% to 81% [6–8], and 77% [6], 80% [8], and 94% [9] of racehorses made at least one start after surgery. There is not enough evidence to determine if the prognosis is better for racing Standardbreds or Thoroughbreds, and there is conflicting evidence on whether the prognosis for racing is better for younger or older horses. There seems to be a trend for horses to drop in class after surgery [8,9]. Differing methodologies among the studies make further inferences difficult.

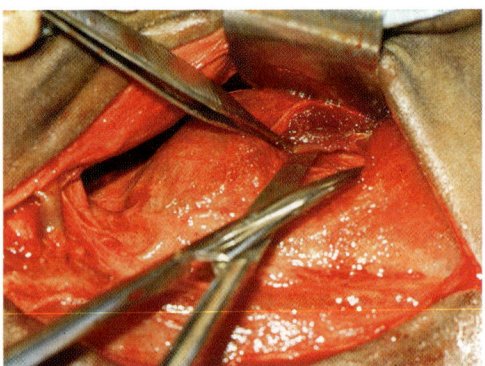

Fig. 1. Intraoperative dissection to expose the muscular process for suture placement during a prosthetic laryngoplasty.

Table 1
Postoperative performance and complications after prosthetic laryngoplasty

No. operated horses	No. horses with follow-up	Percent satisfaction	Exercise intolerance after surgery (%)	Respiratory noise after surgery (%)	Coughing after surgery (%)	Reference
70	55	60	42	47	33	[8]
80	69	70	25	9	—	[7]
230	176	81	—	25	26	[6]
104	79	92	6	21	9	[11]
200	198	86	13	27	—	[10]

Horses engaging in nonracing sports have a much better prognosis. Several studies have reported a successful outcome in 86% [10], 90% [7], 92% [11], and 93% [8] of horses after a laryngoplasty. For racehorses and nonracing horses, exercise intolerance, respiratory noise, and coughing seem to be major complications of the procedure. Unquestionably, prosthetic laryngoplasty is a difficult procedure to perform, and results can vary widely. The fact remains, however, that the procedure has now been performed for 36 years without any serious rival for replacement. This is at least some evidence that the procedure is efficacious to some degree.

Laryngeal reinnervation

The first report on laryngeal reinnervation in ponies appeared in 1989 and demonstrated that the technique was possible [12,13]. A subsequent experimental study using horses with LH induced by transaction of the recurrent laryngeal nerve demonstrated that a nerve-muscle pedicle graft from the first cervical nerve was capable of improving or restoring respiratory variables to baseline values; however, horses were only exercised at 7 m/s [14]. There is only one clinical report of this procedure using 129 Thoroughbreds, of which results were available for 113 horses [15]. Ninety-five percent of horses that raced before surgery started in at least one race after surgery, but only 60% of unraced horses were able to race after surgery. Six of 10 Standardbreds that underwent surgery raced after surgery, and 5 of 7 warmbloods were improved.

This study principally used race records to assess results; thus, comparison with a laryngoplasty in which owner satisfaction was used is impossible. It is tempting to compare race records for laryngeal reinnervation with the prosthetic laryngoplasty race records, but methods used in the various studies were so disparate that meaningful comparisons are impossible. It is also unclear how widely this procedure is performed. In the 16 years since the initial report in experimental horses, there is only one clinical study and two surgeons accounted for all the cases. That study clearly shows that laryngeal reinnervation can be successful; however, a prosthetic laryngoplasty still seems to be the choice of most surgeons.

Arytenoidectomy

It is more difficult to assess a prognosis for return to function after an arytenoidectomy than after a prosthetic laryngoplasty because an arytenoidectomy is performed to treat several conditions, including AC and LH, as well as to treat horses in which a prosthetic laryngoplasty has failed. Two arytenoidectomy techniques are described that differ in the amount of the arytenoid cartilage removed.

A subtotal arytenoidectomy was reported to result in 90% of 20 racehorses returning to racing. Racing performance was reported as excellent or fair in these horses; however, no information about the longevity or success of the racing careers was presented [16]. In 1990, an experimental study in treadmill horses demonstrated that upper airway mechanics did not improve after a subtotal arytenoidectomy to correct LH induced by recurrent laryngeal nerve neurectomy [17]. It is noteworthy that the subtotal arytenoidectomy did not result in improvement in these horses even at a treadmill speed of 7 m/s. Based on the failure of this technique to improve airway mechanics under experimental conditions and the lack of follow-up reports to verify the initial results, this technique has been abandoned.

The initial report on partial arytenoidectomy in 1980 described successful return to function in three quarters of non-racing horses [18]. A subsequent report of 75 cases revealed that 75% of non-racing horses were able to return to their intended use but that only 45% of Thoroughbreds and 20% of Standardbreds were able to return to racing [19]. This report may be overly pessimistic about racehorse performance, because approximately 30% of the racehorses underwent a bilateral arytenoidectomy. A later report demonstrated that 61% of horses that had not previously raced and 78% of horses that had raced were able to race after a partial arytenoidectomy [20]. Research evidence confirms that a partial arytenoidectomy is able to attenuate the detrimental effects on airway mechanics in horses with induced LH at speeds that correlated to 100% of maximal heart rate (HR_{max}) [21,22]. All the clinical studies included horses operated on for AC and LH. The authors attempted to separate the results so that the reader could determine if the prognosis was different between the two conditions; however, group size was too small to allow any inferences to be drawn.

A recent study in treadmill horses with induced LH attempted to determine whether a prosthetic laryngoplasty or a partial arytenoidectomy was superior. Both procedures nearly restored respiratory variables to normal values when horses were exercised at speeds corresponding to HR_{max}, and there was a slight advantage to a prosthetic laryngoplasty. This would seem to indicate that the procedures are comparable for horses exercising at submaximal intensity. The speed corresponding to HR_{max} is still substantially less than racing speed; thus, it cannot be determined from the available evidence whether arytenoidectomy and laryngoplasty are equivalent in racehorses [22].

Respiratory noise

The persistence of respiratory noise is a major complication after all treatments for AC and LH. The initial description of the prosthetic laryngoplasty combined that procedure with a ventriculectomy [1]. In the 1980s, the necessity of the ventriculectomy was questioned. One research study demonstrated that a ventriculectomy alone did not reverse the detrimental effects of induced LH on upper airway mechanics, even when horses only exercised at 7.2 m/s [3]. Subsequent research using microphone recordings of respiratory noise have convincingly demonstrated that a ventriculocordectomy alone is superior to a prosthetic laryngoplasty alone at reducing airway noise [23]. A unilateral laser ventriculectomy was not successful in reducing airway noise using the same methodology [24]. Based on these objective studies using a realistic model, it is reasonable to conclude that the ventriculocordectomy is the most efficacious procedure at eliminating respiratory noise secondary to LH.

Curiously, the academic debate on the necessity of a ventriculectomy was largely ignored by surgeons, because all retrospective studies on prosthetic laryngoplasty and arytenoidectomy performed between 1970 and 2003 combined those procedures with a ventriculectomy or ventriculocordectomy. This is in spite of the fact that clinical studies have been unable to document any improvement in performance with the addition of a ventriculectomy or ventriculocordectomy [6,7]. Clearly, surgeons perceive a benefit, even if it is unsubstantiated by the available evidence. A treadmill study in exercising horses with induced LH demonstrated that a ventriculocordectomy improves upper airway mechanics but is vastly inferior to a prosthetic laryngoplasty [23]. In another study, a ventriculocordectomy did not result in any additional improvement in airway mechanics beyond that provided by a prosthetic laryngoplasty [5]. Recently, a ventriculocordectomy has been reported as the sole treatment for 92 horses with incomplete laryngeal paralysis. Owners or trainers subjectively judged that performance was improved in 59% of horses, and surgery was considered worthwhile by 86% of owners. Twenty-two percent of the horses coughed after surgery, and noise during exercise remained in 21% of horses, which is comparable to the results of studies of a prosthetic laryngoplasty. This study shows that respiratory noise may be decreased and performance improved after a ventriculocordectomy; however, further comparisons with other surgical procedures for LH are not possible, because this report principally consists of horses with incomplete laryngeal paralysis [25].

Dorsal displacement of the soft palate

Little is clear when it comes to analyzing the literature to determine the best treatment for DDSP. The condition is prevalent in racing Standardbreds and Thoroughbreds, and although the incidence is unknown, one prominent authority has estimated the incidence at 10% to 20% [26]. The most accurate method of diagnosis is debated, and diagnostic methods and inclusion criteria vary between studies. Careful reading reveals that many horses in these studies were operated on without a clear diagnosis or for lack of other options. Also, many of the horses in those studies had more than one upper airway condition.

Outcome assessment is difficult for racehorses, and selection of the comparison group can greatly influence results. Use of the horse as its own control is ideal, but there are many reasons why a horse may not race well and horses are often retired (and lost to follow-up) for unrelated reasons. Statistical comparison can be problematic when horses do not race before or after surgery. Further complicating interpretation of results is that the use of random controls can skew results in favor of the study population if that population is an elite one that is not comparable to the average horse.

In addition to these previously acknowledged limitations, there are others that are never mentioned. It is uncommon to be called on to treat a horse at a referral center that has not had some prior medical or surgical treatment performed. Several studies of surgical interventions report the incidence of other known prior surgical interventions in the study population to be 9% [27], 29% [28], 68% [29], and 93% [30], and this probably underestimates the actual incidence, because many horses are presented with no history. The history of prior surgery is a confounding variable that is not addressed in any of the articles. In addition, there is an inherent bias in comparing populations from different referral centers, attributable, in large part, to the quality of the horses, but this fact is widely ignored when comparing studies. These authors believe that the bias introduced by the study population is significant and may account for most of the differences between studies Fig. 2.

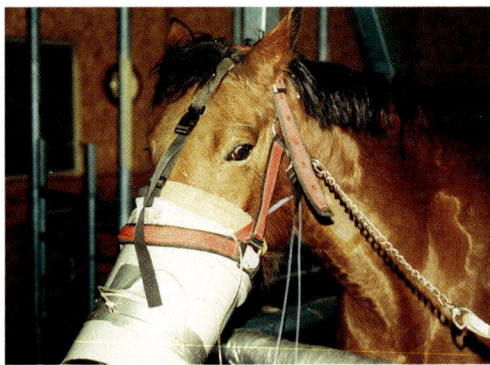

Fig. 2. Horse instrumented with a pneumotachograph and tracheal and pharyngeal catheters for measurement of respiratory variables during treadmill exercise to determine the efficacy of surgical procedures for DDSP in an experimental study.

In light of these problems, is it possible to determine what the best surgical procedure is for DDSP? Actually, even among surgeons, there is no consensus that the best option is surgery [31]. Advocates of nonsurgical therapy cite results similar to the surgical procedures; however, this argument is weakened by the fact that there are few surgical cases in which some form of medical therapy has not been attempted.

In interpreting the success of therapy, objective race data are increasingly being used to determine the success of procedures as opposed to owner satisfaction. Interpretation of these data presents its own challenges, however. Most of the studies report the percentage of racehorses in which racing performance was improved after surgery. The reader of these studies is cautioned to read the fine print, because this figure includes analysis of horses that were able to race a specified number of races (typically one to three races) before and after surgery. In many studies, this results in exclusion from the analysis of greater than 50% of the horses. For example, a study of 209 horses reported 59% and 60% success rates for the procedures being studied; however, these percentages were based on racing data from only 89 horses of the 209 reported [32]. Similar attrition is present in many reports in which the take-home message of percent success is derived from 42% [32], 45% [27], 49% [28,33], and 80% [34] of the operated cases. Reports differ significantly in how well the remaining cases are accounted for.

It has almost become axiomatic that a 60% success rate for DDSP treatment can be expected regardless of what one does. This sentiment has been now repeated so often that it is difficult to attribute the original quote. Complex data from years of surgery are distilled to a single number, the "percent success"; this is then compared with the other surgical options. The reader is cautioned that there is no uniformity in how this number is derived (Table 2) [35,36].

Surgical techniques for dorsal displacement of the soft palate

In brief, DDSP has been proposed to result from caudal retraction of the larynx or an inability of the upper airway to resist the dynamic collapsing forces. Surgical procedures have developed that address each of these mechanisms. The caudal retraction theory gave rise to several variations of the sternothyrohyoidius myectomy [27,34,37,38]. These are probably the most widely performed procedures and have proven to be safe and efficacious (approximately 60%) when performed by many individuals. They are also the basis for combination procedures.

Several procedures have been developed to decrease upper airway compliance and resist dynamic collapse. These include staphylectomy, palatoplasty, thermal cauterization techniques, and epiglottic augmentation. A pitfall of most of the aforementioned techniques is that that research studies designed to validate the basic premise for these procedures have been uniformly unsuccessful. The three different thermal cauterization techniques

Table 2
Results of procedures used to treat dorsal displacement of the soft palate

Procedure	n	Percent success	Criteria for success	Percentage of horses included in percent success	Reference	Year
Midcervical sternothyrohyoidius myectomy	17	58	Subjective assessment	—	[37]	1988
Staphylectomy	69	59	Total earnings: three races before and after	42	[32]	1995
Midcervical sternothyrohyoidius myectomy	80	60	Total earnings: three races before and after	—	[32]	1995
Sternothyrohyoidius and partial omohyoideus myectomy	50	70	Earnings per start	100	[35]	1997
Sternothyroideus tenectomy	41	70	Race times	10	[38]	1997
Variety of surgical and medical	92	64	Earnings per start	49	[28]	2002
Sternothyroideus tenectomy and transnasal laser cauterization	52	92	Subjective assessment	—	[39]	2002
Sternothyroideus tenectomy, staphylectomy, thermoplasty	96	62	Total earnings	80	[34]	2005
Sternothyroideus tenectomy, staphylectomy, oral thermoplasty	102	63	Earnings per start	45	[27]	2005
Sternothyrohyoidius myectomy, staphylectomy, ventriculectomy	53	60	Earnings per start	49	[33]	2004
Tie-forward	116	87	Subjective assessment	—	[29]	2005
Epiglottic augmentation	59	66	Performance index	—	[30]	1997
Conservative	31	61	Earnings per start	—	[36]	2005

reported also include various permutations of a sternothyroideus tenectomy and staphylectomy; thus, their results cannot be attributed solely to the thermal cauterization as the authors suggest [27,34,39].

A newer procedure, the tie-forward, does have credible research that supports the procedure as well as a thorough prospective clinical evaluation [29]. One notable caveat for the tie-forward is that the proposed cause this procedure addresses has not been demonstrated to cause DDSP. Results of the tie-forward procedure have not been confirmed by others because of the newness of the technique.

For all procedures, it remains to be seen if the proposed cause of DDSP is (1) correct or (2) incorrect, with the procedures being beneficial for other reasons, or if the favorable responses are a result of the study population. It is likely that the results obtained from all surgical treatments are more reflective of the hospital population than any differences in the procedures. It is almost unquestionable that the debate is likely to continue for some time.

Epiglottic entrapment

EE occurs much less frequently than LH or DDSP. EE may be persistent or intermittent. The persistent form of EE is readily and accurately diagnosed with upper airway endoscopy, leaving little reason to question the accuracy of the diagnosis in the studies reviewed here. The intermittent condition is easily diagnosed during endoscopy on a high-speed treadmill. It would seem intuitive that the prognosis for surgical correction would be the same for the intermittent and persistent forms of EE; however, studies on EE preceded widespread use of high-speed treadmills for diagnostic purposes, and only 4 of 179 cases examined here were reported to be intermittent [40–43]. The surgical approach to the aryepiglottic fold is through a laryngotomy and resection of the aryepiglottic fold [40] or through transnasal [44] or transoral [41] axial division of the aryepiglottic fold. A laryngotomy has subjectively been demonstrated to have a greatly reduced prognosis for racing (27%) when compared with transoral axial transection in a small number of cases [40].

Two studies have evaluated transendoscopic neodymium:yttrium aluminum garnet (Nd:YAG) transaction of the aryepiglottic fold. Tate and colleagues [42] found that 10 of 11 horses with EE were performing their intended activity after surgery. Tulleners [43] reported that among 57 Standardbreds and 44 Thoroughbreds, 66% to 80% had no change, 10% to 17% improved, and 5% to 17% decreased in racing class after surgery. Transoral transaction of the aryepiglottic fold has resulted in 20 of 20 racehorses returning to racing at their prior level [41]. Transoral division of the aryepiglottic fold was shown by Lumsden and colleagues [40] to result in 82% owner satisfaction, and 75% of these horses demonstrated no change in racing performance. Transnasal transaction of the aryepiglottic fold resulted in 16 of 17 racehorses returning to successful competition [44].

All methods evaluated were effective in correcting the entrapment. Fewer horses had a satisfactory outcome when treated by means of a laryngotomy approach. The transnasal, transoral, and transendoscopic approaches achieve comparable results. It seems that preoperative performance is the best predictor of postoperative performance with EE and that the literature does not suggest that one method is superior to another.

Summary

In spite of the difficulties posed in evaluating surgical techniques of the equine respiratory system, it should be possible to assess procedures and practice critically using evidence-based assessments. The emphasis for future research in equine respiratory surgery needs to be on prospective rather than retrospective studies, on trials instead of case series, and on systematic reviews rather than unsystematic ones. Strategies to improve the quality of the evidence available would include education of surgeons in clinical research methodology, improved funding for research, and compulsory evaluation of new techniques before their general adoption. In addition, if randomized controlled trials are not feasible, alternative designs, such as prospective matched-pair trials, may need to be better developed and used.

References

[1] Marks D, Mackay-Smith MP, Cushing LS, et al. Use of a prosthetic device for surgical correction of laryngeal hemiplegia. J Am Vet Med Assoc 1970;157(1):157–63.
[2] Derksen FJ, Stick JA, Scott EA, et al. Effect of laryngeal hemiplegia and laryngoplasty on airway flow mechanics in exercising horses. Am J Vet Res 1986;47(1):16–20.
[3] Shappell KK, Derksen FJ, Stick JA, et al. Effects of ventriculectomy, prosthetic laryngoplasty, and exercise on upper airway function in horses with induced left laryngeal hemiplegia. Am J Vet Res 1988;49(10):1760–5.
[4] Tate LP, Corbett WT, Bishop BJ, et al. Blood gas tensions, acid-base status, heart rates, and venous profiles in exercising horses with laryngeal hemiplegia before and after corrective surgery. Vet Surg 1993;22(3):177–83.
[5] Tetens J, Derksen FJ, Stick JA, et al. Efficacy of prosthetic laryngoplasty with and without bilateral ventriculocordectomy as treatments for laryngeal hemiplegia in horses. Am J Vet Res 1996;57(11):1668–73.
[6] Hawkins JF, Tulleners EP, Ross MW, et al. Laryngoplasty with or without ventriculectomy for treatment of left laryngeal hemiplegia in 230 racehorses. Vet Surg 1997;26(6):484–91.
[7] Kidd JA, Slone DE. Treatment of laryngeal hemiplegia in horses by prosthetic laryngoplasty, ventriculectomy and vocal cordectomy. Vet Rec 2002;150(15):481–4.
[8] Russell AP, Slone DE. Performance analysis after prosthetic laryngoplasty and bilateral ventriculectomy for laryngeal hemiplegia in horses: 70 cases (1986–1991). J Am Vet Med Assoc 1994;204(8):1235–41.
[9] Strand E, Martin GS, Haynes PF, et al. Career racing performance in Thoroughbreds treated with prosthetic laryngoplasty for laryngeal neuropathy: 52 cases (1981–1989). J Am Vet Med Assoc 2000;217(11):1689–96.
[10] Dixon PM, McGorum BC, Railton DI, et al. Long-term survey of laryngoplasty and ventriculocordectomy in an older, mixed-breed population of 200 horses. Part 2: owners' assessment of the value of surgery. Equine Vet J 2003;35(4):397–401.
[11] Kraus BM, Parente EJ, Tulleners EP. Laryngoplasty with ventriculectomy or ventriculocordectomy in 104 draft horses (1992–2000). Vet Surg 2003;32(6):530–8.

[12] Ducharme NG, Horney FD, Partlow GD, et al. Attempts to restore abduction of the paralyzed equine arytenoid cartilage II. Nerve implantation (pilot study). Can J Vet Res 1989;53(2):210–5.
[13] Ducharme NG, Viel L, Partlow GD. Attempts to restore abduction of the paralyzed equine arytenoid cartilage III. Nerve anastomosis. Can J Vet Res 1989;53(2):216–23.
[14] Fulton IC, Derksen FJ, Stick JA, et al. Treatment of left laryngeal hemiplegia in Standardbreds, using a nerve muscle pedicle graft. Am J Vet Res 1991;52(9):1461–7.
[15] Fulton IC, Stick JA, Derksen FJ. Laryngeal reinnervation in the horse. Vet Clin North Am Equine Pract 2003;19(1):189–208.
[16] Haynes PF, McClure JR, Watters JW. Subtotal arytenoidectomy in the horse: an update. Proceedings of the American Association of Equine Practitioners. 1984;30:21–33.
[17] Belknap JK, Derksen FJ, Nickels FA, et al. Failure of subtotal arytenoidectomy to improve upper airway flow mechanics in exercising Standardbreds with induced laryngeal hemiplegia. Am J Vet Res 1990;51(9):1481–7.
[18] White NA, Blackwell RB. Partial arytenoidectomy in the horse. Vet Surg 1980;9(1):5–12.
[19] Tulleners EP, Harrison IW, Raker CW. Management of arytenoid chondropathy and failed laryngoplasty in horses: 75 cases (1979–1985). J Am Vet Med Assoc 1988;192(5):670–5.
[20] Barnes AJ, Slone DE, Lynch TM. Performance after partial arytenoidectomy without mucosal closure in 27 Thoroughbred racehorses. Vet Surg 2004;33(4):398–403.
[21] Lumsden JM, Derksen FJ, Stick JA, et al. Evaluation of partial arytenoidectomy as a treatment for equine laryngeal hemiplegia. Equine Vet J 1994;26(2):125–9.
[22] Radcliffe CH, Woodie JB, Hackett RP, et al. A comparison of laryngoplasty and modified partial arytenoidectomy as treatments for laryngeal hemiplegia in exercising horses. Vet Surg 2006;35:643–52.
[23] Brown JA, Derksen FJ, Stick JA, et al. Ventriculectomy reduces respiratory noise in horses with laryngeal hemiplegia. Equine Vet J 2003;35(6):570–4.
[24] Brown JA, Derksen FJ, Stick JA, et al. Laser vocal cordectomy fails to effectively reduce respiratory noise in horses with laryngeal hemiplegia. Vet Surg 2005;34(3):247–52.
[25] Taylor SE, Barzaki SZ, Dixon P. Ventriculocordectomy as the sole treatment for recurrent laryngeal neuropathy: long-term results from ninety-two horses. Vet Surg 2006;35:653–7.
[26] Ducharme NG. Equine surgery. In: Auer JA, Stick JA, editors. Equine surgery. 3rd edition. St. Louis (MO): Elsevier Inc.; 2006. p. 544–65.
[27] Smith JJ, Embertson RM. Sternothyroideus myotomy, staphylectomy, and oral caudal soft palate photothermoplasty for treatment of dorsal displacement of the soft palate in 102 Thoroughbred racehorses. Vet Surg 2005;34(1):5–10.
[28] Parente EJ, Martin BB, Tulleners EP, et al. Dorsal displacement of the soft palate in 92 horses during high-speed treadmill examination (1993–1998). Vet Surg 2002;31(6):507–12.
[29] Woodie JB, Ducharme NG, Kanter P, et al. Surgical advancement of the larynx (laryngeal tie-forward) as a treatment for dorsal displacement of the soft palate in horses: a prospective study 2001–2004. Equine Vet J 2005;37(5):418–23.
[30] Tulleners E, Stick JA, Leitch M, et al. Epiglottic augmentation for treatment of dorsal displacement of the soft palate in racehorses: 59 cases (1985–1994). J Am Vet Med Assoc 1997;211(8):1022–8.
[31] Holcombe SJ, Derksen FJ, Stick JA, et al. Pathophysiology of dorsal displacement of the soft palate in horses. Equine Vet J Suppl 1999;30:45–8.
[32] Anderson JD, Tulleners EP, Johnston JK, et al. Sternothyrohyoidius myectomy or staphylectomy for treatment of intermittent dorsal displacement of the soft palate in racehorses: 209 cases (1986–1991). J Am Vet Med Assoc 1995;206(12):1909–12.
[33] Barakzai SZ, Johnson VS, Baird DH, et al. Assessment of the efficacy of composite surgery for the treatment of dorsal displacement of the soft palate in a group of 53 racing Thoroughbreds (1990–1996). Equine Vet J 2004;36(2):175–9.
[34] Dykgraaf S, McIlwraith CW, Baker V, et al. Sternothyroideus tenectomy combination surgery for treatment of dorsal displacement of the soft palate in 96 Thoroughbred racehorses

(1996–2004). Proceedings of the Annual Convention of the American Association of Equine Practitioners 2005;51:323–6.

[35] Duncan D. Retrospective study of 50 Thoroughbred racehorses subjected to radical myectomy for treatment of dorsal displacement of the soft palate. Proceedings of the Annual Convention of the American Association of Equine Practitioners 1997;43:237–8.

[36] Barakzai SZ, Dixon PM. Conservative treatment for Thoroughbred racehorses with intermittent dorsal displacement of the soft palate. Vet Rec 2005;157(12):337–40.

[37] Harrison IW, Raker CW. Sternothyrohyoidius myectomy in horses: 17 cases (1984–1985). J Am Vet Med Assoc 1988;193(10):1299–302.

[38] Llewellyn H, Petrowitz A. Sternothyroideus myotomy for the treatment of dorsal displacement of the soft palate. Proceedings of the Annual Convention of the American Association of Equine Practitioners 1997;43:239–43.

[39] Hogan P, Palmer SE, Congelosi M. Transendoscopic laser cauterization of the soft palate as an adjunctive treatment for dorsal displacement in the racehorse. Proceedings of the Annual Convention of the American Association of Equine Practitioners 2002;48:228–30.

[40] Lumsden JM, Stick JA, Caron JP, et al. Surgical treatment of epiglottic entrapment in horses: 51 cases (1981–1992). J Am Vet Med Assoc 1994;205:729–35.

[41] Ross MW, Gentile DG, Evans LE. Transoral axial division, under endoscopic guidance, for correction of epiglottic entrapment in horses. J Am Vet Med Assoc 1993;203(3):416–20.

[42] Tate LP, Sweeney CL, Bowman KF, et al. Transendoscopic Nd:YAG laser surgery for treatment of epiglottal entrapment and dorsal displacement of the soft palate in the horse. Vet Surg 1990;19:356–63.

[43] Tulleners EP. Transendoscopic contact neodymium:yttrium aluminum garnet laser correction of epiglottic entrapment in standing horses. J Am Vet Med Assoc 1990;196(12): 1971–80.

[44] Honnas CM, Wheat JD. Epiglottic entrapment: a transnasal surgical approach to divide the aryepiglottic fold axially in the standing horse. Vet Surg 1988;17:246–51.

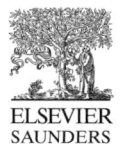

Evidence-Based Gastrointestinal Medicine in Horses: It's Not About Your Gut Instincts

Rose Nolen-Walston, DVM[a],*,
Julia Paxson, PhD, DVM[b], David W. Ramey, DVM[c]

[a]School of Veterinary Medicine, University of Pennsylvania, 382 West Street Road, Kennett Square, PA 19348, USA
[b]Cummings School of Veterinary Medicine, Tufts University, 300 Westboro Road, North Grafton, MA 01536, USA
[c]Ramey Equine, P.O. Box 9114, Calabasas, CA 91372, USA

From the writings of Aspyrtus and Pelagonius in the fourth century, when equine medicine and magic inhabited the same field, to the statistically analyzed randomized clinical trials (RCTs) of today, veterinary literature has made careful examination of the digestive ills of the horse. Unfortunately, this body of data is too large for the practitioner to cover in its entirety yet too incomplete to answer many of the clinical questions that equine practitioners must ask on a daily basis. An ability to sort through a mountain of data, evaluate the quality of findings, and obtain what is useful and relevant is a skill needed by the twenty-first century equine veterinarian as much as the ability to pass a tube or perform a rectal palpation.

This article is organized to reinforce the principle that the cornerstone of evidence-based medicine is the clinical question. Specific questions are further categorized as to topic [1], with epidemiologic risk factors, diagnostic process, clinical examination, differential diagnosis, diagnostic tests, treatment, harm, prognosis, and prevention as general themes. The topics covered in this article are by no means exhaustive but give an example of how the veterinary literature can be used to answer clinically important questions in an evidence-based manner.

---

* Corresponding author.
  E-mail address: rnolenw@vet.upenn.edu (R. Nolen-Walston).

Analgesia for colic

Question 1: treatment

Which analgesic is most effective at treating acute colic pain in the adult horse?

Important questions regarding the choice of analgesic agents for colic include their relative safety and side effects as well as their duration of action, in addition to simply the effectiveness of the analgesia that they provide. No extensive systemic reviews of this topic were identified, although several opinion pieces by experts have been published on the subject [2,3]. There exists a fairly extensive body of literature on the topic, however, including multiple RCTs of naturally occurring (and thus etiologically diverse) colic as well as experimental models of colic induced by visceral balloon distention.

The use of experimental models that fairly accurately mimic naturally occurring disease processes illustrates one of the primary differences between human and veterinary evidence-based medicine (EBM) literature; in human beings, it is generally ethically impossible to perform testing of a new therapy on an experimental group that accurately replicates clinical disease. Thus, laboratory animal studies must often be used to infer efficacy of a particular drug before its use in clinical cases. In veterinary medicine, however, trials may be performed in the target animal (horse) in a highly controlled and standardized manner before their use in a more variable, and thus difficult to analyze, clinical population.

The main categories of therapeutics used in the treatment of gastrointestinal (GI) pain in the horses are the α_2 agonists (detomidine and xylazine), nonsteroidal anti-inflammatory drugs (NSAIDS; flunixin meglumine, ketoprofen, and phenylbutazone), opioids (especially butorphanol), antispasmodics (N-butylscopolammonium [Buscopan]), and nonpharmacologic treatments (especially acupuncture). In a clinical trial using naturally occurring colic, detomidine (20 µg/kg and 40 µg/kg) showed significantly superior pain reduction and a decrease in heart rate and respiratory rate compared with butorphanol, xylazine, and flunixin meglumine [4]. This trial extended to 90 minutes after administration; thus, it did not evaluate long-term duration effects, in which flunixin meglumine might be expected to be superior. A blind crossover design study of nine horses using a cecal balloon dilation model found xylazine to be superior in analgesic effect and duration to the narcotic analgesics butorphanol, meperidine, and pentazocine [5]. Although using fewer horses than the previous study, the ability to compare drugs using the same colic model (as opposed to comparing horse with mild impaction with those with torsion) allows more standardized data.

N-butylscopolammonium was compared with butorphanol using a blind randomized cecal dilation model in eight ponies [6]. Although twice the number of ponies showed a positive analgesic response to N-butylscopolammonium compared with butorphanol (six of eight ponies versus three of eight ponies), the study was underpowered to show a statistical difference.

A single blind controlled study directly compared two different NSAIDS (ketoprofen and flunixin meglumine) in cases of mild to moderate colic. No significant difference was observed in the effect or duration of the two agents [7]. A butorphanol constant rate infusion has been compared with placebo in another good-quality RCT [8] and was found to have a significant positive effect on pain scores, weight loss, and cortisol measurements in postoperative colic cases already receiving flunixin meglumine. This study notes that these effects happen in the absence of any changes in heart rate between the experimental and control groups, showing that it is not a sensitive parameter for postoperative pain control.

Many studies have evaluated nonpharmacologic methods of analgesia in colic, including acupuncture and other forms of alternative treatment. Unfortunately, most of these studies are not effectively controlled or randomized, making the data hard to interpret. A particularly rigorous experiment using sham-treated and nontreated controls and blinded observers did not show any significant analgesic effects of electroacupuncture at the Guan-yuan-shu (similar to BL-21) acupoints bilaterally in a balloon distention model [9]. It is unusual for a single acupoint to be used in practice, however, and further experiments of this quality are needed to evaluate the efficacy of multiple-point acupuncture in a colic model.

Quality of evidence

The number and quality of RCTs in this area of equine medicine are unusual. Perhaps the most significant problem with the studies using clinical cases is that colic is a sign rather than a particular disease. Although most reports compared the baseline clinical data in the experimental and control groups to show that they were approximately equivalent, there is still an important confounder in the fact that horses with mild gas colic are being compared with those that turn out to have colon torsion.

Clinical implications

For short-term colic relief, detomidine is significantly more effective than other agents, with butorphanol showing the least effect of the drugs evaluated (although it was not evaluated in combination with other drugs, as it is most typically used in practice). Data illustrating time points beyond 90 minutes have not been reported, but for postoperative pain control, an intravenous butorphanol infusion seems to add significantly to the analgesia of horses already receiving flunixin meglumine. No convincing data exist for the effectiveness of acupuncture in the treatment of colic pain. Interestingly, there were no data supporting the commonly held view that flunixin meglumine is superior to phenylbutazone for controlling visceral pain, and this would be an interesting avenue for further investigation in the future.

Prokinetic agents

Question 1: treatment

Which prokinetic agent is most effective at treating or preventing ileus in horses?

Ileus is commonly seen in horses after abdominal surgery [10] as well as in inflammatory conditions of the small intestine, such as proximal enteritis [11]. Two recent retrospective analyses have examined populations of horses with postoperative ileus (POI) and identified a wide range of agents currently being used in practice [12]. Although there was no overall improvement in survival associated with their overall use in cases of POI after small intestinal resection [13], the data were not broken down to specific agents, allowing the possibility that some of the drugs were, in fact, effective but that their utility was diluted statistically by the inclusion of ineffective agents.

Intravenous lidocaine infusion has been evaluated in two RCTs using clinical cases after colic surgery. The first evaluated the efficacy of lidocaine constant rate infusion immediately after surgery to prevent POI in 28 horses [14]. The study was blind, and saline was used as a placebo control. Horses receiving lidocaine had less postoperative small intestine dilation and peritoneal fluid as determined by sonography, but no differences were seen in quantity or reflux, or in eventual outcome. The second study considered the use of lidocaine infusion as a treatment for POI or proximal enteritis in 32 clinical cases [15]. Results demonstrated significantly decreased reflux in the lidocaine-treated group when compared with placebo; although no significant difference was seen in the mortality rate between the two groups, the study was underpowered to evaluate this parameter.

Metoclopramide is a serotonin (5-HT) antagonist commonly used as a prokinetic in human medicine. It is used cautiously in equids because of the prevalence of neurologic side effects, and its efficacy is supported by a retrospective analysis of 70 cases of POI. Although the title of the article suggests that it was used to treat POI, in the materials and methods section, it is stated that metoclopramide was given within 30 minutes of recovery from anesthesia, suggesting that its use was actually prophylactic. Three groups were analyzed, including metoclopramide constant infusion, intermittent metoclopramide, and no metoclopramide [16]. Cases that received metoclopramide by constant infusion showed significantly less total reflux and shorter hospital stays and had no evidence of adverse reactions. The mortality rate in this group was 0%, but, again, the numbers were too small to show significance.

Cisapride, currently commercially unavailable in the United States, has been evaluated clinically and experimentally in an intravenous formulation. In an RCT that enrolled 70 postoperative colic cases, cisapride was compared with a saline placebo [17]. Horses receiving placebo had a higher incidence of POI, although this difference was not statistically significant. In another study, cisapride increased GI transit time in an experimental model of POI [18] and was reported as effective in 22 clinical cases. This group was unmatched by controls, however, and firm conclusions about the efficacy of the compound cannot be established from this study.

Using an experimental model of POI in 8 ponies, propanolol, yohimbine, yohimbine plus propanolol, and metoclopramide were evaluated for their effect on transit time of beads and electromechanical activity of various segments of the GI tract of live horses [19]. Although yohimbine and metoclopramide were identified as having therapeutic promise, only two to three animals were used per group, minimizing the utility of these data in making meaningful clinical conclusions.

Quality of evidence

Comprehensive RCTs examining the use of lidocaine and cisapride provide pertinent information about the effects of these two drugs in the treatment and prevention of ileus. Interestingly, in one prospective study [15], 19 cases of ileus were excluded from analysis because of resolution of reflux simultaneously with onset of therapy; this highlights the risk of making post hoc assumptions in clinical medicine, wherein the resolution of a problem that occurs shortly a therapeutic intervention can cause a clinician to attribute the improvement to the therapy rather than to the natural course of the disease.

Clinical implications

Although high-quality data on the use of lidocaine for POI have been published, the data show only mild benefit for prophylactic and therapeutic effects. Metoclopramide as a constant rate infusion seems more promising for prevention of POI, but well-controlled prospective studies need to be performed to confirm this finding, and further data on the incidence of adverse reactions are important. Neostigmine, yohimbine, acepromazine, and erythromycin are all used clinically with some frequency [20], and significant bodies of in vitro data exist on the effects of several of these agents on intestinal motility, but minimal evidence-based data exist to determine their value in a clinical setting.

Renosplenic entrapment of the large colon

Question 1: clinical examination

Is ultrasound superior to rectal examination in the diagnosis of renosplenic entrapment of the large colon?

Although several studies briefly touch on the sensitivity of rectal palpation for the diagnosis of renosplenic entrapment (RSE), only one article specifically addresses the comparison of rectal versus sonographic findings [21]. The experimental design is not clear, although it seems to be a retrospective analysis. The study population included 42 horses with sonographic findings consistent with left dorsal displacement of the large colon and 40 horses considered not to have RSE. In this study, RSE was correctly diagnosed by ultrasound in 88% of cases compared with a definitive diagnosis rate of 32% by rectal palpation alone. False-negative results were rare in both groups, but no data on false-positive results were available for either group, because a "gold standard" (surgical exploration) was not applied to every case included. Two retrospective analyses of RSE in 57 cases [22] and 62 cases [23] reported sensitivities of 61.2% and 95%, respectively, for diagnosis per rectum, but these were not compared sonographic techniques, nor were all the cases examined surgically to define the accuracy of the diagnosis. As a result, it is not possible to use data from these studies to calculate positive and negative predictive values for ultrasound versus rectal examination.

Strength of evidence

This apparent case-control series has good numbers for a veterinary study but does not give detailed explanations of case selection criteria. No statistical analysis of the results was performed. The additional reports of high sensitivity are unconvincing because of the complete lack of comparison with a gold standard.

Clinical significance

There is conflicting evidence regarding the sensitivity of rectal examination for the diagnosis of RSE and no data regarding its specificity. Data do suggest that ultrasonographic diagnosis of RSE is more sensitive than diagnosis made by palpation per rectum, however.

Question 2: treatment

Is nonsurgical therapy of renosplenic entrapment as safe and efficacious as correction by means of celiotomy?

There are two commonly used methods of nonsurgical correction of RSE: "rolling" under general anesthesia [24] and administration of intravenous phenylephrine to reduce splenic size and allow mechanical de-entrapment with exercise [25]. These techniques are frequently combined [26,27]. Five retrospective analyses address rolling [22–24,28,29], one addresses phenylephrine therapy only [30], and two cover both [26,27]. No RCTs addressing this question were identified. A total of 397 cases of RSE were analyzed in these eight reports, and the results are compiled (Table 1).

Strength of evidence

The most significant deficit in most of these studies is method of case selection. Only one study consistently used rectal examination as well as sonographic evidence of RSE for all cases [26]. Considering the questionable accuracy of rectal palpation for the diagnosis of RSE [21], a portion of the cases that resolved nonsurgically may not have been true RSE; thus, the true efficacy of medical

Table 1
Compiled results from eight studies evaluating therapeutic outcome in renosplenic entrapment

	Success rate	Unsuccessful: sent to surgery	Mortality rate
Phenylephrine only	85% (17/20)	15% (3/20)	0% (0/20)
Phenylephrine plus rolling	86% (19/22)	10% (2/22)	5% (1/22)
Rolling only	78% (104/134)	16% (22/134)	4% (6/134)[a]
Surgery after rolling	73% (16/22)	Not applicable	27% (6/22)[a]
Surgery: first treatment	93% (179/192)	Not applicable	7% (13/192)
Spontaneous recovery	11% (32/236)	Not applicable	Not applicable
Total	93% (369/397)	Not applicable	7% (28/397)

[a] Overall mortality rate for horses rolled was 9% (12 of 134 horses).

Data from Mezerova J, Zert Z, Kottman J. [Diagnostic and therapeutic aspects of left dorsal displacement of the large colon in the horse]. Pferdeheilkunde 2003;19:65–74 [in German]; and Hardy J, Minton M, Robertson JT, et al. Nephrosplenic entrapment in the horse: a retrospective study of 174 cases. Equine Vet J 2000;32:95–7.

therapy may be skewed. Also, some reports include cases of left dorsal displacement of the large colon (wherein the colon is not specifically entrapped), whereas others do not specify exact criteria for diagnosis. Because these were retrospective analyses, there was no randomization as to how animals were treated; thus, the excellent outcomes for phenylephrine may be affected by selection bias in that milder (or misdiagnosed) cases could have received the least invasive treatment, thus inflating the apparent success of this group. The strength of evidence, therefore, cannot be considered strong.

Clinical significance

There are limited data that phenylephrine infusion alone may be effective in treating RSE, but until further investigation by means of a prospective study using stringent inclusion criteria and randomized treatment groups and controls, it is difficult to come to a definitive conclusion as to the efficacy of phenylephrine as a stand-alone treatment. Surgery was more efficacious than rolling alone in resolving RSE (93% versus 78%), although rolling after phenylephrine infusion raised the success rate to 86%. The overall mortality rate after rolling is minimally higher with rolling (and subsequent surgery) than with surgery alone (9% versus 7%). Nevertheless, a proportion of the mortality rate in these studies comprised elective euthanasia for humane or financial reasons, thus reducing the potential significance of a small difference.

Fluid therapy in treatment of gastrointestinal disease

Question 1: therapy

Are enteral fluids more effective than intravenous fluids in the treatment of colonic impactions?

Equine GI disease can be associated with significant intravascular fluid shifts. Therefore, before development of a fluid therapy plan, a thorough assessment of the patient's hydration, electrolyte, and acid-base status should be undertaken. In many cases of large colon ingesta impaction, however, horses are presented with only mild signs of systemic dehydration or electrolyte imbalances and the major treatment goal is simply rehydration and passage of the ingesta.

Traditional methods for promoting increased colonic fluid content have included systemic overhydration with intravenous fluids combined with administration of cathartics, such as magnesium sulfate. This treatment is speculated to increase intraluminal osmolality and promote increased colonic fluid content [31]. Alternatively, it has been argued that administration of enteral fluids adequately increases colonic fluid content while simultaneously promoting colonic motility through the gastrocolic reflex [32].

There are two studies with a randomized crossover design in an experimental model that examine colonic fluid content after treatment with intravenous fluids combined with a magnesium sulfate cathartic or enteral fluids. In both studies, colonic fluid content was sampled directly by means of a right dorsal colon fistula. In the first study, administration of an approximately isotonic enteral solution (measured osmolality of ~254 mOsmol/L) was compared with administration of the same volume (60 L) of intravenous lactated Ringer's solution (LRS) combined with orally administered magnesium sulfate (1 g/kg of body weight) in four horses. Horses receiving enteral fluids urinated less and weighed more after the treatment period ended. Although increased ingesta hydration was observed in all four horses, it was greater in horses receiving enteral fluids ($P<.05$). The authors also suggest that the trend toward greater fecal production during treatment with enteral fluids ($P = .0565$) may indicate a greater gastrocolonic response [32]. The second study compared colonic fluid content in seven horses using the same experimental model. The treatments evaluated were intravenous fluids (LRS) and enteral administration of magnesium sulfate, sodium sulfate, water, or a balanced electrolyte solution. Again, in this study, the colonic fluid was sampled by means of a fistula created in the right dorsal colon. The right dorsal colon fluid content as well as the fecal fluid content increased most significantly in horses receiving enteral electrolyte solution ($P<.01$). In addition, these animals seemed to have a faster GI transit time, as assessed by measurement of cobalt (administered enterally at time 0) in the right dorsal colon ($P<.01$) [33].

Strength of evidence

Although these studies are supportive of enteral fluid therapy, RCTs evaluating intravenous versus enteral fluid therapy are necessary to show the effect of these findings on outcome variables of horses with colonic impactions.

Clinical significance

The data suggest that enteral treatment with balanced electrolyte solutions is superior for increasing colonic fluid content. This treatment option should be considered in cases of colonic impaction that are mildly to moderately dehydrated with no significant serum electrolyte imbalances because it shows promise of being less expensive as well as more effective than intravenous hydration.

Salmonellosis

Question 1: diagnostic tests

Is a polymerase chain reaction–based test superior to isolation by culture in the diagnosis of clinical salmonellosis?

Salmonella is a cause of potentially fatal enteric disease in horses, with mortality rates of 42% to 44% for virulent strains [34,35]. The accurate identification of active *Salmonella* shedding in symptomatic and asymptomatic animals is critical to the development of appropriate treatment protocols and in reducing hospital-wide nosocomial outbreaks [34]. In evaluation of studies that compare identification of *Salmonella* by culture versus polymerase chain reaction (PCR) testing, not only are the type and size of the study important but there must be an understanding of the limitations of culture and PCR as well as the methodology used to perform the diagnostic tests.

Evidence-based evaluation of new diagnostic testing methods requires description of the sensitivity and specificity of the new test compared with a known gold standard test. Sensitivity describes the frequency with which a positive test result correlates with a diseased individual. Specificity describes the frequency with which a negative test result correlates with unaffected animals. True evidence-based studies are hard to construct in the diagnosis of salmonellosis, however. Although the traditional gold standard of positive identification by culture decisively demonstrates the presence of that organism, false-negative results can occur [36], thereby reducing the quality of evidence in comparing the sensitivity of any new diagnostic test with isolation by culture. Furthermore, PCR testing can be overly sensitive because it can identify animals that harbor nonviable organisms [37], which has implications for treatment and isolation protocols. False-negative PCR results can also occur, most commonly because of the presence of inhibitory substances in feces (eg, urea, heme [38,39]).

Reliability of fecal PCR-based *Salmonella* testing has been addressed by targeting a variety of genes associated with pathogenic *Salmonella* species and by using a variety of techniques designed to reduce inhibition from urea and bilirubin compounds in feces (eg, inclusion of positive internal controls). PCR targeting of *Salmonella* pathogenicity genes, such as *ompC*, *spaQ*, and *hisJ*, and construction of an appropriate targeted internal control have enabled direct monitoring of inhibition in each PCR reaction [35,40,41]. In these studies, isolation by culture was used as the gold standard and all culture-positive samples were also PCR-positive. In addition, the authors consistently noted a large number of PCR-positive culture-negative samples [35,40,41]. The reported prevalence of PCR-positive hospitalized horses is as high as 75%, with a corresponding positive identification by culture (one or more positive cultures) of 9.5% [35]. Because these numbers are so vastly different, it raises the question of whether testing by PCR is too sensitive, because a positive test result can include animals with nonviable organisms (ie, not actively shedding *Salmonella* at the time of testing). Alternatively, these numbers may reflect the fact that isolation by culture is not a sensitive test. A compromise may be initial screening by PCR testing, because it seems to be vastly superior in sensitivity, followed by multiple cultures on horses with positive PCR test results to identify individuals that are actively shedding *Salmonella*.

Strength of evidence

The strength of evidence that fecal PCR is a sensitive test for the presence of *Salmonella* DNA is robust; however, the correlation between a positive PCR test result and the presence of live (infectious) *Salmonella*, as demonstrated by culture, has been shown to be poor in several studies. Overall, the quality and number of studies in this area are excellent and provide the practitioner with strong tools for clinical decision making for screening and diagnosing *Salmonella* in horses.

Clinical significance

PCR shows evidence of being an excellent screening test for *Salmonella* in horses (and fomites) but may ask the wrong question ("Is there any DNA present" rather than "Are there live infectious organisms present?") for the diagnosis of clinical cases.

Equine gastric ulcer syndrome

Question 1: risk factors

How does exercise intensity affect the prevalence of equine gastric ulcer syndrome?

Equine gastric ulcer syndrome (EGUS) is an extremely prevalent condition in some equine populations. Horses are continuous gastric acid secretors and are prone to ulceration in the squamous portion of the gastric mucosa. The prevalence of gastric ulcers has been reported as high as 94% to 100% among in-training or racing Thoroughbreds [42]. It has been demonstrated that horses exercised on a high-speed treadmill experience marked gastric compression and decreased gastric pH when moving at speeds greater than a walk. The authors suggest that gastric compression during exercise pushes acidic gastric contents into the squamous gastric mucosa, resulting in a higher prevalence of gastric ulcers in horses in intensive training [43].

Studies investigating the effect of exercise on the prevalence of EGUS are confronted with several obstacles. There are many other risk factors that seem to be associated with EGUS, including intermittent feeding, diet, transport stress, stall confinement, and administration of various drugs [44]. Ensuring that these factors are accounted for in study design is difficult. In addition, quantification of exercise intensity is difficult, because most studies are designed to examine real-world competitive horses. Studies comparing a single time point for horses training at different intensities provide only cross-sectional survey information and cannot rule out other compounding factors, but data from these studies are consistent with a greater prevalence in horses undergoing high-intensity training [45,46].

In an RCT comprising 20 horses with no initial gastric ulceration, two randomly allocated groups were used to evaluate the effect of transportation and a simulated show environment versus a control group being maintained on-site. Development of gastric ulcers was significantly more prevalent in the experimental group, suggesting that normal showing is sufficient to cause EGUS in normal horses [47].

Quality of evidence
Multiple studies show evidence that intensity of training is a factor in EGUS in horses. Although the level of evidence of these studies is variable, and minimal data from RCTs exist, the agreement within this body of data shows good evidence that EGUS is related to training intensity.

Clinical implications
These data are useful to veterinarians diagnostically (EGUS should be higher on a list of differential diagnoses in horses at high levels of training) and also in future efforts to reduce morbidity in specific populations.

Question 2: treatment

What is the most efficacious treatment for equine gastric ulcer syndrome in adult horses?
Current therapeutic strategies for treating EGUS focus on blocking gastric acid secretion and raising stomach pH. The best evidence-based research on the efficacy of treatment involves RCTs in which study subjects with EGUS are identified from the target population (usually Thoroughbred racehorses). After the treatment period, the animals are reassessed and scored. For assessment of EGUS, a standard ulcer scoring system has been developed to quantify the condition more systematically [48,49]. The squamous epithelium is scored as 0 (intact epithelium, no mucosal changes), 1 (small single or multifocal lesions), 2 (large single or multifocal lesions or extensive superficial lesions), and 3 (extensive lesions with deep ulceration). Ideally, this somewhat subjective scoring should be reported

by one blinded reviewer at all time points so as to reduce bias. Because ulcer formation is associated with a variety of risk factors, the study animals should also be subjected to similar training and diet during the study period. In most studies, this is hard to achieve, because the study animals are housed, fed, and trained at different sites and evaluated by different personnel.

RCTs comparing length of treatment and dosing of a proprietary omeprazole paste (Gastrogard, Merial, Duluth, Georgia) showed significant improvement in the subjective ulcer score (77% improvement by day 27 of treatment with 4 mg/kg of body weight per day) [50]. An RCT to investigate the minimum effective dose of Gastrogard for prevention of ulcers in healthy horses entering an intensive training regimen compared sham-dosed horses with horses receiving omeprazole at a rate of 1 mg/kg of body weight per day and found that 82% of those treated remained ulcer-free compared with 10% of the sham-dosed horses [51].

In a modified crossover study to compare treatment with omeprazole with treatment with ranitidine, horses with an ulcer score of 1 or greater were randomly allocated to one of three treatment groups. Even though the mean ulcer score for the group treated with omeprazole was initially worse, after 28 days of treatment with omeprazole or ranitidine, those treated with omeprazole showed significantly more improvement in their ulcer score [49]. As with other studies, the major confounding factor in this study is unknown differences in risk factors associated with ulcer formation (although all horses were in active race training).

An important study in this field compares stabilized propriety omeprazole (Gastrogard) with a simple suspension of omeprazole (compounded product). This RCT, comprising 32 horses with EGUS, showed that compounded omeprazole suspension (which is acid-labile, and therefore deactivated in the low pH environment of the stomach) was ineffective at reducing ulcer scores or attaining effective serum concentrations of omeprazole [52].

Quality of evidence

Probably because of the significant costs associated with bringing a new proprietary formulation through the US Food and Drug Administration (FDA) approval process and to the veterinary market, there is a large body of RCT evidence supporting the use of Gastrogard. These trials are well designed and demonstrate convincing data, although many were financially supported by the manufacturer.

Clinical implications

There is strong evidence supporting the superiority of proprietary omeprazole paste (Gastrogard) over oral ranitidine at a dose of 6.6 mg/kg administered three times daily or compounded omeprazole in the treatment of gastric ulcers in racehorses. Ideally, these data should be repeated in trials that are free from any potential conflict of interest.

Colic epidemiology

Question 1: risk factors

What are the risk factors for colic in adult horses?

Colic is one of the most common causes for mortality and morbidity in the horse [53,54], and it has consequently has inspired a large body of research into epidemiologic factors with a goal of reducing the incidence. Colic is not a disease per se, however, but simply a clinical sign of abdominal pain in the horse. It is self-evident that the risk factors for a strangulating lipoma are different from those for gastric ulcers, and this fact has resulted in significant difficulties in study design and data interpretation. Nonetheless, searching for articles on this subject reveals more than 100 citations, most of which address risk factors for specific colics, such as gastric ulcers or ileal impactions, but also include some that address the incidence of colic less specifically. Although the constraints of space do not allow a comprehensive evidence-based evaluation of these data, two review articles have been published in the last 5 years that summarize most of these studies in a thorough and accessible, although not explicitly systematic, manner (with systematic review and meta-analysis representing the pinnacle of evidence-based data).

The most recent article is a review published in 2006 [55], which gives an excellent overview of the data in this field but does not attempt to judge the strength of the evidence qualitatively for each of the risk factors. A second article published in 2002 [56] examines 12 epidemiologic studies on colic in the horse. The review starts by dividing the studies by design, showing which were cohort, case-control, and cross-sectional studies. This provides an excellent tool for evaluating the quality of the data generated and significantly strengthens the EBM characteristics of the article. The summary of these findings is tabulated here (Table 2).

Most of the risk factors identified in these studies demonstrate conflicting data in multiple studies, especially in regard to differences in quantity, type, and frequency of forage feed (no association with colic [53], increased colic with fibrous forage [57], and decrease in horses receiving only forage [54]). A preponderance of evidence suggests that tapeworm infestation is associated with colic [58,59] and that although anthelmintic treatment against *Anoplocephala* spp is probably warranted, caution should be taken in horses with heavy infestations, because deworming has been associated with an increase in colic with some studies[57,60]. A previous history of colic is a significant risk factor in multiple studies [53,54,61], although variable causes make clinical use of these data somewhat complex.

Conflicting or weak evidence exists for the effects of age (other than strangulating lipoma, which increases in older horses [62,63]), gender (other than colic

Table 2
Risk factors for colic in the horse from 12 epidemiologic studies

Risk factor		Reference											
		[99]	[100]	[57]	[60]	[101]	[102]	[58]	[103]	[104]	[54]	[105]	[106]
Feeding practices														
Nature	Forage			X									
	Concentrate										X	X	X
	Whole corn										X	X	X
Changes	Changes of food	X	X	X		X					X	X	
	No regular watering			X	X								
Parasitism														
Type	Taeniasis						X	X					
Deworming	Deworming treatments			X	X					X			
	No deworming program			X									X
Intrinsic factors														
Gender	Stallions				X								
	Geldings	X											
Age	Age to 2 to 8 years			X							X	X	
	Age more than 11 years												X

EVIDENCE-BASED GASTROINTESTINAL MEDICINE IN HORSES 257

Category		Study columns (X indicates risk factor identified)
Breed	Arabians	X ... X
	Thoroughbred horses	X X X
Medical history	Horses with previous colic	X X X X X
	Medical treatment	X X X
Management		
Housing	Indoor stalling	X X X
	Changes in housing	X X X X
Activity	Exercise	X
	Intense activity	X
	Stressing activity	X
	Changes in activity	X X X X
Weather-related factors	December, March, and August	X X
	Weather change	X

From Goncalves S, Julliand V, Leblond A. Risk factors associated with colic in horses. Vet Res 2002;33:646; with permission.

associated with the reproductive tract of mares and stallions), breed, season, weather, work, access to pasture, transportation, and vaccination, and firm conclusions cannot be drawn at this time regarding the importance of these factors.

Quality of evidence

There are several large and well-designed studies evaluating risk factors for colic, but problems with the definition of "colic," combined with the multifactorial nature of abdominal pain, render the data difficult to interpret. A systematic review or meta-analysis of qualifying studies would add greatly to this field.

Clinical implications

Although many risk factors have been identified to be associated with colic in the horse, there are conflicting data in most areas. Not surprisingly, factors associated with feeding seem to be the most consistently found, with evidence suggesting that diet changes, changes in hay type or quality, high levels of concentrate, and reduced access to grazing increase the risk of colic.

Question 2: indications for colic surgery

What clinical tools are most useful in making a determination of whether a horse needs colic surgery?

When field veterinarians are faced with a horse with colic, a critical decision must be made rapidly. When horses are referred to hospitals for colic surgery, many of them are presented having severe GI lesions that can quickly lead to shock and death [64–67]. Furthermore, it has been shown that the survival rate rapidly decreases in inverse proportion to the duration of clinical signs [68]. The percentage of horses undergoing celiotomy for colic-related GI problems that die or are euthanized during surgery because of the advanced state of their disease has been estimated to range from 8% to 24% [69,70]. Thus, it is incumbent on veterinarians referring horses to hospitals for potential colic surgery to ensure that such referrals are made as quickly as possible. To facilitate early treatment, the most efficient method of diagnosis is simply to attempt to distinguish between cases needing surgical intervention, defined as a horse with intestinal lesions (identified during surgery or at necropsy) that require surgical correction or could benefit from surgery, and those treatable with medicine alone.

Experimental [71–74] and clinical research [75,76] document the usefulness of individual clinical and laboratory variables in helping to distinguish between medical and surgical cases of colic. In addition, at least three studies have attempted to develop algorithms for helping to make this important clinical decision. [76–78]. Information obtained from these and other studies can be used to help clinicians understand which information may be most useful in the clinical decision-making process.

Research, as well as clinical experience, has shown that intensity of pain is one of the most important variables in discriminating surgical and medical cases of colic in horses [77–84]. This relation seems to be linear; that is, the more severe the colic pain, the more likely it is that the colic requires surgical correction.

In colic, changes in the horse's body temperature may occur as a result of increased activity caused by pain, local or systemic inflammatory response, or depressed cardiovascular function. At least one analysis suggests that there is an inverse association between temperature and the need for surgical intervention [78]. The authors of that study suggested that a body temperature of 39°C was consistent with symptoms of enteritis or peritonitis, and therefore inconsistent with a surgical lesion. This finding is supported by other studies; for example, a review of reports on peritonitis found that elevated body temperature was present in 57% of the horses [85]. Of course, fever and peritonitis can also be features of colicking horses that have a ruptured viscus, and although the only chance for survival in such cases might be surgery, the prognosis would be expected to be poor. In another study, 20 of 122 horses with acute diarrhea had rectal temperatures higher than 38.6°C [86].

Two studies have suggested that visual evidence of marked abdominal distention is an important indicator identifying horses with colic that need surgical referral [76,84]. Because marked abdominal distention is somewhat subjective, however, it is difficult to make specific recommendations for a general population of horses based on this variable.

Some studies have demonstrated that a decrease or absence of intestinal sounds is associated with a need for surgery; one study indicated that 50% of the horses that needed surgery presented with absent gut sounds [77,87]. Of course, the 50% figure means that 50% of the horses that needed surgery also had gut sounds; thus, clearly, the absence of gut sounds should be interpreted in light of other factors.

Abdominal fluid color and protein are clinically relevant variables that are easily measured in the field and can also provide immediate information without the need for sophisticated laboratory techniques. In cases of surgical colic, peritoneal fluid may darken because of hemolysis and protein levels may increase. Peritoneal fluid color has been shown to be useful in helping to distinguish between surgical and medical cases of colic [85,88,89]. At least two studies suggest that peritoneal fluid color is most useful in helping to determine the status of colicking horses exhibiting milder clinical signs [78,90]. In addition, in horses without significant abdominal distention, and when rectal palpation has revealed no intestinal distention, peritoneal fluid color may help to separate surgical from medical cases [91]. This relation is linear; that is, darkened color increases the likelihood that a horse needs surgery. Nevertheless, results of abdominal fluid analysis cannot be used alone to predict lesion type accurately, whether medical or surgical treatment is needed, or outcome for horses with colic.

Although abdominal fluid sample analysis may contribute to the decision to proceed to surgery, it is not a diagnostic panacea. In two large studies, a few cases were misclassified by peritoneal fluid hemolysis in both studies [76,78]. In addition, color and protein seem to have a greater negative predictive value than positive predictive value. That is, it is more likely that a horse with normal abdominal fluid does not need surgery than it is that a horse with abnormal fluid does need surgery [28]. Unfortunately, peritoneal fluid cannot always be obtained through abdominocentesis. In one study, fluid was unobtainable in 13% of cases, despite several attempts [92].

Variables reflecting the condition of the cardiovascular system are associated with the prognosis and treatment needed [74,85,93]. A weak peripheral pulse has been reported to increase the risk that surgery is necessary [77]. In another study, the probability that surgical treatment was necessary increased when high packed cell volumes were present [78] Mucous membrane color seems to be a fairly poor predictor of the need for surgery at first examination [87].

When a specific diagnosis has not been made, lack of response or resumption of colic after analgesic administration should be considered as a positive indicator of the need for surgery [84,87]. The presence of constant pain after analgesic administration does not always indicate a need for surgery, however. Conversely, the response to analgesic administration seems to have significant negative predictive value; that is, if a horse responds to analgesic treatment and pain does not return, surgery is likely not to be indicated.

The existing scientific literature supports the diagnostic benefits of rectal examination in colicking horses, although with some considerable differences between studies. Specific diagnoses can occasionally be made on rectal examination; however, more often, the recognition of intestinal distention or dislocation by rectal palpation is an indication that a case belongs to a certain diagnostic category [76,77,93–95]. One study suggested that rectal examination had positive and negative predictive values of 68% and 91%, respectively [96]; that is, 32% of horses classified as surgical cases did not require surgical intervention (false-positive predictive value) and 9% of horses classified as nonsurgical cases actually needed surgical correction (false-negative predictive value). In another study, the positive and negative predictive values of rectal examination were reported as 90% and 99%, respectively [76]. Yet another study reported a sensitivity and specificity of rectal palpation of 50% and 98%, respectively [77].

Conversely, one study has indicated that abnormal rectal examination findings do not necessarily increase the risk for surgery [87]. There may also be some differences in the accuracy of rectal examination for specific types of colic; for example, some horses with small intestinal lesions may be incorrectly classified with false-negative findings by rectal examination [97]. Furthermore, because a significant portion of the abdominal cavity cannot be assessed per rectum, rectal examination may be of limited value in some cases. Still, rectal examination can sometimes help to make a specific diagnosis and may be helpful in determining whether surgery is necessary in individual cases [93].

Although results have been rarely reported, ultrasonographic evaluation of the abdomen has been shown to be useful in helping to delineate between surgical and medical cases of colic. One study reported a sensitivity and specificity of abdominal ultrasonography of 100%, respectively, in cases of horses with acute abdominal pain [98].

Strength of evidence

The evidence pertaining to the relation of particular diagnostic tests to the need for colic surgery is quite strong, because the evidence is routinely evaluated by a gold standard of diagnostic support; that is, the utility of the diagnostic test is supported or refuted by subsequent colic surgery or the problem resolves. As such, this information can be used by practitioners with confidence.

Clinical implications

No single diagnostic test has been shown to predict the need for colic surgery with 100% accuracy. Nevertheless, certain tests seem to be strongly predictive of the need for surgery, including response to analgesia, abdominal ultrasonography, degree of pain, and abdominal fluid color and protein. When present, abdominal distention may be a strong positive predictor. Elevated body temperature seems to have significant negative predictive value. Conversely, such commonly used procedures as rectal examination, auscultation of the abdominal cavity, and assessment of the cardiovascular system seem to be of somewhat more limited value generally but may be of some use in individual cases.

Summary

The use of an evidence-based approach allows veterinary clinicians to assess questions that are clinically relevant to the diagnosis and treatment of equine GI tract disease. This approach involves formulating a clinical question, searching the literature, and answering the question with the best available evidence, with the results summarized as a clinical "bottom line." Additional reports written using such an approach to evaluate specific topics pertinent not only to the equine GI tract but to all areas of clinical medicine would be of considerable value to equine clinicians.

Acknowledgments

The authors thank Heather Trout for her assistance in researching this article.

References

[1] P.Cockcroft MAH. Handbook of evidence-based veterinary medicine. 1st edition. USA: Blackwell Science; 2003.
[2] Gibson K. Equine colic: the choice of analgesics. Aust Equine Vet 1992;10:34–6.
[3] Becht JL. Analgesics for pain management in the horse with colic. 24–5.
[4] Jochle W, Moore JN, Brown J, et al. Comparison of detomidine, butorphanol, flunixin meglumine and xylazine in clinical cases of equine colic. Equine Vet J 1989;7:111–6.
[5] Muir WW, Robertson JT. Visceral analgesia: effects of xylazine, butorphanol, meperidine, and pentazocine in horses. Am J Vet Res 1985;46:2081–4.
[6] Boatwright CE, Fubini SLF, Grohn YT, et al. A comparison of N-butylscopolammonium bromide and butorphanol tartrate for analgesia using a balloon model of abdominal pain in ponies. Can J Vet Res 1996;60:65–8.
[7] Betley M, Sutherland SF, Gregoricka MJ, et al. The analgesic effect of ketoprofen for use in treating equine colic as compared to flunixin meglumine. Equine Practice 1991;13:11–6.
[8] Sellon DC, ROberts MC, Blikslager AT, et al. Effects of continuous rate intravenous infusion of butorphanol on physiologic and outcome variables in horses after celiotomy. J Vet Intern Med 2004;18(4):555–63.
[9] Merritt AM, Xie HS, Lester GD, et al. Evaluation of a method to experimentally induce colic in horses and the effects of acupuncture applied at the Guan-yuan-shu (similar to BL-21) acupoint. Am J Vet Res 2002;63:1006–11.
[10] Cohen ND, Lester GD, Sanchez LC, et al. Evaluation of risk factors associated with development of postoperative ileus in horses. J Am Vet Med Assoc 2004;225:1070–8.
[11] Cohen ND, Faber NA, Brumbaugh GW. Use of bethanechol and metoclopramide in horses with duodenitis/proximal jejunitis: 13 cases (1987–1993). J Equine Vet Sci 1995;15:492–4.
[12] van Hoogmoed LM, Boscan PL. In vitro evaluation of the effect of the opioid antagonist N-methylnaltrexone on motility of the equine jejunum and pelvic flexure. Equine Vet J 2005;37:325–8.
[13] Smith MA, Edwards GB, Dallap BL, et al. Evaluation of the clinical efficacy of prokinetic drugs in the management of post-operative ileus: can retrospective data help us? Vet J 2005; 170:230–6.
[14] Brianceau P, Chevalier H, Karas A, et al. Intravenous lidocaine and small-intestinal size, abdominal fluid, and outcome after colic surgery in horses. J Vet Intern Med 2002;16:736–41.
[15] Malone E, Ensink J, Turner T, et al. Intravenous continuous infusion of lidocaine for treatment of equine ileus. Vet Surg 2006;35:60–6.
[16] Dart AJ, Peauroi JR, Hodgson DR, et al. Efficacy of metoclopramide for treatment of ileus in horses following small intestinal surgery: 70 cases (1989–1992). Aust Vet J 1996;74:280–4.
[17] Velden MA, van der, Klein WR. The effects of cisapride on the restoration of gut motility after surgery of the small intestine in horses; a clinical trial. Vet Q 1993;15:175–9.
[18] Gerring EL, King JN. Cisapride in the prophylaxis of equine post operative ileus. Equine Vet J 1989;52–5.
[19] Gerring EE, Hunt JM. Pathophysiology of equine postoperative ileus: effect of adrenergic blockade, parasympathetic stimulation and metoclopramide in an experimental model. Equine Vet J 1986;18:249–55.
[20] Van Hoogmoed LM, Nieto JE, Snyder JR, et al. Survey of prokinetic use in horses with gastrointestinal injury. Vet Surg 2004;33:279–85.
[21] Santschi EM, Slone DE, Frank WM. Use of ultrasound in horses for diagnosis of left dorsal displacement of the large colon and monitoring its nonsurgical correction. Vet Surg 1993;22:281–4.
[22] Baird AN, Cohen ND, Taylor TS, et al. Renosplenic entrapment of the large colon in horses: 57 cases (1983–1988). J Am Vet Med Assoc 1991;198:1423–6.

[23] Mezerova J, Zert Z, Kottman J. [Diagnostic and therapeutic aspects of left dorsal displacement of the large colon in the horse]. Pferdeheilkunde 2003;19:65–74 [in German].
[24] Kalsbeek HC. Further experiences with non-surgical correction of nephrosplenic entrapment of the left colon in the horse. Equine Vet J 1989;21:442–3.
[25] van Harreveld PD, Cox J, Biller DS. Phenylephrine HCl as a treatment of nephrosplenic entrapment in a horse. Equine Vet Educ 1999;11:282–4.
[26] Abutarbush SM, Naylor JM. Comparison of surgical versus medical treatment of nephrosplenic entrapment of the large colon in horses: 19 cases (1992–2002). J Am Vet Med Assoc 2005;227:603–5.
[27] Hardy J, Minton M, Robertson JT, et al. Nephrosplenic entrapment in the horse: a retrospective study of 174 cases. Equine Vet J Suppl 2000;32:95–7.
[28] Sivula NJ. Renosplenic entrapment of the large colon in horses: 33 cases (1984–1989). J Am Vet Med Assoc 1991;199:244–51.
[29] Boening KJ, Saldern FC. [Treatment of left dorsal displacement of the large colon in horses by rolling, under general anaesthesia]. Tierarztl Umsch 1985;40:252–4, 257 [in German].
[30] Harreveld PD van, Gaughan EM, Valentino LW. A retrospective analysis of left dorsal displacement of the large colon treated with phenylephrine hydrochloride and exercise in 12 horses (1996–98). N Z Vet J 1999;47:109–111.
[31] White NA 2nd, Dabareiner RM. Treatment of impaction colics. Vet Clin North Am Equine Pract 1997;13:243–59.
[32] Lopes MA, Walker BL, White NA 2nd, et al. Treatments to promote colonic hydration: enteral fluid therapy versus intravenous fluid therapy and magnesium sulphate. Equine Vet J 2002;34:505–9.
[33] Lopes MA, White NA 2nd, Donaldson L, et al. Effects of enteral and intravenous fluid therapy, magnesium sulfate, and sodium sulfate on colonic contents and feces in horses. Am J Vet Res 2004;65:695–704.
[34] Schott HC 2nd, Ewart SL, Walker RD, et al. An outbreak of salmonellosis among horses at a veterinary teaching hospital. J Am Vet Med Assoc 2001;218:1152–9.
[35] Ward MP, Alinovi CA, Couetil LL, et al. Evaluation of a PCR to detect salmonella in fecal samples of horses admitted to a veterinary teaching hospital. J Vet Diagn Invest 2005;17:118–23.
[36] Cohen ND, Martin LJ, Simpson RB, et al. Comparison of polymerase chain reaction and microbiological culture for detection of salmonellae in equine feces and environmental samples. Am J Vet Res 1996;57:780–6.
[37] Ewart SL, Schott HC 2nd, Robison RL, et al. Identification of sources of salmonella organisms in a veterinary teaching hospital and evaluation of the effects of disinfectants on detection of salmonella organisms on surface materials. J Am Vet Med Assoc 2001;218:1145–51.
[38] Wilson IG. Inhibition and facilitation of nucleic acid amplification. Appl Environ Microbiol 1997;63:3741–51.
[39] Sachse K. Specificity and performance of diagnostic PCR assays. Methods Mol Biol 2003;216:3–29.
[40] Amavisit P, Browning GF, Lightfoot D, et al. Rapid PCR detection of salmonella in horse faecal samples. Vet Microbiol 2001;79:63–74.
[41] Kurowski PB, TraubDargatz JL, Morley PS, et al. Detection of salmonella spp in fecal specimens by use of real-time polymerase chain reaction assay. Am J Vet Res 2002;63:1265–8.
[42] Murray MJ, Schusser GF, Pipers FS, et al. Factors associated with gastric lesions in Thoroughbred racehorses. Equine Vet J 1996;28:368–74.
[43] Lorenzo-Figueras M, Merritt AM. Effects of exercise on gastric volume and pH in the proximal portion of the stomach of horses. Am J Vet Res 2002;63:1481–7.
[44] Buchanan BR, Andrews FM. Treatment and prevention of equine gastric ulcer syndrome. Vet Clin North Am Equine Pract 2003;19:575–97.

[45] Bezdekova B, Jahn P, Vyskoil M, et al. Gastric ulceration and exercise intensity in Standardbred racehorses in Czech Republic. Acta Vet Brno 2005;74:67–71.
[46] Hartmann AM, Frankeny RL. A preliminary investigation into the association between competition and gastric ulcer formation in nonracing performance horses. J Equine Vet Sci 2003;23:560–1.
[47] McClure SR, Carithers DS, Gross SJ, et al. Gastric ulcer development in horses in a simulated show or training environment. J Am Vet Med Assoc 2005;227:775–7.
[48] Orsini JA, Haddock M, Stine L, et al. Odds of moderate or severe gastric ulceration in racehorses receiving antiulcer medications. J Am Vet Med Assoc 2003;223:336–9.
[49] Lester GD, Smith RL, Robertson ID. Effects of treatment with omeprazole or ranitidine on gastric squamous ulceration in racing Thoroughbreds. J Am Vet Med Assoc 2005;227: 1636–9.
[50] Andrews FM, Sifferman RL, Bernard W, et al. Efficacy of omeprazole paste in the treatment and prevention of gastric ulcers in horses (equine gastric ulceration). Equine Vet J 1999;29:81–6.
[51] McClure SR, White GW, Sifferman RL, et al. Efficacy of omeprazole paste for prevention of gastric ulcers in horses in race training. J Am Vet Med Assoc 2005;226:1681–4.
[52] Nieto JE, Spier S, Pipers FS, et al. Comparison of paste and suspension formulations of omeprazole in the healing of gastric ulcers in racehorses in active training. J Am Vet Med Assoc 2002;221:1139–43.
[53] TraubDargatz JL, Kopral CA, Seitzinger AH, et al. Estimate of the national incidence of and operation-level risk factors for colic among horses in the United States, spring 1998 to spring 1999. J Am Vet Med.Assoc USA 2001;219:67–71.
[54] Tinker MK, White NA, Lessard P, et al. Prospective study of equine colic incidence and mortality. Equine Vet J 1997;29:448–53.
[55] Archer DC, Proudman CJ. Epidemiological clues to preventing colic. Vet J 2006;172:29–39.
[56] Goncalves S, Julliand V, Leblond A. Risk factors associated with colic in horses. Vet Res 2002;33:641–52.
[57] Cohen ND, Gibbs PG, Woods AM. Dietary and other management factors associated with colic in horses. J Am Vet Med Assoc 1999;215:53–60.
[58] Proudman CJ, French NP, Trees AJ. Tapeworm infection is a significant risk factor for spasmodic colic and ileal impaction colic in the horse. Equine Vet J 1998;30:194–9.
[59] Barrett EJ, Blair CW, Farlam J, et al. Postdosing colic and diarrhoea in horses with serological evidence of tapeworm infection. Vet Rec 2005;156:252–3.
[60] Kaneene JB, Miller R, Ross WA, et al. Risk factors for colic in the Michigan (USA) equine population. Prev Vet Med 1997;30:23–36.
[61] Cohen ND. Epidemiology of colic. Vet Clin North Am Equine Pract 1997;13:191–201.
[62] Freeman DE, Schaeffer DJ. Age distributions of horses with strangulation of the small intestine by a lipoma or in the epiploic foramen: 46 cases (1994–2000). J Am Vet Med Assoc 2001;219:87–9.
[63] Garcia-Seco E, Wilson DA, Kramer J, et al. Prevalence and risk factors associated with outcome of surgical removal of pedunculated lipomas in horses: 102 cases (1987–2002). J Am Vet Med Assoc 2005;226:1529–37.
[64] White NA. Epidemiology and etiology of colic. In: White NA, editor. The equine acute abdomen. London: Lea & Febiger; 1990. p. 49–64.
[65] Ebert R. Prognostische Parameter bei der Kolik des Pferdes. Tierärztl Prax 1994;23:256–63 [in German].
[66] Blikslager AT, Roberts MC. Accuracy of clinicians in predicting site and type of lesion as well as outcome in horses with colic. J Am Vet Med Assoc 1995;207:1444–7.
[67] Thoefner MB, Ersbøll AK, Hesselholt M. Prognostic indicators in a Danish hospital based population of colic horses. Equine Vet J 2000;32:11–8.
[68] Parks AH, Doran RE, White NA, et al. Ileal impaction in the horse: 75 cases. Cornell Vet 1989;79:83–91.

[69] Ducharme NG, Hacket RP, Ducharme GR. Surgical treatment of colic: results in 183 horses. Vet Surg 1983;12:206–9.
[70] Pascoe PJ, McDonnell WN, Trim CM, et al. Mortality rate and associated factors in equine colic operations—a retrospective study of 341 operations. Can Vet J 1983;24:76–85.
[71] Turner AS, McIlwraith CW, Trotter GW, et al. Biochemical analysis of serum and peritoneal fluid in experimental colonic infarction in horses. Proceedings. Equine Colic Research Symposium University of Georgia, USA, 1982. p. 79–87.
[72] Puotunen-Reinert A, Huskamp B. Experimental duodenal obstruction in the horse. Vet Surg 1986;15:420–8.
[73] Ruggles AJ, Freeman DE, Acland HM, et al. Changes in fluid composition on the serosal surface of jejunum and small colon subjected to venous strangulation obstruction in ponies. Am J Vet Res 1993;54:333–40.
[74] Parry BW, Gay CC, Anderson GA. Assessment of the necessity for surgical intervention in cases of equine colic: a retrospective study. Equine Vet J 1983;15:216–21.
[75] Arden WA, Stick JA. Serum and peritoneal fluid phosphate concentrations as predictors of major intestinal injury associated with equine colic. J Am Vet Med Assoc 1988;193: 927–31.
[76] Ducharme NG, Pascoe PJ, Lumsden JH, et al. A computer-derived protocol to aid in selecting medical versus surgical treatment of horses with abdominal pain. Equine Vet J 1989;21: 447–50.
[77] Reeves MJ, Curtis CR, Salman MD, et al. Multivariable prediction model for the need for surgery in horses with colic. Am J Vet Res 1991;52:1903–7.
[78] Martin B, Thoefner BK, Ersbøll NJ, et al. Diagnostic decision rule for support in clinical assessment of the need for surgical intervention in horses with acute abdominal pain. Can J Vet Res 2003;67(1):20–9.
[79] Karlsbeek HC. Indications for surgical intervention in equine colic. J S Afr Vet Assoc 1975; 46:101–5.
[80] Scrutchfield WL, Taylor T. Clinical parameters and indices that determine medical or surgical treatment of colic patients. Proceedings of the 27th Annual Convention of the American Association of Equine Practitioners 1981;27:277–83.
[81] Reeves MJ, Curtis CR, Salman MD, et al. Descriptive epidemiology and risk factors indicating the need for surgery and evaluation of prognosis. The Morris Animal Foundation Colic Study. Proceedings of the 33rd Annual Convention of the American Association of Equine Practitioners 1987;33:83–94.
[82] Edwards GB. Equine colic: the decision for surgery. Equine Vet Educ 1991;3:19–23.
[83] Mair T, Edwards B. Medical treatment of equine colic. In Practice 1998;20:578–84.
[84] Peloso JG, Cohen ND, Taylor TS, et al. When to send a horse with signs of colic; is it surgical, or is it referable; a survey of the opinions of 117 equine veterinary specialists. Proceedings of the American Association of Equine Practitioners 1996;42:250–3.
[85] Hillyer MH, Wright CJ. Peritonitis in the horse. Equine Vet Educ 1998;9:136–42.
[86] Cohen ND, Woods AM. Characteristics and risk factors for failure of horses with acute diarrhea to survive: 122 cases (1990–1996). J Am Vet Med Assoc 1999;214:382–90.
[87] White NA, Elward A, Moga KS, et al. Use of Web-based data collection to evaluate analgesic administration and the decision for surgery in horses with colic. Equine Vet J 2005; 37(4):347–50.
[88] Freden GO, Provost PJ, Rand WM. Reliability of using results of abdominal fluid analysis to determine treatment and predict lesion type and outcome for horses with colic: 218 cases (1991–1994). J Am Vet Med Assoc 1998;213:1012–5.
[89] Swanwick RA, Wilkinson JS. A clinical evaluation of abdominal paracentesis in the horse. Aust Vet J 1976;52:109–17.
[90] Matthews S, Dart AJ, Reid SW, et al. Predictive values, sensitivity and specificity of abdominal fluid variables in determining the need for surgery in horses with an acute abdominal crisis. Aust Vet J 2002;80(3):132–6.

[91] Siex MT, Wilson JH. Morbidity associated with abdominocentesis—a prospective study. Equine Vet J 1992;13:23–5.
[92] Parry BW, Anderson GA, Gay CC. Prognosis in equine colic: a study of individual variables used in case assessment. Equine Vet J 1983;15:337–44.
[93] Adams SB, McIlwraith CW. Abdominal crisis in the horse: a comparison of presurgical evaluation with surgical findings and results. Vet Surg 1978;7:63–9.
[94] White NA. Determining the diagnosis and prognosis of the acute abdomen. In: White NA, editor. The equine acute abdomen. London: Lea & Febiger; 1990. p. 116–24.
[95] Huskamp B, Kopf N. Pathologische Befunde. In: Huskamp B, editor. Die rektale Untersuchung beim Kolik Pferd. München (Germany): Wak; 1995. p. 15–96.
[96] Henken AM, Graat EAM, Casal J. Measurement of disease frequency. In: Noordhuizen JPTM, Frankena K, van der Hoofd CM, et al, editors. Application of quantitative methods in veterinary epidemiology. Wageningen (The Netherlands): Wageningen Pers; 1997. p. 76.
[97] Vachon AM, Fischer AT. Small intestinal herniation through the epiploic foramen: 53 cases (1987–1993). Equine Vet J 1995;27(5):373–80.
[98] Klohnen A, Vachon AM, Fischer A. Use of diagnostic ultrasonography in horses with signs of acute abdominal pain. J Am Vet Med Assoc 1996;209:1597–601.
[99] Cohen ND, Peloso JG. Risk factors for history of previous colic and for chronic, intermittent colic in a population of horses. J Am Vet Med Assoc 1996;208:697–703.
[100] Cohen ND, Matejka PL, Honnas CM, et al. Case-control study of the association between various management factors and development of colic in horses. J Am Vet Med Assoc 1995;206:667–73.
[101] Proudman CJ. A two years survey of equine colic in general practice. Equine Vet J 1991;24:90–3.
[102] Proudman CJ, Edwards GB. Are tapeworms associated with equine colic? A case control study. Equine Vet J 1993;25:224–6.
[103] Reeves MJ, Gay JM, Hilbert BJ, et al. Association of age, sex and breed factors in acute equine colic: a retrospective study of 320 cases admitted to a veterinary teaching hospital in the USA. Prev Vet Med 1989;7:149–60.
[104] Reeves MJ, Salman MD, Smith G. Risk factors for equine acute abdominal disease (colic): results from a multi-center case-control study. Prev Vet Med 1996;26:285–301.
[105] Tinker MK, White NA, Lessard P, et al. Prospective study of equine colic risk factors. Equine Vet J 1997;29:454–8.
[106] White NA, Lessard P. Risk factors and clinical signs associated with cases of equine colic. Equine Pract Proc, 32nd Annual Convention of the American Association 1986;63:744.

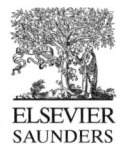

Evidence-Based Gastrointestinal Surgery in Horses

Tim S. Mair, PhD, MRCVS[a,*],
Luisa J. Smith, MRCVS[a,b],
Ceri E. Sherlock, MRCVS[a,c]

[a]Bell Equine Veterinary Clinic, Mereworth, Maidstone, Kent, ME18 5GS, United Kingdom
[b]Royal Veterinary College, Hawkshead Campus, Hawkshead Lane, North Mymms, Hatfield, Hertfordshire, AL9 7TA, United Kingdom
[c]University of Georgia, College of Veterinary Medicine, Athens, GA 30602-7385, USA

Equine gastrointestinal surgery, especially surgery for colic, has become a routine procedure at many hospitals around the world. Although most cases of colic resolve spontaneously or with simple medical treatment, a few (up to 10%) prove fatal unless treated surgically [1]. Over the past 35 years, advances in our understanding of the pathophysiologic mechanisms in equine colic and advances in diagnostic techniques, anesthetic techniques, and postoperative care have contributed to an impressive improvement in survival rates over those obtained during the 1970s and 1980s [2–4]. This has been aided by many other factors, such as the development of residency training programs in medicine, surgery, and anesthesia, and the open sharing of findings from research and clinical case studies by means of forums, such as the Equine Colic Research Symposia [5].

Despite the considerable improvements in the management of surgical colic, the procedure still carries relatively high mortality and complication rates. In a large part, this can be explained by wide variations in the type and severity of the underlying disease and the seriousness of the resultant insult to the intestines, the time delay between onset of disease and surgical treatment, and the extraintestinal effects of hypovolemia and endotoxemia, for example. Variations in surgical techniques and complementary treatments almost certainly affect these rates as well. Careful monitoring and analysis of the survival and complication rates of colic surgery not only provide insights into risk factors for the development of negative outcomes but

---

* Corresponding author.
  E-mail address: tim.mair@btinternet.com (T.S. Mair).

identify areas in which individual surgeons or clinics can improve their success rates [6].

Although many advances in the treatment of equine colic have come from basic research and experimental models, clinical evidence of the effectiveness and complications of treatment procedures, including surgical techniques, is particularly important to clinicians "on the front line" who have to treat colicky horses and advise owners about treatment options. This type of objective evidence-based information aids clinicians in making informed decisions about treatments that are not reliant on anecdote or personal experience [6,7]. Surgery is notoriously difficult to evaluate scientifically, and many studies are anecdotal and based on case series [8]. Although prospective studies are likely to generate more useful and scientifically robust data about survival and postoperative complications [9,10], retrospective studies are also helpful and provide valuable information on which future prospective studies can be based. This review focuses on studies that have addressed survival rates and complications after colic surgery; preoperative assessment and postoperative intensive care are not discussed.

Survival rates

Although there have been several published studies of survival rates of horses undergoing colic surgery (Table 1) [2–4,11–25], many of these originate from the 1970s and 1980s and a few are recent studies. A small number of these studies have considered long-term survival and complication rates, and few have attempted to identify factors that might affect the outcomes. Direct comparison of the results of different studies of survival after colic surgery is difficult because of variations in the inclusion criteria and categorization of cases. In addition, differences in decisions about whether to progress to exploratory celiotomy or euthanasia in horses presenting with advanced cardiovascular compromise are likely to have marked effects on the success rates.

The pattern of postoperative survival has been documented in detail [9,10]. This pattern shows a high mortality rate in the first few days after surgery and continuing mortality at a lower rate up to 100 to 120 days after surgery, followed by a low level of mortality. Short-term survival rates (ie, survival to discharge from the hospital) therefore give an incomplete and possibly unrealistic picture of postoperative survival. The high mortality rates in the immediate postoperative periods and the incidence of the different complications that are recorded in these periods provide valuable information on which future efforts to improve survival rates may be based, however.

Different studies have frequently shown contradicting results with respect to the correlation between survival after colic surgery and pre-, intra-, and postoperative factors. For example, several studies have indicated that old

Table 1
Published survival rates of colic surgery

Reference	Years	N	Survival rate
Tennant et al, 1972 [2]	1958–1968	95	46.5%[a]
Tennant, 1975 [3]	1969–1971	36	71.2%[a]
Pearson et al, 1975 [4]	Before 1975	82	28.0%[a]
Pascoe et al, 1983 [11]	1974–1980	300	50.0%[d]
White and Lessard, 1986 [12]	1979–1984	2055	48.0%[a]
Huskamp, 1982 [13]	1979–1981	724	74.3%[c]
Ducharme et al, 1983 [14]	1976–1981	181	62.8%[d]
Ducharme et al, 1983 [14]	1976–1981	181	45.5%[b]
Parry et al, 1983 [15]	Before 1983	44	38.6%[a]
Reeves et al, 1986 [16]	1974–1984	145	44.0%[a]
Shires et al, 1986 [20]	1982–1985	138	53.6%[d]
McCarthy and Hutchins, 1988 [21]	Before 1988	74	34.0%[d]
Phillips and Walmsley, 1993 [22]	1987–1991	151	72.2%[d]
Phillips and Walmsley, 1993 [22]	1987–1991	151	66.2%[b]
Santschi et al, 2000 [23]	1968–1990	206	85.0%[d,e]
Van der Linden et al, 2003 [24]	1999–2000	183	54.0%[d]
Van der Linden et al, 2003 [24]	1999–2000	183	47.0%[f]
Abutarbush et al, 2005 [25]	1992–2002	277	73.5%[d]
Mair and Smith, 2005 [17]	1994–2001	300	70.3%[d]
Mair and Smith, 2005 [19]	1994–2001	293	65.5%[f]

[a] Time scale not specified.
[b] Survival longer than 7 months.
[c] Survival longer than 3 weeks.
[d] Survival means discharge from hospital.
[e] Juvenile horses less than 2 years of age only.
[f] Survival longer than 12 months.

age is a risk factor for the development of colic and is associated with a poorer prognosis for survival compared with younger horses [11,16,26]. Another study [17] found no association between survival from colic surgery and age, however. Breed has also been found to be associated with the risk of mortality; in one study, draft horses, Thoroughbreds, and Thoroughbred-cross horses carried a significantly worse prognosis than other breeds [26]. The influence of the surgeon has also shown variable results. Although some studies have suggested that experience of the primary surgeon has no influence on outcome [10], others have shown that different surgeons and different levels of surgical experience have a major effect on outcome [20,27,28]. A trend for decreasing survival rates with increasing surgery time has been identified [10,17,22], which suggests that speed of surgery, which may be influenced by surgical experience, is an important issue. The nature of the lesion and the surgical techniques required also have major effects on the duration of surgery, however.

The most common postoperative complications in one recent study were postoperative ileus (18.2%), persistent pain (32.1%), and endotoxemic shock (13.9%) [17,18]. All these complications seemed to have a significant effect on survival and death rates. The prevalence of these complications is, in turn, related to the nature of the original lesion and the duration of disease before surgery. Numerous studies have shown that short-term survival rates are poorest in horses showing the most severe pain and the poorest cardiovascular status at the time of surgery [10,15–17,24,26,29–37]. The importance of cardiovascular status demonstrates that the speed of referral and the decision to undertake surgery are likely to have a major effect on the outcome in those horses with strangulating obstructions that rapidly develop cardiovascular compromise.

Short-term survival after small intestinal surgery

Short-term survival rates tend to be poorer with small intestinal obstructions compared with large intestinal obstructions [11,12,15,17,22]. A recent study [17] demonstrated a higher short-term survival rate for horses with simple obstructions of the small intestine (79.6%) compared with strangulating obstructions of the small intestine (54.8%). These findings are in agreement with those from one study [11] but differ from those of several other studies [14,22,27]. As long ago as 1961 [38], it was demonstrated that the prognosis for small intestinal obstructions is favorable only for 6 hours and deteriorates after 12 hours. The speed of diagnosis and referral are thus extremely important in achieving a successful outcome in such cases [27]. The use of diagnostic abdominal ultrasonography has been shown to improve the accuracy of the diagnosis of small intestinal obstructions [39], and this procedure has proved to be a valuable adjunct to the evaluation of horses with colic. The identification of small intestinal distention, edema, and lack of motility are consistent findings in horses with small intestinal obstruction, and this can permit earlier surgical intervention, especially when distended small intestine cannot be palpated per rectum.

The survival rates for published series of horses affected by small intestinal obstructions are summarized in Table 2 [40–46]. Short-term survival rates for small intestinal surgery (excluding horses that died under anesthesia) reported over the past 15 years range from approximately 50% to approximately 85%. Numerous factors may influence these recovery rates, and this makes it difficult to compare the results between different studies directly. The presence of other underlying diseases (eg, grass sickness) also influences the apparent recovery rates after small intestinal surgery. Multiple pre-, intra-, and postoperative factors affect the short-term survival for horses with small intestinal disease, but one study identified the following factors to be most influential on survival: postoperative ileus, necessity for repeat celiotomy, and elevated heart rate and low total plasma protein concentration in the initial 24-hour postoperative period [47]. Postoperative ileus was the factor that placed horses at the greatest risk of nonsurvival in that and other studies [18]. In one study, [47], horses that developed

Table 2
Survival rates after small intestinal surgery

Reference	Years	Overall short-term recovery (%)	Survival after recovery from anesthesia (%)	Long-term survival (%)
Pascoe et al, 1983 [11]	1974–1980	39[a]	49[a]	—
Huskamp, 1982 [13]	1979–1981	69[b]	82[b]	—
Ducharme et al, 1983 [14]	1976–1981	—	—	34[c]
Hunt et al, 1986 [63]	1970–1984	47[a]	55[a]	—
Kersjes et al, 1988 [40]	1976–1985	49[a]	65[a]	—
MacDonald et al, 1989 [49]	1968–1986	—	49[d]	24[d]
Van der Velden and Klein, 1993 [41]	1990–1991	67[a]	76[a]	—
Phillips and Walmsley, 1993 [22]	1987–1991	—	—	52[e]
Engelbert et al, 1993 [42]	1983–1992	74[f]	88[f]	—
Singer and Livesey, 1997 [43]	1987–1992	—	56[g]	34[g]
Vachon and Fischer, 1995 [120]	1987–1993	66[h]	79[h]	70[h]
Freeman et al, 2000 [27]	1994–1999	66[a]	85[a]	68[a]
Freeman et al, 2000 [27]	1994–1999	63[b]	84[b]	—
Fugaro and Cote, 2001 [44]	1988–1997	—	81[i]	56[i]
Fugaro and Cote, 2001 [44]	1988–1997	—	65[j]	47[j]
Van den Boom and Van der Velden, 2001 [45]	1993–1996	50[b]	68[b]	61[b]
Semevolos et al, 2002 [114]	1989–2000	—	88[m]	57[m]
Stephen et al, 2004 [51]	1988–2000	80[n]	—	—
Mair and Smith, 2005 [17–19]	1994–2001	64[a]	76[a]	57[a]
Mair and Smith, 2005 [17–19]	1994–2001	55[b]	70[b]	55[b]
Mair and Smith, 2005 [17–19]	1994–2001	69[d]	69[d]	59[d]
Freeman and Schaeffer, 2005 [57]	1994–2003	64[b]	89[b]	—
Garcia-Seco et al, 2005 [28]	1987–2002	60[k]	80[k]	64[k]
Archer et al, 2004 [46]	1991–2001	69[l]	84	—

Overall short-term survival includes horses that were subjected to euthanasia under anesthesia because of financial constraints or poor prognosis or died under general anesthesia or in recovery.

Long-term survival excludes horses that that were subjected to euthanasia under anesthesia because of financial constraints or poor prognosis or died under general anesthesia or in recovery.

[a] Small intestinal obstruction; long-term survival 1 year.
[b] Small intestinal strangulation obstruction only.
[c] Small intestinal obstruction only; long-term survival.
[d] Small intestinal resection and anastomosis only.
[e] Small intestinal obstruction; survival longer than 7 months.
[f] Epiploic foramen obstructions only; survival for 1 month.
[g] Survival in horses less than 25 months old; survival longer than 60 days.
[h] Epiploic foramen only (n = 53).
[i] Small intestinal anastomosis with or without resection.
[j] Small intestinal anastomosis with resection.
[k] Pedunculated lipomas only.
[l] Epiploic foramen obstructions only.
[m] Jejunal resection and anastomosis only.
[n] Small intestinal volvulus only; short-term survival.

postoperative ileus were 29.7 times less likely to survive than horses that did not develop ileus. In a study of factors affecting long-term survival after small intestine surgery, the risk of death was found to be associated with high preoperative packed cell volume (PCV), low total plasma protein, increased duration of surgery, and repeat celiotomy [48].

The influence of different surgical techniques on short-term survival has been assessed by several workers. Jejunocecostomy has been associated with a reduced survival rate and higher complication rates (compared with horses having other forms of small intestinal surgery) [27,28,49–51]. Reduced survival rates associated with this procedure have been attributed to the inability to resect all the ileum, necessitating persistence of devitalized bowel in some horses, and an increased rate of postoperative ileus after jejunocecostomy [27]. Jejunocecostomy has also been associated with an increased likelihood of mechanical complications that require early repeat celiotomy [52]. Potential reasons why jejunocecostomy may be prone to short-term complications include the fact that horses requiring this procedure may have more severe forms of intestinal disease than others [53]. Also, jejunocecostomy results in the creation of a sharp transition between intestinal segments of dissimilar function. The jejunum must overcome intracecal pressure to empty [54] without the coordinating mechanism of the ileum and the ileocecal valve [27,55,56]. Although several studies have suggested that jejunocecostomy is associated with more complications and a lower survival rate than other forms of intestinal anastomosis, the type of jejunocecostomy could have a significant effect on the outcome [57–59], and this could lead to a wide range of survival rates between different hospitals and different surgeons. Jejunoileal anastomosis seems to result in a postoperative complication rate similar to that reported after jejunojejunostomy procedures and is preferred over jejunocecostomy whenever possible [60,61].

Survival after large intestinal surgery

Despite the fact that diseases affecting the large intestine are a common cause of surgical colic, few studies have detailed survival and complication rates after large intestinal surgery. In a long-term study of 275 horses undergoing surgery for large intestinal diseases, age, heart rate before surgery, PCV, bowel resection, and repeat celiotomy were all associated with an increased risk of postoperative death [62].

Complications after exploratory celiotomy

As the rate of postoperative survival has increased over the past 3 decades, complications after exploratory celiotomy for abdominal pain in the horse have become more apparent [27,62]. These postoperative complications are coming under increasing scrutiny as their relative importance increases in terms of the overall cost of treatment and the length of time to recovery.

The main postoperative complications documented after colic surgery include the following [9,10,14,17,18,22,27,63,64]:

1. Incisional infection, herniation, and dehiscence
2. Jugular vein thrombophlebitis
3. Postoperative ileus
4. Recurrent episodes of colic or pain
5. Postoperative shock
6. Laminitis
7. Colitis or diarrhea
8. Anastomotic leakage
9. Septic peritonitis

Although the nature of postoperative complications identified in these studies was similar, there was marked variation in the prevalence of the complications between different studies.

Although many postoperative complications are amenable to medical management, some are potentially life threatening. The most common causes of euthanasia in the immediate postoperative period include postoperative ileus [17,18,63], anastomotic leakage [49], septic peritonitis [22], postoperative pain [17], and shock [14]. In some instances of postoperative ileus and pain, the decision for euthanasia is influenced by economic constraints [17].

Even with complications associated with low mortality, the increased postoperative morbidity results in an increase in the length of hospitalization of the patient [17,18], increasing the overall cost of the treatment and prolonging the eventual return to work. There has also been a direct link recognized between some of the more minor complications, for example, incisional infections, and some of the more serious complications, such as incisional hernias [64,65]. For these reasons, much research is now being directed at the identification of risk factors contributing to postoperative complications [9,18,47,64,66,67] and strategies that may help to avoid these complications from developing [68–70].

Incisional complications after exploratory celiotomy

Incisional complications play a large role in postoperative morbidity and mortality [65,66,71–74] and are a major cause of nonfatal complications after colic surgery [75,76]. Complications include swelling or edema, drainage, wound infection, suture sinuses, hematoma formation, dehiscence, and hernia formation. Numerous factors have been identified that affect the occurrence and rates of these complications, including patient age, anemia, chronic illness, shock and hypovolemia, postoperative leukopenia, hypoproteinemia, concurrent infection, increased fibrinogen concentration in peritoneal fluid, neoplasia, increased intra-abdominal pressure, muscle strain, size, postoperative ileus, postoperative mobilization of protein and lipid, nutritional status, type of incision, type of suture material, method of wound closure, surgical trauma, length of surgery, repeat celiotomy, protective wound dressings, and quality of the anesthetic recovery [65,66,71–74,77–82]. Using the classification system proposed by the Committee on Trauma of the National Research Council, few colic operations are classified as "clean" surgical procedures, with many procedures being classified as "clean-contaminated" or even "contaminated." Clean-contaminated or contaminated procedures are associated with an increased likelihood of exposure of the incision to contamination, which is likely to contribute to the increased rate of incisional infections seen after an emergency celiotomy [22,77].

A higher incidence of incisional complications after clean-contaminated emergency surgical procedures has been reported in Equidae compared with other species, with rates of 5% [83,84] and 15% [85] reported for small animals and cattle, respectively, compared with 24% in horses [86]. Incisional complications, ranging from edema and drainage to more serious complications, including infection, acute dehiscence, and hernia formation, occur relatively commonly after exploratory celiotomy [66,71]. Some studies have associated this high incidence rate with intraoperative incisional trauma, primarily from the manipulation and evacuation of the large colon [22].

Any form of drainage from the celiotomy incision is frequently considered to be synonymous with incisional infection, even when a bacterial culture of the fluid has not been performed. Previous studies [66,77] have shown that a large proportion of celiotomy incisions that are draining any fluid, be it serous, serosanguineous, or purulent, yield a positive bacterial culture. Incisional drainage may not just be evidence of incisional infection but is also associated with the more serious incisional complications that could occur (hernia or dehiscence) (Fig. 1) [19,64].

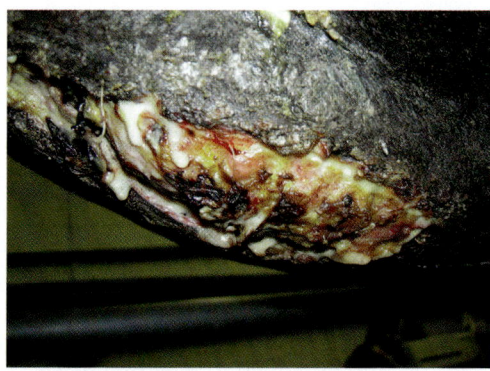

Fig. 1. Partial dehiscence of a ventral celiotomy wound 8 days after colic surgery.

The prevalence of incisional infections after celiotomy in horses is variable, with proportions from 4% [18] to 9.9% [66], 24% [86], 25.4% [77], and 27% [71] reported. The wide variation in these figures may be attributable to the differences in the definition of "wound infection," which range from any incisional drainage [71,86] to purulent incisional drainage with associated heat and pain on palpation [18] or to positive bacterial culture [77]. Similarly, although some studies were restricted to celiotomies for colic [18,66,77], other studies included all forms of abdominal surgery [71], which would alter the expected rate of incisional complications. An increased occurrence of incisional complications between 57% [87] and 87.5% [66] was also reported after repeat celiotomies [22,66,87].

Risk factors for incisional complications

Many studies have identified risk factors that may be associated with incisional complications after exploratory celiotomy. These risk factors can be broadly divided into three categories: systemic, local, and mechanical factors.

1. Systemic factors: increased serum total bilirubin and decreased serum calcium, inorganic phosphorus, and α-globulin concentrations on day 1 after surgery [78]; increased serum urea and triglyceride concentrations and decreased venous PCO_2 during days 1 to 7 after surgery [78]; the development of postoperative ileus [88]; and the development of postoperative endotoxemia
2. Local factors: horses weighing more than 300 kg (43%) in comparison to horses weighing less than 300 kg (8%) [71]; overall surgery time [71,89]; increased intra-abdominal pressure during recovery from general anesthesia, during rectal palpation, or during exercise [90]; manipulation of the gastrointestinal tract traumatizing the incisional edges [22,77]; and exposure of the incision to potential sources of contamination during routine enterotomy or gastrointestinal resection [22,77]
3. Mechanical factors: includes factors relating to the location of the incision and the suture material, placement, and pattern used in closure

Ventral celiotomies are most commonly performed through the linea alba, and numerous studies have addressed factors affecting the healing of this layer of the body wall. The equine linea alba is capable of withstanding the high tensions of sutures within a ventral midline incision because of the perpendicular orientation of the fibers in relation to the force of the suture tension [82]. In normal horses, it is thicker (approximately 1 cm) and has a greater breaking strength at the umbilicus compared with the cranial abdomen (where it is approximately 0.3 cm thick) [82,91]. The reduced breaking strength cranially has been suggested to be attributable to a combination of not only the thinner linea alba here but the shape of the equine abdomen, which concentrates the load of the abdominal contents cranially [91]. When the incised linea alba heals normally, however, the entire length of the wound heals uniformly, such that the cranial end is not thinner or weaker [91].

Suture materials and patterns

The incised linea alba is significantly weaker 2 weeks after closure with interrupted cruciate sutures than the unincised linea alba [91]. By 8 weeks, histologic examination demonstrates mature collagen bundles within the incision and the incised linea alba is no longer significantly weaker than the unincised linea alba [91]. This dictates the importance of the suture material retaining its tensile strength for a minimum of 2 weeks after surgery, but it does not need to retain tensile strength after 8 weeks. Suture material should be as small as possible to achieve the desired strength within the tissue [81]. In vitro studies suggest that suture failure is more likely than fascial failure [82], even with large-diameter materials [92]. It is unsurprising that larger suture materials (eg, number 7 polydioxanone, number 6 polyglactin 910) have significantly higher breaking strengths than smaller materials (eg, number 2 polydioxanone, number 3 polyglactin 910), however [92].

Synthetic nonabsorbable suture materials, such as polypropylene, are infrequently used in closure of the linea alba because they have been associated with the formation of suture abscesses and sinuses [93]. The high memory of these materials and associated poor knot security [94] necessitate the use of multiple throws to prevent knot slippage. This increases the volume of suture material needed within the wound and may cause inflammation and mechanical irritation [93], which can predispose to weakening of the incision or infection [95,96].

Monofilament synthetic absorbable suture materials (eg, polydioxanone, polyglyconate) may be used in closure of the linea alba, but they are susceptible to rough handling (eg, with instruments), which damages the outer core of the material [82]. This decreases suture diameter, and thus strength [82].

Multifilament synthetic absorbable suture materials (eg, polyglycolic acid, lactomer 9:1, polyglactin 910) are less susceptible to rough handing than the monofilament materials [82]. They do not stretch as much as monofilament materials, and they have less memory [82]. Their structure causes more tissue drag (minimized by their coating), however, and there are potential crevices for bacterial colonization and replication, which are thought to be protected from the host immune response and the effect of any systemic antimicrobials administered [82].

Number 3 polyglactin 910 is the largest diameter, absorbable, single-suture material currently available, and in vitro studies demonstrated comparable or increased strength to most other suture materials used in clinical cases to close celiotomy incisions [82]. Polyglactin 910 has been reported as the suture material of choice when closing the abdomen, unless an excessive amount of contamination has occurred [14]. In one study, however, the use of polyglactin 910 in the closure of the linea alba was associated with a greater number of wound infections, using univariable and multivariable analyses, when compared with polydioxanone and polyglycolic acid [77]. It was proposed that the contamination resulting from an enterotomy may leave sufficient numbers of bacteria remaining in the abdomen to contaminate the suture material, thereby allowing establishment of postoperative wound infections [77]. Polyglycolic acid has a slightly higher breaking strength than that of polyglactin 910 [82], and it has been demonstrated to retain its high breaking strength up to 28 days after implantation within subcutaneous tissues, although its mechanical performance at this time is inferior to that of polydioxanone [97]. Double-stranded, number 2, braided lactomer 9:1 (copolymer of glycolide and lactide) demonstrated comparable bursting strengths to polyglactin 910 in vitro [98]; however, clinical evidence of any superiority is currently lacking.

Although monofilament stainless steel is not generally used in an uncomplicated closure because of its poor handling qualities, its use has been advocated in horses with wound dehiscence, especially if infection is present [99]. This is attributable to the absence of wicking and excellent strength and knot security [100].

Some investigation into surgical techniques used in line alba closure has been performed. The knot has been demonstrated to be the weakest point in a suture loop, because it undergoes shear stress when tension is applied to the loop or suture line [82,101]. One study [102] demonstrated the mode of failure to be associated with the knot in 100% of inverted cruciate closures and 71% of simple continuous closures. Knot failure may be related to knot slippage because of poor knot formation or insufficient throws per knot [103]. Poor knot formation can itself alter the structural properties of monofilament suture materials [94].

Knot formation to prevent slippage can be difficult in the linea alba, because the wound edges are often under tension. Measures necessary for adequate knot security vary depending on knot types and suture materials used [103]. The end of a continuous suture line of polyglactin 910 requires six throws for maximum security [103]. Other absorbable suture materials also require six throws for maximum security [104], again potentially causing mechanical irritation and suture sinus formation [93]. A square knot preserves the properties of the suture material best but does not maintain tissue apposition under tension [105,106]. A surgeon's knot, an asymmetric square knot (sliding half-hitch), or clamping the first throw can assist in prevention of knot slippage but may alter the structural properties of the suture material depending on the material used [94].

An alternative to commencing a line of continuous interrupted suture with a knot has been described recently [98]. Number 2, braided, lactomer 9:1 loop material was used to create a double-stranded continuous pattern. The first suture was secured by passing the swaged needle and suture material through the loop instead of tying a knot. Loop failure was attributed to

7% of failure modes in this study [98], and bursting strength was comparable to results of previous cadaveric studies using number 3 polyglactin 910 in a simple continuous pattern.

The advantages of this method include the potential for quicker closure times, a reduction in the number of knots, and having two strands of suture material; however, the increased volume of suture material in the wound and the difficulties when tying a four-stranded knot must be acknowledged. A striking finding in this study was that suture failure caused 29% of wound failures and fascial failure caused 71% of the failures [98]. In an earlier study using a similar experimental model and comparing simple continuous suture with inverted cruciate sutures in polyglactin 910, suture failure caused 86% of wound failures and fascial failure caused 14% of failures [102]. This difference in the number of wound failures between the two studies may be attributable to the overall increased diameter of the suture material increasing the overall strength of the suture material, including the knot or, it may be associated with increased damage to the incision because of increased fiber disruption with a wider diameter suture material.

The use of a near-far-far-near suture pattern when closing the linea alba has been associated with an increased incidence of incisional complications [66]. It has been proposed that the dead space created when undermining tissue to place the sutures contributed to this increased occurrence of incisional infection [66]. Nevertheless, a later study that investigated the influence of suture pattern as a factor in the development of incisional infection did not find the use of a near-far-far-near suture pattern statistically associated with an increased incidence of incisional complications [77]. In that study, however, no undermining of tissues occurred before the placement of the sutures, thereby minimizing the dead space created at the incision. It was proposed that the lack of dead space when using this suture pattern helped to avoid the development of incisional infection [77]. A more recent study [18] found that when the fascial tissues were dissected from the linea alba before closure, horses were almost four times more likely to experience postoperative wound complications than those in which no dissection occurred, although all horses in this study had their linea alba closed using a simple continuous suture pattern. This more recent report concurs with the earlier studies [66,77], in which it was proposed that the increased incidence of complications may be associated with the undermining of tissues and creation of dead space as opposed to the specific suture pattern used. Inverted cruciate sutures were demonstrated to have a significantly lower (17%) bursting strength than simple continuous sutures in vitro using the same suture material (number 3 polyglactin 910 with one surgeon's throw and five square throws); suture failure was the main failure mode [102].

A continuous suture pattern using a synthetic absorbable suture material seems to be a proven and practiced method of linea alba closure in horses [107,108]. This has been attributed to even tension distribution across the entire length of the wound, decreasing tension concentration on the knots

[96,102]. Distribution of tension is most pertinent during periods of abdominal distention. In human patients, abdominal distention may cause a 30% increase in wound length [109]. A continuous suture line is able to accommodate the lengthening of the linea alba during abdominal distention through small adjustments of position [95,96,109]. In human patients, a suture length/wound length ratio of 4:1 is recommended to ensure there is a sufficient length of material to accommodate this wound lengthening during periods of increased intra-abdominal pressure [109]; however, these values have not been established in horses. Continuous closure is also considered faster than interrupted closure, and retention of suture material within the wound is reduced [102,107]. Simple interrupted sutures were demonstrated to have a similar clinical appearance, histologic findings, and breaking strength as simple continuous sutures in a study examining clinical survival, however [108].

Whether using a continuous pattern or an interrupted pattern, attaining optimal tension on the wound edges is essential. An excessively tight linea alba closure can cause foci of necrosis at the wound edges [110]. A 15-mm bite size provides maximum strength [82] and avoids incorporation of the rectus muscle and sheath. In human patients, tissue bite size should approximate suture interval [109]. There was no significant difference in bursting strength or method of failure using a 1- or 1.5-cm suture interval in a simple continuous pattern of number 2 double-stranded lactomer 9:1 in a cadaveric study.

The methods used to test suture pattern and material in vitro are somewhat artificial because they do not take cyclic strains and inflammatory changes within the tissue into consideration. This highlights the necessity to perform prospective controlled randomized trials and retrospective studies to optimize surgical techniques.

One prospective study compared a two-layer closure technique (linea alba and skin) and a conventional three-layer method (linea alba, subcutaneous tissues, and skin) [69]. The study found that the two-layer closure provided a safe means of achieving ventral midline abdominal closure. Increased rates of wound complications were not seen. A lower prevalence of wound infection was observed in horses with the two-layer closure (18.7%) compared with the three-layer closure (23.9%), although the difference was not statistically significant.

Incisional bandages

In a study investigating preoperative preparation of the linea alba and risk factors for incisional drainage, an increase in numbers of bacterial colony-forming units after recovery from anesthesia increased the likelihood of subsequent incisional drainage. The authors of this study suggested that adhesive drapes may protect against contamination in the recovery stall [68].

In one prospective randomized controlled study [70], the use of an abdominal bandage (belly band) in the immediate postoperative period was investigated. It was found that using a belly band, although not 100% effective at preventing incisional complications, did reduce the incidence and severity of incisional complications after colic surgery at 14 and 30 days after discharge from the hospital. Those horses that had a belly band applied had the risk of developing a postoperative incisional complication reduced by 45% when compared with those horses that did not have a belly band applied.

Repeat celiotomy

Horses that undergo a second celiotomy early in the postoperative period (before discharge from the hospital) have a significantly higher likelihood of developing postoperative incisional complications than those horses that have a single surgical procedure [18,19,22,53]. It has been proposed that the increased incidence of incisional infection after repeat celiotomy may be caused by the transfer of bacteria from the raw edges of the wound and diminished resistance in the friable and edematous tissues [53]. In one large retrospective study, the prevalence of incisional drainage after a repeat celiotomy was 57% compared with only 29% after a single celiotomy [18]. Similarly, the likelihood of developing an incisional hernia increased after a repeat celiotomy (through the same incision) from 7.2% to 25% [18]. For this reason, some surgeons prefer to perform a second celiotomy through a new (paramedian) incision. One study demonstrated that incisional complications were more commonly encountered in horses after approaches through the muscular body wall (88%) than in ventral midline approaches (40%), however [71]. This was attributed to the increase in dead space and muscular necrosis secondary to surgical trauma or overly tight suture materials; however, no large-scale study exists comparing these approaches in horses undergoing exploratory celiotomy for colic.

Postoperative ileus

Postoperative ileus is a common complication and an important reason for undertaking a repeat celiotomy (Fig. 2) or euthanasia in the immediate postoperative period [18,64,87]. The prevalence of postoperative ileus in previously reported case series is summarized in Table 3 [111]. The large variation in the reported rates can be at least partly explained by the criteria used to define postoperative ileus. There is also a tremendous difference in the death rates for postoperative ileus recorded in different studies and in the prevalence rate of postoperative ileus in all horses that die after surgery. Diversity in the management of cases between different clinics may partly explain some of these inconsistencies. A variable proportion of the fatal cases of postoperative ileus have been euthanized at the owner's request because of economic considerations and concerns over the welfare of affected horses, and it is likely that the death rate from postoperative ileus could be

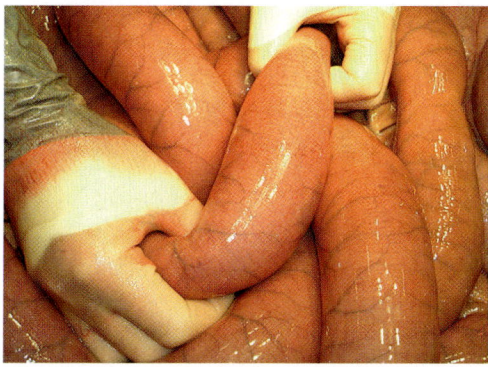

Fig. 2. Postoperative ileus. Distended small intestine identified at repeat celiotomy 3 days after small intestinal resection and anastomosis.

reduced significantly if intensive treatment was maintained for longer (although this could be associated with an increased rate of other complications, such as wound infection [88], intra-abdominal adhesions, and jugular thrombophlebitis). Such factors are virtually impossible to control in clinical cases, and it is impossible to compare these influences between different studies.

Factors that seem to be associated with the development of postoperative ileus include the duration and severity of colic at admission, heart rate, capillary refill time, PCV and total plasma protein, presence of gastric reflux, duration of anesthesia and surgery, small intestinal lesions, and presence of small bowel distention at surgery [18,64,67,88,112]. Taken together, all these factors suggest that the development of postoperative ileus is more likely in long-standing small intestinal obstructions. This, once again, emphasizes the importance of early diagnosis and treatment of horses with small intestinal obstructions.

In some studies, a clear association between strangulating obstruction of small intestine and the development of postoperative ileus has been demonstrated [27,113], whereas simple and strangulating obstructions have been implicated in others [18,67,112]. One study [64] demonstrated that the risk of postoperative ileus in its population of cases was specifically associated with pedunculated lipoma obstruction. This study found no association between ileus and age, and the reason why pedunculated lipoma obstruction is associated with ileus more commonly than other forms of small intestinal strangulation is unclear. The varying prevalence of this condition in different hospitals may be one reason for the varying rates of postoperative ileus encountered in different clinics, however.

Pelvic flexure colotomy has been shown to reduce the risk of postoperative ileus in at least two studies [18,67]. This suggests that evacuation of the colon should be considered as a routine procedure in all horses believed to be at risk of developing postoperative ileus. Further evaluation of this

Table 3
Prevalence and death rates of postoperative ileus

Reference	Prevalence of POI (% cases at risk)	Prevalence of fatal POI (% cases at risk)	Deaths from POI (% all deaths)	Deaths in horses with POI (affected)
Ducharme et al, 1983 [14]	—	3.6[a]	9.8[a]	—
Ducharme et al, 1983 [14]	—	8.8[b]	23.5[b]	—
Edwards and Hunt, 1985 [113]	16[c]	14[c]	—	86[c]
Hunt et al, 1986 [63]	14[c]	—	43[a]	86[a]
MacDonald et al, 1989 [49]	16[d]	8.6[d]	17[d]	52[d]
DeGeest et al, 1991 [111]	12[e]	—	25[e]	50[e]
Van der Velden and Klein, 1993 [41]	27[e]	7[f]	—	25[f]
Van der Velden and Klein, 1993 [41]	40[g]	10[g]	36[f,g]	25[g]
Proudman et al, 2002 [9]	9.6[a]	2.9[a]	8.6[a]	30.0[a]
Phillips and Walmsley, 1993 [22]	—	4.7[e]	25[a]	—
Blikslager et al, 1994 [112]	47[e]	2.7[e]	40[a]	13[a]
Vachon and Fischer, 1995 [120]	16[h]	—	—	—
Freeman et al, 2000 [27]	10[e]	1.4[e]	9[e]	14[e]
Semevolos et al, 2002 [114]	53[d]	—	—	—
Cohen et al, 2004 [88]	19	16	59	41
Mair and Smith, 2005 [18]	18.2[a]	9.5[a]	55.8[a]	52.2[a]
Mair and Smith, 2005 [18]	34.1[e]	17.1[e]	72.4[e]	50.0[e]
Garcia-Seco et al, 2005 [28]	34[i]	—	—	—

Data have been corrected as needed to relate the short-term (hospitalization) period to horses that recovered from general anesthesia.
Abbreviation: POI, postoperative ileus.
[a] All colics, ileus only.
[b] All colics, ileus and gastric rupture combined.
[c] Small intestine only, excluding ileus caused by devitalized bowel or peritonitis.
[d] Small intestinal resection and anastomosis only.
[e] Small intestinal surgery only.
[f] Small intestinal surgery with prophylactic cisapride.
[g] Small intestinal surgery without cisapride.
[h] Small intestinal surgery for strangulation in epiploic foramen.
[i] Pedunculated lipoma cases only.

technique in a prospective controlled clinical trial is required before it can be recommended as a standard prophylactic treatment, however.

There is evidence from some studies to suggest that the type of small intestinal anastomosis performed may influence the rates of postoperative ileus, indicating that the anastomosis may provide some mechanical contribution to a functional problem [27]. In one study [27], postoperative ileus was shown to occur more frequently after jejunocecostomy than after other forms of small intestinal anastomosis. In a comparison of three different techniques for jejunal resection and anastomosis, the stapled side-to-side anastomotic technique was found to result in a significantly shorter duration of postoperative ileus than hand-sewed end-to-end and stapled functional end-to-end techniques [114].

Intestinal ischemia, distention, peritonitis, electrolyte imbalance, endotoxemia, traumatic handling of intestine, resection and anastomosis, and general anesthesia have all been proposed as potential contributing factors to the development of postoperative ileus [115]. Endotoxin, which is released from damaged and ischemic intestine, has been shown to cause aberrations in intestinal motility [116]. Ileus has also been experimentally induced by abrading segments of small intestine [117], and it is likely that surgical trauma associated with decompression of small intestine could predispose to ileus [113]. Both of these factors are likely to attain a greater significance in longer standing cases of small intestinal obstruction.

Repeat celiotomy and postoperative ileus

Repeat celiotomy is now widely accepted as a treatment option in the management of postoperative ileus and postoperative colic [118]. Reported rates of repeat celiotomy during the immediate postoperative period are 9.6% [9], 12.5% [118], 10.6% [87], 15% (small intestinal herniation through the epiploic foramen only) [119], 19% (small intestinal obstruction only) [53], 27% (small intestinal herniation through the epiploic foramen only) [120], and 28% (jejunocecostomy only) [52]. Postoperative ileus and epiploic foramen entrapment were found to be significant risk factors associated with repeat celiotomy in one study [64]. In another study [9], 53% of the horses that underwent repeat celiotomy died or were subjected to euthanasia within the study period, with a median time to death of 11 days. The median survival time in that study was 77 days, and the incidence of postoperative colic in these horses was 0.65 episodes per horse-year at risk. Other reported short-term survival rates after repeat celiotomy are 64% [53], 56% [118], 50% [120], 49% [121], 48.1% [87], and 36.4% [47]. Financial considerations may contribute to some of the differences in survival rates reported in these studies. The need for repeat celiotomy seems to be associated with an 18-fold increased risk of mortality in the postoperative period [47]. Repeat celiotomies are associated with an increased rate of wound complications.

Long-term survival and complications

Relatively few studies have assessed long-term survival and complication rates after colic surgery (see Table 1). The most frequently recorded long-term postoperative complication is colic [19], and a history of colic after discharge is associated with a higher death rate. One study [9] reported a prevalence of postoperative colic of 32%, with an incidence of 0.55 episodes per horse-year at risk. Most first postoperative bouts of colic occurred within 100 days, but some cases occurred up to 1 year after surgery. Although many horses had at least one colic episode, only 5% had three or more episodes. The incidence of colic was 2.8 to 7.6 times higher in horses that had undergone colic surgery than in the general horse population. Multivariable modeling indicated that two variables were significantly associated with postoperative colic, namely, large colon volvulus ($>360°$) and repeat celiotomy [53]. In another study [19], no association between postoperative colic and large colon volvulus could be identified. In fact, horses with small bowel obstructions had a significantly higher rate of postoperative colic than horses with large bowel obstructions, and there were apparent associations between the rates of colic and resection of bowel and the development of postoperative ileus.

It is likely that a proportion of horses that develop recurrent colic after discharge do so because of intra-abdominal adhesions. The precise rate of adhesion formation is impossible to predict, because the exact cause of recurrent or severe colic after discharge from the hospital is frequently not determined. In addition, many adhesions are probably clinically "silent" [122]. Adhesions only become a clinical problem when they mature to restrictive fibrous adhesions that compress or anatomically distort the intestine (Fig. 3) and cause obstruction. Adhesions may also lead to intestinal incarceration, strangulation, or volvulus, predisposing the patient to severe or recurrent signs of intestinal

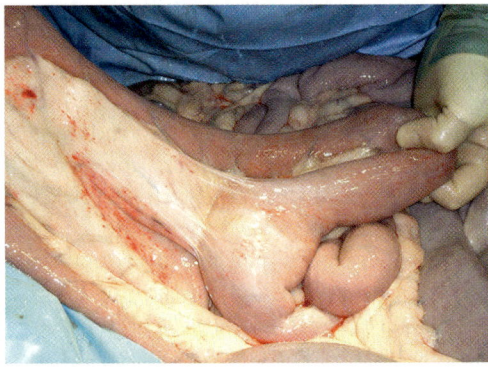

Fig. 3. Surgical appearance of mesenteric adhesions causing a "U-bend" in the jejunum. This horse had colic surgery 18 months previously and was affected by recurrent episodes of colic. Resection of the adhesions resulted in resolution of the recurrent colic.

obstruction. Published rates of adhesion formation after colic surgery have varied widely, probably as a result of such uncertainties. Previous reports have estimated prevalence rates of adhesions of 8.9% [19], 14% [22], 22% [123], 26% (small intestinal obstructions only) [49], 6% (small intestinal surgery only) [27], and 6% (epiploic foramen entrapments only) [120].

The primary method of minimizing postoperative adhesions is the application of meticulous atraumatic surgical technique [122,124]. Intraperitoneal administration of heparin has been shown to reduce adhesion formation in laboratory animals [125,126], and the results of one study suggest that its use in horses might reduce the rates of confirmed adhesion formation and the rate of postoperative colic [19]. These findings need to be confirmed with a controlled prospective study, however. The systemic administration of heparin was shown in one small experimental study to reduce the rates of abdominal adhesions in ponies [121]; however, a recent experimental study of ischemia-induced small intestinal adhesions in foals showed that systemic heparin treatment had minimal beneficial effects [127].

The use of a bioresorbable hyaluronate-carboxymethylcellulose membrane (Seprafilm, Genzyme Co., Cambridge, Massachusetts) has been shown to reduce postoperative adhesion formation significantly in horses, with no adverse effects on intestinal or peritoneal healing [128,129]. Other reported techniques that have been used in an attempt to reduce the rate of postoperative adhesions include postoperative peritoneal lavage [130] and omentectomy [131]. Sodium carboxymethylcellulose solution has also been used in equine abdominal surgery to act as a protective tissue coating and has been shown to reduce the rate of adhesion formation [132,133], with no effect on abdominal wound healing [134].

Summary

The monitoring of results by individual clinicians and clinics and attention to detail are of vital importance if the quality of care is to be optimized and if clinicians are to aspire to "best practice." These principles underlie the concept of "clinical audit," which is currently gaining acceptance in veterinary practice as a quality improvement tool. Clinical auditing seeks to establish protocols for dealing with particular problems based on documented evidence when it is available, monitoring the effectiveness of these protocols once they have been put into effect and modifying them as appropriate. It should be an ongoing upward spiral of appraisal and improvement [135]. Conducting a clinical audit means that you are comparing your actual performance in a defined area of clinical practice against targets and guidelines (which should be evidence based) to see whether you are consistently achieving best practice (ie, whether you are meeting your targets and guidelines). If you are not meeting the targets, you then have to investigate why not, create an action plan to amend any shortcomings, implement the actions, and re-audit once these have been successfully implemented.

As the interest in evidence-based medicine grows in veterinary science, so application of its principles to specific areas of equine surgery is starting to take place. The aim of evidence-based surgery should be to encourage sound research to improve diagnosis, treatment, and skills of the individual clinician [6]. In human surgery, these objectives are attained while emphasizing the importance of listening to the patient, taking an excellent history, performing a thorough physical examination, and coming to the best and most sensible conclusions from the patient's point of view [136]. In equine surgery, the interests of the owner or trainer must also be balanced with the welfare implications to the horse. In many areas of surgical practice, anecdote influences the choice of techniques. The techniques that surgeons learn during their training tend to become the accepted practice and are perpetuated over the years. The concept of challenging a well-accepted surgical tenet has tended to be foreign to the discipline. The search for evidence-based surgery should not, of course, lead to the wholesale abandonment of treatments that have been hallowed by time yet have little or no scientific basis. Rather, such procedures should be discarded only when indicated by evidence-based surgery [136].

References

[1] Hillyer MH, Taylor FGR, French NP. A cross-sectional study of colic in horses on Thoroughbred training premises in the British Isles in 1997. Equine Vet J 2001;33:380–5.

[2] Tennant B, Wheat JD, Meagher DM. Intestinal obstruction in the horse. Some aspects of differential diagnosis in equine colic. Proceedings of the 18th Annual Convention of the American Association of Equine Practitioners 1972;18:251–2.

[3] Tennant B. Intestinal obstructions in the horse. Some aspects of differential diagnosis in equine colic. Proceedings of the 21st Annual Convention of the American Association of Equine Practitioners 1975;21:426–39.

[4] Pearson H, Pinsent PJN, Denny HR, et al. The indications for equine laparotomy—an analysis of 140 cases. Equine Vet J 1975;7:131–6.

[5] Moore JN. Five decades of colic: a view from thirty-five years on. Equine Vet J 2005;37: 285–6.

[6] Mair TS, White NA. Improving quality of care in colic surgery: time for international audit? Equine Vet J 2005;37:287–8.

[7] Mair TS. Contributions to an evidence-based medicine approach to colic surgery. Equine Vet J 2002;34:428–9.

[8] Horton R. Surgical research or comic opera: questions, but few answers. Lancet 1996;347: 984–5.

[9] Proudman CJ, Smith JE, Edwards GB, et al. Long-term survival of equine surgical colic cases. Part 1: patterns of mortality and morbidity. Equine Vet J 2002;34:432–7.

[10] Proudman CJ, Smith JE, Edwards GB, et al. Long-term survival of equine surgical colic cases. Part 2: modelling postoperative survival. Equine Vet J 2002;34:438–43.

[11] Pascoe PJ, McDonell WN, Trim CM, et al. Mortality rates and associated factors in equine colic operations—a retrospective study of 341 operations. Can Vet J 1983;24:76–85.

[12] White NA, Lessard P. Risk factors and clinical signs associated with cases of equine colic. Proceedings of the 23rd Annual Convention of the American Association of Equine Practitioners 1986;23:637–43.

[13] Huskamp B. Diagnosis and treatment of acute abdominal conditions in the horse: various types and frequency seen at the animal hospital in Hochmoor. Proceedings of the 1st Equine Colic Research Symposium 1982;1:261–72.
[14] Ducharme NG, Hackett RP, Ducharme GR, et al. Surgical treatment of colic. Results in 181 horses. Vet Surg 1983;4:206–9.
[15] Parry BW, Anderson GA, Gay CC. Prognosis in equine colic: a comparative study of variables used to assess individual cases. Equine Vet J 1983;15:211–5.
[16] Reeves MJ, Hilbert BJ, Morris RS. A retrospective study of 320 colic cases referred to a veterinary teaching hospital. Proceedings of the 2nd Equine Colic Research Symposium 1986; 2:242–50.
[17] Mair TS, Smith LJ. Survival and complication rates of 300 horses undergoing surgical treatment of colic. Part 1. Short-term survival following a single laparotomy. Equine Vet J 2005; 37:296–302.
[18] Mair TS, Smith LJ. Survival and complication rates of 300 horses undergoing surgical treatment of colic. Part 2. Short-term complications. Equine Vet J 2005;37:303–9.
[19] Mair TS, Smith LJ. Survival and complication rates of 300 horses undergoing surgical treatment of colic. Part 3. Long-term complications and survival. Equine Vet J 2005;37:310–4.
[20] Shires GM, Kaneps AJ, Wagner PC, et al. A retrospective review of 219 cases of equine colic. Proceedings of the 2nd Equine Colic Research Symposium 1986;2:239–41.
[21] McCarthy RN, Hutchins DR. Survival rates and post-operative complications after equine colic surgery. Aust Vet J 1988;65:40–3.
[22] Phillips TJ, Walmsley JP. Retrospective analysis of the results of 151 exploratory laparotomies in horses with gastrointestinal disease. Equine Vet J 1993;25:427–31.
[23] Santschi EM, Slone DE, Embertson RM, et al. Colic surgery in 206 juvenile Thoroughbreds: survival and racing results. Equine Vet J Suppl 2000;32:32–6.
[24] Van der Linden MA, Laffont CM, Sloet van Oldruitenborgh-Oosterbaan MM. Prognosis in equine medical and surgical colic. J Vet Intern Med 2003;17:343–8.
[25] Abutarbush SM, Carmalt JL, Shoemaker RW. Causes of gastrointestinal colic in horses in western Canada: 604 cases (1992–2002). Can Vet J 2005;46:800–5.
[26] Proudman CJ, Dugdale AH, Senior JM, et al. Pre-operative and anaesthesia-related risk factors for mortality in equine colic cases. Vet J 2006;171:89–97.
[27] Freeman DE, Hammock P, Baker GJ, et al. Short- and long-term survival and prevalence of post-operative ileus after small intestinal surgery in the horse. Equine Vet J Suppl 2000; 32:42–51.
[28] Garcia-Seco E, Wilson DA, Kramer J, et al. Prevalence and risk factors associated with outcome of surgical removal of pedunculated lipomas in horses: 102 cases (1987–2002). J Am Vet Med Assoc 2005;226:1529–37.
[29] Greatorex JC. Observations on the diagnosis of gastrointestinal disorders in the horse. Ir Vet J 1972;26:229–37.
[30] Eikmeier H. Diagnostik und therapie der koliken beim pferd. Tierarztl Prax 1973;1:61–5 [in German].
[31] Kalsbeek HC. Indications for surgical intervention in equine colic. J S Afr Vet Assoc 1975; 46:101–5.
[32] Berggren PC, Reinertson EL. Evaluation of the acute abdominal crisis in the equine. Iowa State Univ Vet 1977;39:46–9.
[33] Parry BW, Anderson GA, Gay CC. Prognosis in equine colic: a study of individual variables used in case assessment. Equine Vet J 1983;15:337–44.
[34] Puotunen-Reinert A. Study of variables commonly used in examination of equine colic cases to assess prognostic value. Equine Vet J 1986;18:275–7.
[35] Orsini JA, Elser AH, Galligan DT, et al. Prognostic index for equine acute abdominal crisis (colic). Am J Vet Res 1988;49:1969–71.
[36] Furr MO, Lessard P, White NA. Development of a colic severity score for predicting the outcome of equine colic. Vet Surg 1995;24:97–101.

[37] Thoefner MB, Ersboll AK, Hesselholt M. Prognostic indicators in a Danish hospital-based population of colic horses. Equine Vet J Suppl 2000;32:11–8.
[38] Schebitz H. Ileus—chirurgerie beim pferde. Berl Munch tierarztl Wschr 1961;74:165–70 [in German].
[39] Klohnen A, Vachon AM, Fischer AT. Use of diagnostic ultrasonography in horses with signs of acute abdominal pain. J Am Vet Med Assoc 1996;209:1597–601.
[40] Kersjes AW, Bras GE, Nemeth F, et al. Results of operative treatment of equine colic with special reference to surgery of the ileum. Vet Q 1988;10:17–25.
[41] Van der Velden MA, Klein WR. The effects of cisapride on the restoration of gut motility after surgery of the small intestine in horses: a clinical trial. Vet Q 1993;15:175–9.
[42] Engelbert TA, Tate LP, Bowman KF, et-al. Incarceration of the small intestine in the epiploic foramen: report of 19 cases (1983–1992). Vet Surg 1993; 13: 158–166.
[43] Singer ER, Livesey MA. Evaluation of exploratory laparotomy in young horses: 102 cases (1987–1992). J Am Vet Med Assoc 1997;211:1158–62.
[44] Fugaro MN, Cote NM. Survival rates for horses undergoing stapled small intestinal anastomosis: 84 cases (1988–1997). J Am Vet Med Assoc 2001;218:1603–7.
[45] Van den Boom R, Van der Velden MA. Short- and long-term evaluation of surgical treatment of strangulating obstructions of the small intestine in horses: a review of 224 cases. Vet Q 2001;23:109–15.
[46] Archer DC, Proudman CJ, Pinchbeck G, et al. Entrapment of the small intestine in the epiploic foramen in horses: a retrospective analysis of 71 cases recorded between 1991 and 2001. Vet Rec 2004;155:793–7.
[47] Morton AJ, Blikslager AT. Surgical and postoperative factors influencing short-term survival of horses following small intestinal resection: 92 cases (1994–2001). Equine Vet J 2002; 34:450–4.
[48] Proudman CJ, Edwards GB, Barnes J, et al. Factors affecting long-term survival of horses recovering from surgery of the small intestine. Equine Vet J 2005;37:360–5.
[49] MacDonald MH, Pascoe JR, Stover SM, et al. Survival after small intestinal resection and anastomosis in horses. Vet Surg 1989;18:415–23.
[50] Bladon BM, Hillyer MH. Effect of extensive ileal resection with a large resulting mesenteric defect and stapled ileal stump in horses with a jejunocaecostomy: a comparison with other anastomotic techniques. Equine Vet J Suppl 2000;32:52–8.
[51] Stephen JO, Corley KT, Johnston JK, et al. Factors associated with mortality and morbidity in small intestinal volvulus in horses. Vet Surg 2004;33:340–8.
[52] Pankowski RL. Small intestinal surgery in the horse: a review of ileo and jejunocecostomy J Am Vet Med Assoc 1987;190:1609.
[53] Freeman DE, Rotting AK, Inoue OJ. Abdominal closure and complications. Clin Tech Equine Pract 2002;1:174–87.
[54] Huskamp B. Ileum-resektion und jejunocaecostomie beim pferd. Berl Münch Tierarztl Wochenschr 1973;86:161–3 [in German].
[55] Ross MW, Cullen KK, Rutkowski JA. Myoelectric activity of the ileum, caecum and right ventral colon in ponies during interdigestive, nonfeeding, and digestive periods. Am J Vet Res 1990;51:561–6.
[56] Roger YT, Malbert CH. Caracteristique anatomo-fonctionelles de la jonction ileocaecale du poney. Rev Med Vet 1989;140:851–5 [in French].
[57] Freeman DE, Schaeffer DJ. Short-term survival after surgery for epiploic foramen entrapment compared with other strangulating diseases of the small intestine in horses. Equine Vet J 2005;37:292–5.
[58] Blackwell R. Jejunocecostomy in the horse: a comparison of two techniques. Proceedings of the 1st Equine Colic Research Symposium 1982;1:288.
[59] Röcken M, Ross MW. Vergleichsstudie über die jejunocaecostomie als end-zu-seitanastomose und seit-zu-seitanastomose. Pferdheilkunde 1994;10:311–5 [in German].

[60] Loesch DA, Rodgerson DH, Haines GR, et al. Jejunoileal anastomosis following small intestinal resection in horses: seven cases (1999–2001). J Am Vet Med Assoc 2002;221:541–5.
[61] Rendle DI, Wood JLN, Summerhays GES, et al. End-to-end jejuno-ileal anastomosis following resection of strangulated small intestine in horses: a comparative study. Equine Vet J 2005;37:356–9.
[62] Proudman CJ, Edwards GB, Barnes J, et al. Modelling long-term survival of horses following surgery for large intestinal disease. Equine Vet J 2005;37:366–70.
[63] Hunt JM, Edwards GB, Clarke KW. Incidence, diagnosis and treatment of postoperative complications in colic cases. Equine Vet J 1986;18:264–70.
[64] French NP, Smith J, Edwards GB, et al. Equine surgical colic: risk factors for postoperative complications. Equine Vet J 2002;34:444–9.
[65] Gibson KT, Curtis CR, Turner AS, et al. Incisional hernias in the horse. Incidence and predisposing factors. Vet Surg 1989;18:360–6.
[66] Kobluk CN, Ducharme NG, Lumsden JH, et al. Factors affecting incisional complication rates associated with colic surgery in horses: 78 cases (1983–1985). J Am Vet Med Assoc 1989;195:639–42.
[67] Roussel AJ, Cohen ND, Hooper RN, et al. Risk factors associated with development of postoperative ileus in horses. J Am Vet Med Assoc 2001;219:72–8.
[68] Galuppo LD, Pasoce JR, Jang SS, et al. Evaluation of iodophor skin preparation techniques and factors influencing drainage from ventral midline incisions in horses. J Am Vet Med Assoc 1999;215:963–9.
[69] Coomer RP, Edwards GB, Proudman CJ. Preliminary results of a randomised, controlled trial to evaluate the effect of subcutaneous sutures on the prevalence of laparotomy wound infection. Proceedings of the 8th Equine Colic Research Symposium 2005;8:186–7.
[70] Smith LJ, Mair TS. Incisional complications following exploratory celiotomy: does a belly band reduce the risk? Proceedings of the 8th Equine Colic Research Symposium 2005;8:199–200.
[71] Wilson DA, Baker GJ, Boero MJ. Complications of celiotomy incisions in horses. Vet Surg 1995;24:506–14.
[72] McIlwraith CW. Complications of laparotomy incisions in the horse. Proceedings of the 24th Annual Convention of the American Association of Equine Practitioners 1978;24:209–18.
[73] Robertson-Smith R, Adams SB. Management of postoperative complications following equine abdominal surgery. Compend Contin Educ Pract Vet 1986;8:844–9.
[74] White NA. Incisional hernia after abdominal surgery in the horse. Equine Vet Educ 1996;8:308–12.
[75] Traub-Dargatz JL, George JL, Dargatz DA. Survey of complications and antimicrobial use in equine patients at veterinary teaching hospitals that underwent surgery because of colic. J Am Vet Med Assoc 2002;220:1359–65.
[76] Wiemer P, Bergman HJ, van der Veen H, et al. Colic surgery in the horse: a retrospective study of 272 patients. Tijdschr Diergeneeskd 2002;127:682–6.
[77] Honnas CM, Cohen ND. Risk factors for wound infection following celiotomy in horses. J Am Vet Med Assoc 1997;210:78–81.
[78] Protopapas K, Marr CM, Archer FJ, et al. Ultrasonographic assessment and factors associated with incisional infection and dehiscence following celiotomy in horses. Vet Surg 2000;29:289.
[79] Stone WC, Lindsay WA, Masonn DF, et al. Factors associated with acute wound dehiscence following equine abdominal surgery. Proceedings of the 4th Equine Colic Research Symposium 1990;4:52.
[80] Cook G, Bowman KF, Bristol DG, et al. Ventral midline herniorrhaphy following colic surgery in the horse. Equine Vet Educ 1996;8:304–7.
[81] Trostle SS. Surgical approaches to the equine abdomen—procedures and complications. Proceedings of the 8th Annual American College of Surgery Symposium 1998;8:173–5.

[82] Trostle SS, Wilson DG, Stone WC, et al. Study of the biomechanical properties of the adult linea alba—relationship of tissue bite size and suture material to breaking strength. Vet Surg 1994;23:435–41.
[83] Vasseur PB, Paul HA, Enos LR, et al. Infection rates in clean surgical procedures: a comparison of ampicillin prophylaxis vs a placebo. J Am Vet Med Assoc 1985;187:825–7.
[84] Vasseur PB, Levy J, Dowd E, et al. Surgical wound infection rates in dogs and cats. Data from a teaching hospital. Vet Surg 1988;17:60.
[85] Desrochers A, St-Jean G, Anderson DA. Comparative evaluation of two surgical scrub preparations in cattle. Vet Surg 1996;25:336.
[86] Ingle-Fehr JE, Baxter GM, Howard RD, et al. Bacterial culturing of ventral median celiotomies for prediction of postoperative incisional complications in horses. Vet Surg 1997;26: 7–13.
[87] Mair TS, Smith LJ. Survival and complication rates of 300 horses undergoing surgical treatment of colic. Part 4. Early (acute) re-laparotomy. Equine Vet J 2005;37:315–8.
[88] Cohen ND, Lester GD, Sanchez LC, et al. Evaluation of risk factors associated with development of postoperative ileus in horses. J Am Vet Med Assoc 2004;225:1070–8.
[89] Trostle SS, Hartmann FA. Surgical infection. In: Auer JA, Stick JA, editors. Equine surgery. Philadelphia: Saunders Co.; 1999. p. 47–54.
[90] Kirker-Head CA, Kerwin PJ, Steckel RR, et al. The in vivo biodynamic properties of the intact equine linea alba. Equine Vet J Suppl 1989;7:98–106.
[91] Chism PN, Latimer FG, Patton CS, et al. Tissue strength and wound morphology of the equine linea alba after ventral median celiotomy. Vet Surg 2000;29:145–51.
[92] Fierheller EE, Wilson DG. An in vitro biomechanical comparison of the breaking strength and stiffness of polydioxanone (sizes 2, 7) and polyglactin 910 (sizes 3, 6) in the equine linea alba. Vet Surg 2005;34:18–23.
[93] Trostle SS, Hendrickson DA. Suture sinus formation following closure of ventral midline incisions with polypropylene in three horses. J Am Vet Med Assoc 1995;207: 742–5.
[94] Huber DJ, Egger EL, James SP. The effect of knotting method on the structural properties of large diameter nonabsorbable monofilament sutures. Vet Surg 1999;28:260–7.
[95] Poole GV Jr. Mechanical factors in abdominal wound closure: the prevention of fascial dehiscence. Surgery 1985;97:631–40.
[96] Poole GV Jr, Meredith JW, Kon ND, et al. Suture technique and wound-bursting strength. Am Surg 1984;50:569–72.
[97] Campbell EJ, Bailey JV. Mechanical properties of suture materials in vitro and after in vivo implantation in horses. Vet Surg 1992;21:355–61.
[98] Hassan K, Galuppo LD, van Hoogmoed LM. An in vitro comparison of two suture intervals using braided absorbable loop suture in the equine linea alba. Vet Surg 2006;35:310–4.
[99] Tulleners EP, Donawick WJ. Secondary closure of infected abdominal incisions in cattle and horses. J Am Vet Med Assoc 1983;182:1377–9.
[100] Schumacher J, Hanselka D, Adams G, et al. Stainless steel closure of the equine linea alba. Equine Pract 1981;3:47–53.
[101] Carlson MA. Acute wound failure. Surg Clin North Am 1997;77:607–36.
[102] Magee AA, Galuppo LD. Comparison of incisional bursting strength of simple continuous and inverted cruciate suture patterns in the equine linea alba. Vet Surg 1999;28:442–7.
[103] Rosin E, Robinson GM. Knot security of suture materials. Vet Surg 1997;18:269–73.
[104] Bourne RB, Bitar H, Andreae PR, et al. In-vivo comparison of four absorbable sutures: Vicryl, Dexon Plus, Maxon and PDS. Can J Surg 1988;31:43–5.
[105] Herrmann JB. Tensile strength and knot security of surgical suture materials. Am Surg 1971;37:209–17.
[106] Thacker JG, Rodeheaver G, Moore JW, et al. Mechanical performance of surgical sutures. Am J Surg 1975;130:374–80.

[107] Turner AS, Yovich JV, White NA, et al. Continuous absorbable suture pattern in the closure of ventral midline abdominal incisions in horses. Equine Vet J 1988;20:401–5.
[108] Looysen BS, De Bowes RM, Clem MF, et al. Comparison of simple interrupted and simple continuous patterns for closure of the equine linea alba. Vet Surg 1988;17:36.
[109] Jenkins TPN. The burst abdominal wound: a mechanical approach. Br J Surg 1976;63: 873–6.
[110] Sanders RJ, Di Clementi D. Principles of abdominal wound closure. I. Animal studies. Arch Surg 1976;112:1184–7.
[111] DeGeest J, Vlaminck K, Muylle E, et al. A clinical study of cisapride in horses after colic surgery. Equine Vet Educ 1991;3:138–42.
[112] Blikslager AT, Bowman KF, Levine JF, et al. Evaluation of factors associated with postoperative ileus in horses: 31 cases (1990–1992). J Am Vet Med Assoc 1994;205:1748–52.
[113] Edwards GB, Hunt JM. An analysis of the incidence of post-operative ileus (POI) and an assessment of the predisposing factors. Proceedings of the 2nd Equine Colic Research Symposium 1985;2:307–12.
[114] Semevolos SA, Ducharme NG, Hackett RP. Clinical assessment and outcome of three techniques for jejunal resection and anastomosis in horses: 59 cases (1989–2000). J Am Vet Med Assoc 2002;220:215–8.
[115] Hardy J, Rakestraw PC. Postoperative management for colics. Clin Tech Equine Pract 2002;1:188–97.
[116] King JN, Gerring EL. The action of low dose endotoxin on equine bowel motility. Equine Vet J 1991;23:11–7.
[117] Gerring EL, Hunt JM. Pathophysiology of equine post-operative ileus: effect of adrenergic blockade, parasympathetic stimulation and metoclopramide in an experimental model. Equine Vet J 1985;18:249–55.
[118] Huskamp B, Bonfig H. Relaparotomy as a therapeutic principle in postoperative complication of horses with colic. Proceedings of the 2nd Equine Colic Research Symposium 1985;2: 317–21.
[119] Scheidemann W. Beitrag zur diagnostik und therapie der kolik des pferdes. Die hernia\ foraminis omentalis. DMV thesis, Muenchen 1989 [in German].
[120] Vachon AM, Fischer AT. Small intestinal herniation through the epiploic foramen: 53 cases (1987–1993). Equine Vet J 1995;27:373–80.
[121] Parker JE, Fubini SL, Car BD, et al. Prevention of intraabdominal adhesions in ponies by low-dose heparin therapy. Vet Surg 1987;16:459–62.
[122] Mueller POE. Advances in prevention and treatment of intra-abdominal adhesions in horses. Clin Tech Equine Pract 2002;1:163–73.
[123] Baxter GM, Broome TE, Moore JN. Abdominal adhesions after small intestinal surgery in the horse. Vet Surg 1989;18:409–14.
[124] Southwood LL, Baxter GM, Hutchison JM, et al. Survey of diplomates of the American College of Veterinary Surgeons regarding postoperative intra-abdominal adhesion formation in horses undergoing abdominal surgery. J Am Vet Med Assoc 1997;211:1573–6.
[125] Diamond MP, Linsky CB, Cunningham T, et al. Synergistic effects of Interceed (TC 7) and heparin in reducing adhesion formation in the rat uterine horn model. Fertil Steril 1991;55: 389–94.
[126] Sahin Y, Saglam A. Synergistic effects of carboxymethylcellulose and low molecular weight heparin in reducing adhesion formation in the rat uterine horn model. Acta Obstet Gynecol Scand 1994;73:70–3.
[127] Sullins KE, White NA, Lundin CS, et al. Prevention of ischaemia-induced small intestinal adhesions in foals. Equine Vet J 2004;36:370–5.
[128] Mueller POE, Hay W, Harmon B, et al. Evaluation of a bioresorbable hyaluronate-carboxymethylcellulose membrane for prevention of experimentally induced adhesions in horses. Vet Surg 2000;18:415–23.

[129] Mueller POE, Eggleston RB, Peroni JF. How to apply a bioresorbable hyaluronate membrane for the prevention of postoperative adhesions in horses. Proceedings of the 47th Annual Convention of the American Association of Equine Practitioners 2001;47:428–32.
[130] Hague BA, Honnas CM, Berridge BR, et al. Evaluation of peritoneal lavage in standing horses for prevention of experimentally induced abdominal adhesions. Vet Surg 1998;27: 122–6.
[131] Kuebelbeck KL, Slone DE, May KA. Effect of omentectomy on adhesion formation in horses. Vet Surg 1998;27:132–7.
[132] Moll HD, Schumacher J, Wright JC, et al. Evaluation of sodium carboxymethylcellulose for prevention of experimentally induced abdominal adhesions in ponies. Am J Vet Res 1991;52:88–91.
[133] Hay WP, Mueller POE, Harmon BG, et al. One percent sodium carboxymethylcellulose prevents experimentally induced adhesions in horses. Vet Surg 2001;30:223–7.
[134] Mueller POE, Hunt RJ, Allen D, et al. Intraperitoneal use of sodium carboxymethylcellulose in horses undergoing exploratory celiotomy. Vet Surg 1995;24:112–7.
[135] Viner B. Clinical audit in veterinary practice—the story so far. Vet Rec Suppl. In Practice 2005;27:215–8.
[136] McColl I. Evidence-based surgery in the United Kingdom. In: Evidence-based surgery. Hamilton (Canada): B.C. Decker Inc.; 2000. p. 89–102.

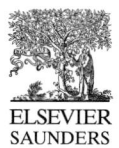

Evidence-Based Medicine in Equine Critical Care

Daniela Bedenice, Dr med vet

Department of Clinical Sciences, Cummings School of Veterinary Medicine, Tufts University, 200 Westboro Road, North Grafton, MA 01536, USA

Evidence-based medicine (EBM) is the integration of best research evidence with clinical expertise and patient values—David Sackett [1].

As highlighted elsewhere in this issue (see the article by Holmes and Ramey elsewhere in this issue), the practice of evidence-based medicine (EBM) is established through the careful integration of well-designed unbiased research and clinical expertise, while requiring incorporation of client values and understanding in determining optimal interventions. This definition acknowledges that not all research evidence is considered equal but necessitates careful interpretation when evaluating therapeutic options [2].

One of the fundamental skills required for practicing EBM is the development of a well-built clinical question, which specifies the patient group or problem, intervention, and outcome of interest. The objective of EBM is to maximize the help and minimize the harm we do to patients, by basing our clinical decisions on the types of evidence that are least likely to be incorrect [3]. For this purpose, various "levels of evidence" (Table 1) have been developed in the human literature, which rank the validity of evidence. Our established conclusions and advice are thus supported by specific "grades of recommendations" as listed in Table 2, which are intended to give an indication of the "strength" of a clinical recommendation [3].

The following article was compiled with these principles in mind. We may also have to consider Dr. Sydney Burell's sardonic statement carefully, however: "Half of what we are taught as medical students will in 10 years have been shown to be incorrect. The trouble is that none of your teachers knows which half..." [4].

Advanced management of critically ill equine patients is commonly influenced by developments in the human literature, because veterinary studies in this field are not as prevalent, often encompass small patient numbers, and

E-mail address: daniela.bedenice@tufts.edu

Table 1
Levels of evidence

Evidence	Grading definitions in the human literature	Extrapolated grading of the veterinary literature
Level 1a	Systematic review of randomized controlled clinical trials	Systematic review of randomized controlled trials
Level 1b	Individual randomized controlled clinical trials	Individual randomized controlled trials (incorporating clinical patients or disease models in the same species)
Level 2	Prospective, controlled, nonrandomized cohort studies	Retrospective nonrandomized cohort or case-control studies
Level 3	Retrospective nonrandomized cohort or case-control studies	Case series
Level 4	Case series (report on a series of patients with an outcome of interest, control group is lacking)	Research model in the same or a related mammalian species
Level 5	Expert opinion without explicit critical appraisal or based on physiology, bench research, or "first principles"	In vitro testing or theoretic physiologic justification

are restricted by limited financial support. This approach has distinct limitations, because even though general physiologic principles are often extrapolated from related mammalian species, using critical judgment, there are cross-species differences. Nevertheless, a good example of the influence of developments in the human literature on equine critical care is the application of "early goal-directed therapy" (EGDT) to veterinary patients as discussed here.

The information presented in this article is based on an extensive PubMed literature search from January 1966 to December 2006, with a specific focus on preexisting systematic reviews of the human literature as well as on independent key word searches, including but not limited to the following terms: equine, horses, foals, outcome, mortality, prognosis, fluid therapy, saline, lactated Ringer's, hetastarch, HES, colloids, crystalloids, sepsis, septic shock, endotoxemia, resuscitation, lactate, anion gap (AG), hypoxia, catecholamine, vasopressin (VP), dopamine, dobutamine, norepinephrine (NE), and phenylephrine.

Table 2
Grades of recommendation

A	Consistent level 1 studies
B	Consistent level 2 or 3 studies or extrapolations from level 1 studies
C	Level 4 studies or extrapolations from level 2 or 3 studies
D	Level 5 evidence or troublingly inconsistent or inconclusive studies of any level

Adapted from Ball C, Sackett D, Philips B, et al. Levels of evidence and grades of recommendations. Oxford Centre for Evidence-based Medicine, 2001. Available at: http://www.cebm.net/index.aspx?o=1025. Accessed November 2006.

Question 1: does early goal-directed therapy designed to improve tissue oxygenation reduce mortality attributable to sepsis?

EGDT designed to improve tissue oxygenation reduces the mortality attributable to sepsis, with a recommendation grade of level B in human beings. Sepsis is one of the most common clinical diagnoses of neonatal foals admitted to referral centers [5,6] and is usually associated with marked disturbances of the cardiovascular system that can result in inadequate tissue oxygen delivery, abnormalities in oxygen extraction, and myocardial depression. Fluid therapy is generally the first line of treatment to improve oxygen delivery by increasing circulating volume, and thus venous return and cardiac output (CO). If fluid therapy is inadequate to restore tissue oxygenation, vasoactive agents (eg, vasopressors, inotropes) are used to support the cardiovascular system [7].

Accurate hemodynamic assessment of the critically ill patient is challenging, however, and commonly needs to go beyond standard physical examination, hematology, central venous pressure (CVP), and urinary output measurements [8]. Human studies have shown that a more definitive resuscitation strategy involves goal-oriented manipulation of cardiac preload (circulating volume), afterload (peripheral resistance), and cardiac contractility to achieve a balance between systemic oxygen delivery and oxygen demand [9]. This type of EGDT is a cardiovascular support protocol aimed at early hemodynamic optimization [8] (Fig. 1). The protocol is initiated as soon as sepsis-induced hypoperfusion is identified on admission and targets end points of resuscitation derived from hemodynamic monitoring, including CVP, mean arterial pressure (MAP), lactate concentration, pH, and central venous oxygen saturation ($Scvo_2$) as a surrogate of the oxygen supply/demand balance [10,11]. An elevated serum lactate level may identify tissue hypoperfusion in patients at risk but not yet hypotensive [12], thus assisting the early recognition of hemodynamic derangements in human beings and horses.

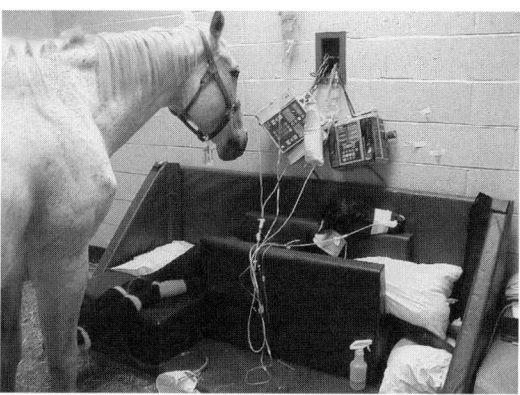

Fig. 1. Septic neonatal foal undergoing early goal directed fluid therapy and vasopressor treatment during neonatal intensive care.

Human patients

An evidence-based review of goal-directed resuscitation, including a comprehensive MEDLINE literature search from 1966 through 2003, was published in 2004 [12]. This scientific review recommended that resuscitation of patients with sepsis-induced tissue hypoperfusion should begin immediately on recognition of the syndrome. During the first 6 hours of resuscitation, the treatment goals should include all the following: CVP of 8 to 12 mm Hg, MAP of 65 mm Hg or greater, urine output of 0.5 mL/kg/h or greater, and ($Scvo_2$) or mixed venous oxygen saturation (Svo_2) saturation of 70% or greater.

Evidence for the usefulness of this approach was documented in a randomized, controlled, predominantly blind study of 263 patients presenting with severe sepsis or septic shock who maintained a systolic blood pressure (BP) of less than 90 mm Hg after a crystalloid challenge of 20 to 30 mL/kg or a blood lactate level of greater than 4 mmol/L [8,12]. The patients were randomly assigned to receive 6 hours of standard therapy or 6 hours of EGDT before admission to the intensive care unit.

The control group was treated according to a standard hemodynamic support protocol, which aims to ensure that the patients had a CVP between 8 and 12 mm Hg, a MAP greater than 65 mm Hg, and a urine output of greater than 0.5 mL/kg/min through crystalloid, colloid, and vasopressor use. The treatment aims of the EGDT group were the same, except that an $ScvO_2$ greater than 70% (measured by means of a central venous catheter) also needed to be achieved through the use of transfused red blood cells (RBCs) and positive inotropes as well as through sedation and mechanical ventilation to reduce oxygen demand as needed.

During the first 6 hours of therapy, the EGDT group received more intravenous fluid (5.0 versus 3.5 L; $P<.001$), RBC transfusions ($P<.001$), and inotropic therapy ($P<.001$). During the subsequent 66 hours, however, the control group required more RBC transfusions ($P<.001$), vasopressors ($P=.03$), mechanical ventilation ($P<.001$), and pulmonary artery catheterization ($P=.04$). The in-hospital mortality rate was significantly higher in the control group than in the EGDT group (46.5% versus 30.5%, respectively; $P=.009$) and maintained through to day 28 ($P=.01$) and day 60 ($P=.03$) of follow-up [8,12].

An earlier study of goal-directed hemodynamic therapy had failed to demonstrate improved morbidity or mortality rates in critically ill patients for whom supranormal cardiac index (CI) values or normal values for Svo_2 were achieved compared with a control group treated to achieve a normal CI [13]. A more recent study evaluated the impact of initiating "standard operating procedure" (SOP) for management of severe sepsis and septic shock, including early EGDT, glycemic control, administration of stress doses of hydrocortisone, and use of recombinant human activated protein C (rhAPC) on measures of organ dysfunction and outcome [14].

Organ failure scores were significantly reduced in the SOP group for liver ($P = .015$), cardiovascular ($P = .030$), and central nervous system ($P = .050$) subscores on days 2, 6, and 8. Additionally, mortality was reduced from 53% in the historical control group to 27% after implementation of SOP ($P < .05$) in this study.

The current Surviving Sepsis Campaign guidelines further endorse the use of EGDT for the management of severe sepsis and septic shock [15]. For the purpose of hemodynamic monitoring, this consensus panel judged $Scvo_2$ and Svo_2 measurements to be equivalent. In mechanically ventilated patients, the panel recommended a higher target CVP of 12 to 15 mm Hg to account for the increased intrathoracic pressure. Similar consideration may be warranted in circumstances of increased abdominal pressure. A decrease in elevated pulse with fluid resuscitation was also regarded as a useful marker of improving intravascular filling [15]. Although lactate measurements were considered clinically useful, they were believed to lack precision as a measure of tissue metabolic status. Several studies have suggested that elevated lactate levels may result from cellular metabolic failure rather than from global hypoperfusion in sepsis [16]. The prognostic value of raised blood lactate levels has been well established in patients with septic shock, however, especially if the high levels persist [17]. It has been further noted that blood lactate levels are of greater prognostic value than oxygen-derived variables [18].

Clinical relevance

The human literature strongly supports the logical recommendation that resuscitation should start as early as possible to prevent further organ dysfunction and failure. The longer resuscitation is delayed, the less likely it is that a beneficial effect is going to be achieved [12]. Once cellular dysfunction and death have evolved, the resuscitation strategies designed to improve tissue oxygenation are unlikely to be helpful. Based on the human literature, we should therefore provide resuscitation to our equine patients at the earliest possible stage, because it is unclear when the transition from reversible to irreversible cellular dysfunction occurs [12]. Furthermore, resuscitation should be patient specific, using markers of hemodynamic and metabolic status (MAP, lactate, urine output, CVP, and Svo_2) in human and veterinary patients (Fig. 2).

Equine patients

The potential significance of EGDT has not been critically evaluated in equine patients to date. Several small studies have attempted to determine the outcome significance of various hemodynamic and metabolic markers in horses, however, and support the following statements.

Hyperlactemia is associated with mortality in critically ill neonatal foals

Hyperlactemia is associated with mortality in critically ill neonatal foals, with a level of evidence of veterinary grade 2 [19–21]. A recent equine study demonstrated the association between low blood lactate concentrations on

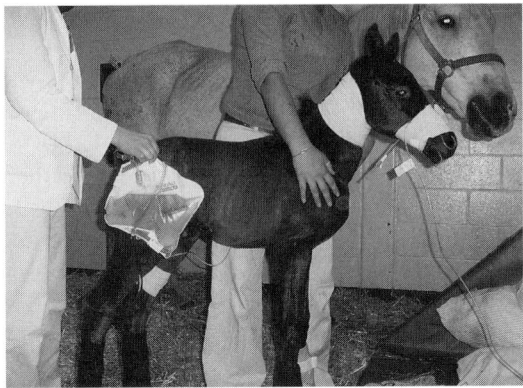

Fig. 2. Measurement of urine output in the recovering septic neonatal foal in Fig. 1.

patient admission and after 24 hours of hospitalization with survival in critically ill neonatal foals [19]. This retrospective cohort analysis of 72 intensive care foals investigated the association of blood lactate with clinical and metabolic parameters. In this study, 61 (85%) of 72 foals had a lactate concentration greater than 2.5 mmol/L on presentation, which was significantly lower in foals that survived (mean lactate: 4.4 ± 0.6 mmol/L) than in those that did not (mean lactate: 9.3 ± 0.9 mmol/L) ($P < .001$). Similarly, lactate concentrations at 18 to 36 hours were 3.2 ± 0.5 mmol/L in survivors versus 9.1 ± 0.7 mmol/L in nonsurviving foals ($P < .001$). Although low admission lactate levels predicted survival well (negative predictive value = 94%, 95% confidence interval: 88–100), death was poorly predicted by hyperlactemia (lactate ≥2.5 mmol/L, positive predictive value = 45%, 95% confidence interval: 32–57) [19].

Subset analysis further demonstrated that foals with a blood lactate level greater than 5 mmol/L (32 [44%] of 72) and concurrent pH of 7.35 or lower were less likely to survive than those without acidemia ($P = .012$). The authors postulated that the ability to compensate acid-base derangements affords some level of protection or is related to less severe physiologic derangements [19]. A significant association of admission lactate with MAP further supported the premise that blood lactate is mainly an indicator of cardiovascular status. Bacteremic foals (mean lactate: 7.3 ± 5 mmol/L) also had greater mean admission lactate levels than those with a negative blood culture (mean lactate: 5 ± 4 mmol/L). Similarly, foals with perinatal asphyxia syndrome (PAS) showed a high mean admission lactate (8.5 mmol/L), suggesting severe cardiovascular disturbances in this patient group. The authors concluded that measuring lactate at and 18 to 36 hours after admission is clinically relevant in neonatal foals [19].

Similarly, decreased partial pressure of venous oxygen (Pvo_2; $P = .0342$) and increased AG ($P = .0047$) were relevant indicators of poor prognosis in critically ill neonates with a variety of primary problems in another study [20]. High AGs occur if there are increased serum concentrations of unmeasured anions (volatile fatty acids, lactate, pyruvate, sulfates, and phosphates) or decreases in the concentration of unmeasured cations (calcium and magnesium) [22]. However, the major unidentified anion in critically ill horses is expected to be lactate [23]. Similar to hyperlactemia, AG increases may reflect decreased tissue oxygen delivery or defective oxygen use. Nonsurvival increased 11.3-fold (95% confidence interval: 3.3–39.4; $P<000.1$) in 58 of 67 foals with radiographic evidence or lung disease that had an admission AG of 20 mEq/L or greater in one study [6]. Another study showed that mean lactate values (but not AGs) were significantly different between surviving and nonsurviving critically ill neonatal foals. Only a moderate correlation of the AG with lactate concentration (correlation coefficient = 0.69; $P<.001$) was observed in this study [19]. Because the AG correlated better with lactate in foals with a negative admission blood culture, the authors suggested that nonketone unidentified anions contribute to the AG in endotoxemia and sepsis [24,25].

Decreased venous oxygen saturation, hyperlactemia, and decreased blood pressure are clinically relevant indicators of nonsurvival in horses with colic

Decreased venous oxygen saturation, hyperlactemia, and decreased BP are clinically relevant indicators of nonsurvival in horses with colic, with a level of evidence of veterinary grade 2 [26–29]. A retrospective cohort analysis of 165 horses admitted for acute abdominal disease attempted to determine the impact of 32 physical examination and laboratory variables on patient survival. Four variables, including heart rate, peritoneal fluid total protein, blood lactate concentration, and abnormal mucous membranes, were significantly associated with poor outcome in the stepwise logistic regression analysis. Mean lactate was 58.3 ± 2.7 mg/dL in nonsurvivors versus 23.9 ± 1.9 in surviving horses ($P<.001$), although lactate values alone were not considered accurate predictors of outcome [26]. Nonetheless, this study supported earlier findings that associated a blood lactate value greater than 75 mg/dL with high mortality in equine colic [30]. Another study further determined that systolic BP, blood lactate concentration, oral mucous membrane capillary refill time, diastolic pressure, and arterial pulse amplitude were able to discriminate between survival and nonsurvival in 73 equine patients with colic (in order of decreasing merit). Combined assessment of systolic pressure, blood lactate concentration, blood urea concentration, and hematocrit permitted accurate classification of 93% (68 of 73) of the cases examined [27].

Svo_2 was evaluated as a predictor of tissue injury in a 1995 prospective study performed in seven anesthetized clinically healthy horses subjected to 3 hours of localized large colon ischemia. The purpose of the study was to determine abnormalities in local colonic coagulation, fibrinolysis, and oxygenation for purposes of making a rapid indirect assessment of colonic mucosal injury. Venous lactate, Svo_2, and Pvo_2 were the most significant predictors of the severity of histologic damage within the ischemic colons ($R^2 = 0.661$) [28]. More specifically, venous oxygen saturation was significantly reduced in ischemic colon segments compared with control segments throughout the period of ischemia but returned to preischemic values after re-establishment of blood flow. The increase in Svo_2 with reperfusion was attributed to increased oxygen delivery or inability of damaged cells to extract oxygen from arterial blood [28]. In a second study, five anesthetized ponies were subjected to 2.5 hours of complete ischemia of the left dorsal and ventral colon [29]. Median venous oxygen saturation and median Pvo_2 were significantly lower ($P<.001$) in the experimental ponies at the end of 2 hours of ischemia but were significantly increased during the reperfusion phase ($P<.05$), similar to the 1995 report [28].

Question 2: should colloid solutions be used in preference to crystalloids for the initial resuscitation of hypovolemic patients?

It is currently uncertain, with a recommendation grade of level B in human beings, whether colloid solutions should be used in preference to crystalloids for the initial resuscitation of hypovolemic patients.

Human patients

Meta-analyses comparing mortality in crystalloid versus colloid resuscitated human patients have yielded conflicting results. An evidence-based clinical practice guideline on fluid resuscitation in human neonatal and pediatric hypovolemic shock was published in 2006 [31]. These guidelines and recommendations were developed by a national multidisciplinary committee and based on a comprehensive search and analysis of the pediatric literature.

Premature and full-term human neonates

Only one randomized controlled trial was included in the 2006 resuscitation guidelines [32]. Other studies focused on prophylactic fluid administration after birth [31,33–35] or failed to analyze hypovolemic neonates separately [36]. In the former study, a randomized controlled clinical trial evaluated the efficacy of a colloid (ie, 5% albumin) versus a crystalloid (ie, isotonic saline) in the treatment of 63 hypotensive preterm neonates. Outcomes, as assessed by mortality (relative risk [RR] = 1.36, 95% confidence interval: 0.69–2.66), chronic lung disease (RR = 0.48, 95% confidence interval: 0.13–1.87), or intraventricular hemorrhage (RR = 1.52, 95% confidence interval: 0.91–4.87) did not differ significantly between the groups [32]. However, the reviewers suggested that this study was underpowered based on the presence of wide 95% confidence intervals [31].

Adult human beings

To date, seven meta-analyses of randomized controlled trials [37–45] have been published on the use of colloids versus crystalloids in fluid resuscitation of critically ill human patients. Systematic reviews of poor methodologic quality and those that did not analyze hypovolemic patients separately [45] were excluded from the analyses. Two reviews documented a 6% increase in mortality in critically ill human patients receiving albumin compared with crystalloids [37,38], although a meta-analysis observed no difference between crystalloid and colloid resuscitation with respect to the incidence of pulmonary edema (pooled $RR = 0.84$ [range: 0.25–2.45]), mortality (pooled $RR = 0.86$ [range: 0.63–1.17]), and length of hospital stay [43]. In the 2006 meta-analysis, however, the authors emphasized that the power of the aggregated data was insufficient to detect small but potentially clinically important differences [31]. Subgroup analysis of this study showed a statistically significant reduction in the mortality rate of patients with trauma receiving crystalloid versus colloid resuscitation ($RR = 0.39$, 95% confidence interval: 0.17–0.89).

Recently, a large randomized controlled trial known as the Saline versus Albumin Fluid Evaluation (SAFE) study was conducted in 6997 adult human patients who required fluid administration to maintain or increase intravascular volume [46]. The relative mortality risk of patients randomly assigned to receive 4% albumin compared with those given isotonic saline was 0.99 (95% confidence interval: 0.91–1.09), which indicated no difference in outcome. A subgroup analysis supported the notion that patients with trauma might benefit more from resuscitation with saline than patients without trauma, however. The increased relative mortality risk among patients with trauma receiving albumin ($RR = 1.36$, 95% confidence interval: 0.99–1.87) as compared with those without trauma resulted from a small excess number of deaths among patients who had traumatic brain injury. It has been speculated that albumin may induce greater hemodilution than saline or increased blood loss because of transient alterations in coagulation. In contrast, a comparison of the relative mortality risk among septic patients provided limited evidence of a treatment effect that favors albumin in patients with severe sepsis ($RR = 0.87$, 95% confidence interval: 0.74–1.02). The benefit of albumin or saline in the treatment of highly selected populations of critically ill patients still requires further study, however [46].

According to another meta-analysis, one type of colloid solution was not more effective or safer than another when comparing albumin versus hydroxyethyl starch (HES; $RR = 1.17$, 95% confidence interval: 0.91–1.50) and albumin versus gelatin ($RR = 0.99$, 95% confidence interval: 0.69–1.42) [42]. Again, the 95% confidence intervals in this study are wide, and the results do not exclude clinically relevant differences among colloids [31].

Clinical relevance

The evaluated human studies fail to show an advantage of colloid over crystalloid resuscitation in critically ill hypovolemic patients when survival rates are considered [31]. Although crystalloids and colloids restore tissue perfusion to the same degree when titrated to a similar level of filling pressure [47], approximately three times greater crystalloid volumes are required because of their rapid distribution throughout the entire extracellular space (25% intravascular and 75% interstitial). Some clinicians therefore favor synthetic colloids after initial crystalloid resuscitation in patients with refractory hypovolemia and significant hemodynamic changes (eg, severe sepsis) [31]. Interestingly, the SAFE study showed that to maintain stable circulation, the volume ratio of infused albumin to isotonic saline was only 1:4 [46].

Crystalloids are generally regarded as first-line fluids for the hemodynamically stable patient, and colloids are often administered in addition to rather than in lieu of crystalloids in human and veterinary patients. These two groups of fluids are largely indistinguishable in terms of their effects on cardiac preload, recruitable stroke volume (SV), and oxygen delivery in human beings, however [48].

The essence of the crystalloid-colloid controversy is the importance of plasma colloid oncotic pressure (COP) in modulating extravascular fluid movement [49]. In the presence of increased hydrostatic pressures (end points of fluid resuscitation), COP becomes a determinant of extravascular fluid flux, and colloids may be associated with a reduced incidence of pulmonary edema in these situations [47,50]. In contrast to results of the recent SAFE study, a 6% increased mortality rate after albumin resuscitation was reported by earlier studies [37,38]. Reviewers speculated that an accelerated distribution of small-molecular-weight colloids (albumin, 60 kDa) across the capillary membranes in the face of inflammation [51] may facilitate edema formation. These systematic reviews have inherent limitations, however, in that the effects of crystalloids and colloids on pulmonary edema and the contribution of hydrostatic pressure to edema formation cannot be delineated from the data [49]. Contrary to earlier concerns, colloids do not increase the severity of pulmonary edema in permeability states if equivalent filling pressures are maintained [52]. Furthermore, evidence confirms neither greater safety nor efficacy of one colloid over another when clinically relevant outcomes are considered [31].

Equine patients

To date, the effect of colloids on hemodynamic variables has only been evaluated in a limited number of critically ill horses and foals. Nonetheless, the current literature supports the following statements.

Oncotic effects of a high-molecular-weight hydroxyethyl starch in healthy horses last longer than those of pentastarch and hypertonic saline

Oncotic effects of a high-molecular-weight HES in healthy horses last longer than those of pentastarch and hypertonic saline, with a level of evidence of veterinary grade 1b [53–55]. Pentastarch (HES of 200 kDa) is a synthetic colloid with a higher osmotic pressure than hetastarch (HES of 450 kDa), allowing a more rapid [56] but less sustained plasma volume expansion. The magnitude and duration of the oncotic effects of HES depend on the number and vascular retention of osmotically active polymers [57]. The overall elimination rate is influenced by species-specific differences in plasma amylase activity, which hydrolyzes larger HES polymers [53]. In healthy horses, the initial phase half-life ($T_{1/2}$) of pentastarch was documented as 5.6 hours, with effects on packed cell volume (PCV), total solids (TS), and plasma viscosity lasting for 12 to 24 hours [53]. In contrast, the higher molecular weight hetastarch (infusions of 10 and 20 mL/kg) showed prolonged increases in COP compared with baseline over a 5-day study period in healthy ponies [55]. Administration of hypertonic saline (2400 mOsm/L) at 5 mL/kg in normal horses increased plasma volume (12.3 ± 1%) and decreased mean plasma protein concentration (−12.1 ± 1%) and PCV (11.9 ± 0.7%) transiently, similar to isotonic saline solution (300 mOsm/L) [54].

Cardiovascular responses to hydroxyethyl starch and hypertonic saline infusion may be shorter and inferior in horses with systemic illness compared with healthy controls

Cardiovascular responses to HES and hypertonic saline infusion may be shorter and inferior in horses with systemic illness compared with healthy controls, with levels of evidence of veterinary grade 1b [54,58,59] and grade 2 [60]. In hypoproteinemic horses, significant oncotic effects of Hespan (6.2% hetastarch in 0.9% sodium chloride) were sustained for 24 hours [60]. In contrast, the clinical effects of hypertonic saline (↑SV, ↑CO, ↓systemic vascular resistance [SVR]) have been documented to only persist for 1 to 2 hours in hemorrhagic [59] and endotoxic [54] shock models in anesthetized ponies and awake horses, respectively. Similarly, significant increases in CI and SV after a 10% pentastarch infusion at a rate of 4 mL/kg were limited to 2.5 hours and 1 hour, respectively, in clinical equine patients undergoing colic surgery. Interestingly, hypertonic saline infusion (4 mL/kg) did not induce any significant increases in mean CI or SV from baseline throughout the course of the latter study [58].

Early administration of pentastarch results in better anesthetic hemodynamics, based on a higher cardiac index and stroke volume, than hypertonic saline in horses undergoing colic surgery

Early administration of pentastarch results in better anesthetic hemodynamics, based on a higher CI and SV, than hypertonic saline in horses undergoing colic surgery, with a level of evidence of veterinary grade 1b [58]. The effect of 7.2% hypertonic saline at a dose of 4 mL/kg versus an isovolume 10% pentastarch solution has been evaluated in 30 cardiovascularly compromised horses requiring colic surgery [58]. In this study, hemodynamic measurements, including CO and SV, were recorded every 30 minutes during anesthesia. Results showed that preoperative administration of pentastarch resulted in better SV and CO than hypertonic saline for 1 and 2.5 hours after anesthetic induction, respectively. The study was not designed to investigate effects on mortality, however, and no conclusions can be drawn regarding the efficacy of either treatment in preventing death. The authors infer that at least 1403 study horses would be required to detect an increase from 80% [61] to 86% postoperative survival, with a power of 80% and $P \leq .05$ [58].

Hypertonic saline produces significant hemodynamic improvements in anesthetic-induced hypotension and in hemorrhagic and endotoxic shock in horses

Hypertonic saline produces significant hemodynamic improvements in anesthetic-induced hypotension and in hemorrhagic and endotoxic shock in horses, with a level of evidence of veterinary grade 1b [54,59,62]. The hemodynamic effects of small-volume hypertonic saline resuscitation were evaluated in 12 adult anesthetized horses for 2 hours using a controlled hemorrhagic shock model. In contrast to low-volume isotonic saline infusion (3.8–4.5 mL/kg of body weight), treatment with an isovolume of 7.2% hypertonic saline produced rapid improvements in hemodynamic function (↑CO, ↑SV, ↑cardiac contractility, ↑mean systemic and pulmonary arterial pressures, and ↑urine output) and was accompanied by expansion of plasma volume and decreased peripheral vascular resistance [59]. This study supports the concept that hypertonic saline produces transient hemodynamic improvements in experimentally induced hemorrhagic shock in horses. The authors postulated that the administration of hypertonic saline only served as a temporary measure and did not eliminate the need to continue supportive therapy, monitoring, and fluid administration [59].

Similarly, the cardiovascular responses to sublethal endotoxin infusion (*Escherichia coli*) were measured in five standing horses that received a hypertonic or isotonic sodium chloride solution at a rate of 5 mL/kg in a crossover design after endotoxin challenge. CO was significantly increased and total peripheral vascular resistance was significantly decreased during the hypertonic trial [54]. Both studies [54,59] used low-dose isotonic crystalloids as controls in equal volumes as the hypertonic test fluid. Because of the lower tonicity, however, the crystalloid volume used as a control was completely inadequate for patient resuscitation and does not reflect current fluid therapy recommendations [59]. Thus, the studies may have been designed essentially so as to guarantee failure of the controls. Therefore, no conclusion can be drawn on the comparative efficacy of hypertonic saline versus isotonic crystalloids from either equine study. Rather, the authors solely evaluated the cardiovascular effects of hypertonic solutions and may have only indicated that hypertonic saline treatment is superior to inadequate crystalloid therapy.

In contrast, the cardiovascular responses of six anesthetized horses to preinduction infusion of 7.5% hypertonic saline solution (4.0 mL/kg administered intravenously) and equal osmotic loads of lactated Ringer's solution

(20.0 mL/kg administered intravenously) were compared in another study. During anesthesia, an increase in mean arterial BP was observed in the lactated Ringer's solution (BP: 76 ± 3 mm Hg) and hypertonic saline (BP: 73 ± 3 mm Hg) groups compared with control values (BP: 63 ± 2 mm Hg). This change was associated with an increase in CI over baseline (CI = 53 ± 4 mL/min/kg) in horses receiving hypertonic saline (68 ± 4 mL/min/kg), indicating enhanced myocardial contractility. At the time of recovery, however, the hemodynamic variables in treated horses were no longer significantly different from the respective control values. As expected, increased BP and SVR values were apparent for all treatment groups over those observed during anesthesia. Results of this study indicate that lactated Ringer's solution and hypertonic saline solution are effective in maintaining BP during a potential cardiovascular-depressive anesthetic regimen in healthy horses [62].

Clinical relevance of the colloid-crystalloid debate

It has been well established that high-molecular-weight colloids, such as hetastarch, result in a longer duration of plasma volume expansion than low-molecular-weight colloids in healthy animals [53,55]. In contrast, hypertonic saline only transiently increases plasma volume in healthy horses similar to isotonic saline solutions, presumably because of rapid electrolyte clearance [54]. In the clinical setting, it is important to remember that the duration of action of colloids and crystalloids is reduced by systemic illness, such as endotoxic and hemorrhagic shock [54,59]. The type and extent of fluid therapy therefore need to be tailored to the individual patient and based on achieving specific resuscitation targets. Clinically relevant resuscitation goals may include stabilization of vital signs and normalization of cardiovascular parameters (eg, lactate, Svo_2, PCV), adequate COP, and end-organ perfusion (eg, appropriate urination, warm extremities).

The colloid pentastarch demonstrated superior cardiovascular stabilization of horses undergoing colic surgery compared with hypertonic saline [58]. Small-volume fluid resuscitation with hypertonic saline is considered a viable temporary measure to resuscitate adult hypovolemic horses as long as continued supportive care, including subsequent fluid therapy, can be ensured [54,59]. Equal osmotic loads of hypertonic and isotonic fluids seem to have comparable cardiovascular effects, at least in healthy anesthetized horses [62]. The objective comparison of small-volume hypertonic with equal osmotic isotonic and colloid resuscitation, however, requires further investigation in horses.

Question 3: should vasopressin be used for the treatment of refractory hypotension in septic patients?

VP should be used for the treatment of refractory hypotension in septic patients, with a recommendation grade of level B to C in human beings.

Human patients

VP is an endogenously released stress hormone with potent vasopressor activity that has been demonstrated to improve organ perfusion in septic shock [63]. The rationale of its use is based on a relative VP deficiency in advanced circulatory shock and the ability of exogenous VP administration to restore vascular tone in vasoplegic (catecholamine-resistant) shock states. VP is known to act through activation of V_1 receptors, regulation of arterial tone by blocking K_{ATP} channels, modulation of nitric oxide through reduction of intracellular cyclic guanosine monophosphate (cGMP), and potentiation of adrenergic and other vasoconstrictor agents [64,65]. Because VP causes arterial smooth muscle cell contraction through a noncatecholamine receptor pathway, it represents an attractive adjunct therapy of septic shock, especially when catecholamines are ineffective [65]. Available studies on VP in the management of septic shock mainly consist of case series [66,67], retrospective analyses [68,69], and several relatively small randomized controlled trials [70–73]. Nonetheless, literature evidence supports several conclusions on the role of VP in septic shock.

Established septic shock in adult human patients is associated with a vasopressin deficiency

Established septic shock in adult human patients has been associated with a VP deficiency [74]. In 2003, relative VP deficiency (<3.6 pg/mL) was diagnosed in 16 of 62 human patients with late septic shock associated with hyponatremia or a systolic BP of less than 100 mm Hg [75]. Although VP levels were consistently increased (4.3–21 pg/mL) in the early phases of shock, most patients exhibited relative VP deficiency by 36 hours from shock onset. Similarly, another study reported that patients with vasodilatory septic shock had reduced VP levels (3.1 ± 1.0 pg/mL compared with 22.7 ± 2.2 pg/mL in patients with cardiogenic shock) and demonstrated a marked response to exogenous VP infusion of 0.01 to 0.04 U/min [66].

Catecholamine-resistant vasodilatory shock is responsive to a combined infusion of low-dose vasopressin and norepinephrine

Catecholamine-resistant vasodilatory shock was evaluated in 48 human patients prospectively randomized to receive a combined infusion of VP (0.067 U/min) and NE or NE infusion alone [70]. In this study, patients treated with VP had a significantly lower heart rate, NE requirements, and incidence of tachyarrhythmias than patients treated solely with NE. MAP, CO, and SV were also significantly higher in the VP plus NE group. The authors concluded that the combined infusion of low-dose VP and NE proved to be superior to infusion of NE alone in the treatment of cardiocirculatory failure in catecholamine-resistant vasodilatory shock [70].

A 2003 study further demonstrated that low-dose VP infusion (0.02 U/min) prolonged survival in septic sheep after cecal perforation [76]. Although survival times were significantly higher in all three treatment groups (VP + NE, NE alone, and VP alone) compared with controls, infusion with VP alone or with VP plus NE was superior to infusion with NE alone. CO increased in all groups after the induction of peritonitis, consistent with a hyperdynamic model of sepsis. CO was significantly lower in the VP group compared with the VP plus NE group, however. Gastric perfusion (measured by gastric tonometry) was better preserved in the VP plus NE group compared with all other groups, whereas urine output was higher in purely VP-treated sheep than in the NE-treated or control group [76]. A subsequent study in sheep demonstrated that high-dose VP infusion alone (0.052 U/min in healthy 35-kg sheep and 0.04 U/min in endotoxemic ewes) decreased CI, compromised oxygen delivery by decreasing oxygen consumption per unit time (Vo_2) and overall oxygen delivery (Do_2), and increased oxygen extraction ratio (O_2-ER) and the pulmonary vascular resistance index. The authors suggested that these side effects may limit VP use as a sole vasopressor during sepsis. When NE was infused along with VP, the decrease in CI was ameliorated [77].

Vasopressin infusion improves renal function in patients with severe septic shock

The effects of intravenous NE (0.2 µg/kg/min) and VP (0.08 U/min) infusions on systemic, splanchnic, and renal circulation were evaluated in anesthetized dogs weighing 20 kg under basal conditions and during endotoxic shock. In contrast to NE, administration of VP effectively restored renal blood flow and Do_2, with comparable systemic and splanchnic hemodynamic and metabolic effects in endotoxin-induced circulatory shock. The authors suggested that observed improvements in renal blood flow were related to nitric oxide–mediated afferent arteriolar vasodilatation and selective efferent arteriolar vasoconstriction [78]. Similarly, the short-term effects of VP (0.02 U/kg/h) and NE (2 µg/kg/min) were examined in a rat model of endotoxic normokinetic shock. In this study, both test drugs restored MAP without changing renal blood flow. Nevertheless, in contrast to NE, VP improved endotoxin-induced renal dysfunction by attenuating declines in diuresis and insulin clearance, decreasing renal lactate, and normalizing renal ATP [79].

The first double-blind randomized study comparing the effects of NE alone (n = 11) and NE plus VP (0.01–0.08 U/min, n = 13) in human patients with severe septic shock was reported in 2002 [73]. Diuresis and creatinine clearance were significantly improved in patients treated with NE plus VP in contrast to the group treated with NE alone. Because diuresis increased in patients whose MAP remained constant, this finding supports an intrarenal effect of VP. Furthermore, VP infusion spared conventional vasopressor use by allowing a reduction of NE from 25 to 5.3 µg/min in the NE plus VP group by 4 hours of treatment ($P < .001$). Similar results were obtained in 48 patients in a previously mentioned study [70].

High-dose vasopressin worsens gastrointestinal perfusion in septic shock

An observational study of 13 NE-dependent patients with septic shock demonstrated that continuous infusion of VP at a rate of 0.04 U/min significantly increased the difference between gastric and arterial carbon dioxide (CO_2) partial pressure, compatible with gastrointestinal hypoperfusion. VP infusion resulted in an increase in MAP without a decrease in CI [80]. High-dose VP infusion (mean dose of 0.47 U/min) in patients with septic shock has also been shown to redistribute gastrointestinal blood flow to the disadvantage of the mucosa. Global oxygen delivery and CI were significantly decreased at these doses [81]. Similarly, in a porcine model of hypodynamic shock (associated with decreased CO), high-dose VP (0.04 U/min in 30-kg animals) reversed hypotension but decreased gut and systemic blood flow. These effects were associated with hyperlactatemia, signs of visceral dysoxia, and jejunal luminal lactate release [82].

High-dose vasopressin infusion is associated with ischemic skin lesions in patients with septic shock

In a retrospective study of 64 critically ill patients with catecholamine-resistant vasodilatory shock, VP infusion (dose range: 0.067–0.1 U/min) was associated with ischemic skin lesions (ISLs) in 19 (30%) of 63 patients, predominantly located to the distal limbs (68%), trunk (21%), and tongue (26%) [83]. Multiple logistic regression analysis demonstrated that preexistent peripheral arterial occlusive disease and the presence of septic shock were significant independent risk factors for the development of ISLs during VP infusion [74]. In a subsequent prospective study comparing NE with combined VP plus NE infusion in otherwise refractory cardiovascular failure, however, the incidence of ISLs was not significantly different between study groups (incidence of ISL: 25% versus 29.2%, respectively; $P = 1$) [70].

Veterinary patients

The role of select vasopressors has been investigated in equine and small animal patients to evaluate drug efficacy and indications of pressor use in the critical care setting. The following statements are supported by the current literature.

Dobutamine increases cardiac output and blood pressure at therapeutic doses during anesthetic-induced hypotension in healthy horses: the effects on systemic vascular resistance are dose dependent

Dobutamine exerts its effects by direct stimulation of α_1-, β_1-, and β_2-adrenergic receptors [84]. Several studies have consistently documented a significant dose-dependent (1.5–10 µg/kg/min) increase in BP (diastolic arterial pressure [DAP], MAP, systolic arterial pressure [SAP]) and CI in anesthetized horses treated with dobutamine [84,85]. Peripheral vascular resistance was decreased (thus decreasing afterload) [84] or not affected [85].

Thus, dobutamine has the ability to increase SAP by increasing CO in healthy horses [85]. At lower doses, increases in CO seem to be associated with increased SV, whereas the greater CO at higher dobutamine doses may be attributable to increased heart rate [84]. Furthermore, a significant increase in intramuscular blood flow has been demonstrated with dobutamine at a dose of 2.5 to 10 µg/kg/min and in PCV at a dose of 5 µg/kg/min (suggesting α_1 stimulation) [84].

Cardiac arrhythmias are the most commonly reported side effects of dobutamine. In a study of 200 anesthetized horses (receiving dobutamine at a dose of 1.5–3.2 µg/kg/min), the incidence of arrhythmias was 28%, including sinus bradycardia (17%), atrioventricular block (9%), atrial premature contractions (1%), and atrioventricular dissociation (1%) [86]. Dobutamine-induced bradycardia was attributed to increased BP, triggering a vagally mediated sinus bradycardia, or to direct stimulation of myocardial α_1 adrenoreceptors. Sinus tachycardia [84,85] and atrioventricular block [85] were observed in some horses receiving dobutamine at higher doses (>5 µg/kg/min) in separate studies, although cardiac rhythms reverted to normal within 5 minutes of cessation of infusion [84]. By contrast, another study observed positive chronotropic effects of dobutamine at a dose of 2.5 to 10 µg/kg/min [84]. All studies concluded that intravenous infusion was an effective treatment for hypotension in anesthetized horses.

Dopamine increases cardiac output, with variable effects on arterial blood pressure and systemic vascular resistance, during anesthetic-induced hypotension in healthy horses

Dopamine predominantly activates dopaminergic and β_1 receptors, with α-adrenergic receptor stimulation at higher doses. In most studies, dopamine infusion has been documented to enhance myocardial contractility by increasing CO in healthy anesthetized horses [84,85,87,88]. The effects on SAP are dose dependent, with significant increases in SAP, MAP, and DAP reported at a dose of 10 µg/kg/min but not at a dose of 3 to 5 µg/kg/min [85]. However, the same study also showed that the positive inotropic effects and increases in CO were achieved by infusion rates of dobutamine (3 µg/kg/min) lower than those of dopamine (5–10 µg/kg/min).

The effects of dopamine on SVR are variable. One study reported a significant decrease in SVR at a dose of 1 to 10 µg/kg/min [84], whereas a different study only documented significant decreases of total peripheral vascular resistance with an infusion at 5 µg/kg/min, which returned to baseline at an infusion at 10 µg/kg/min, possibly because of increased α_1-adrenergic activity at high doses [85].

The development of cardiac arrhythmias is a complication of dopamine and dobutamine, particularly when higher doses are used (>5 µg/kg/min). The tendency to increase sinus rate was enhanced by increasing dopamine infusion rates in a previously mentioned study [85], with greater chronotropic activity of dopamine compared with dobutamine. Both drugs induced sinus slowing and second-degree atrioventricular block in some horses at the low infusion rates [85].

Phenylephrine fails to improve intramuscular blood flow and cardiac output, despite increases in systemic blood pressure during anesthetic-induced hypotension in healthy horses

Phenylephrine is a pure α-adrenoagonist that reportedly increases MAP, CVP, peripheral vascular resistance, and SVR in a dose-dependent manner (infusion at 0.5–2 μg/kg/min) in halothane-anesthetized horses [84]. Heart rate, intramuscular blood flow, and CO remained unchanged in this study, thus documenting that improvement in muscle blood flow does not merely depend on arterial BP in anesthetized horses. The authors suggest that phenylephrine should not be used routinely for the treatment of anesthetic-induced hypotension in this species [84].

Norepinephrine and dobutamine are better alternatives than vasopressin for restoring cardiovascular function and maintaining splanchnic circulation during isoflurane-induced hypotension in healthy neonatal foals

One study compared the effects of high- and low-dose dobutamine (4 and 8 μg/kg/min), NE (0.3 and 1.0 μg/kg/min), and VP (0.3 and 1.0 mU/kg/min) on cardiovascular function and gastric mucosal perfusion in six anesthetized foals (1–5 days of age) during isoflurane-induced hypotension [89]. Dobutamine administration significantly improved BP and CI (through an increase in heart rate and SV) at either dose, whereas SVR was decreased at the high infusion rate (8 μg/kg/min) only. Furthermore, oxygen delivery increased in a dose-dependent manner, and oxygen consumption was decreased by dobutamine. In contrast, NE administration increased CI (through greater SV), SVR, and oxygen delivery compared with baseline. Although BP was increased by all treatments, the BP effects of NE and dobutamine were superior to those of VP at lower doses, whereas NE was superior to either drug at high-dose levels. The oxygen extraction ratio was decreased after NE and dobutamine treatments compared with baseline. The use of NE to increase MAP through its α-adrenergic effects in septic foals refractory to dobutamine treatment is being investigated. A recent study confirmed that the combined infusion of NE and dobutamine significantly increases arterial BP and SVR, although decreasing heart rate and CI, as compared with a saline control in healthy sedated neonatal foals [90].

VP has been shown to increase BP in hypotensive neonatal foals through increased SVR [89]. CI and SV were significantly lower in the VP group compared with NE and dobutamine therapy at either dose, however. Similarly, oxygen delivery was significantly lower and the oxygen extraction ratio was higher in patients treated with VP compared with NE and dobutamine. Endogenous VP is released to compensate for dehydration in horses [91] and hypotension caused by inhalation anesthesia [92]. Peak endogenous

VP concentrations were observed approximately 10 minutes after induction of hypotension in 1- to 2-week-old foals [93]. The modest cardiovascular effects of exogenous VP observed by investigators may thus be attributable to the fact that endogenous VP release was already maximized during hypotension in foals. If VP depletion occurs during sepsis in horses, however, exogenous VP may prove more effective in restoring cardiovascular function [89].

VP significantly increased the gastric-to-arterial CO_2 gap (ΔCO_2) at high infusion rates in neonatal foals [89], indicating decreased gastric mucosal blood flow. This can be attributed to local vasoconstriction, despite the fact that SVR was similarly increased after NE versus VP administration. NE and dobutamine administration did not result in significant changes in the ΔCO_2. The authors concluded that NE and dobutamine are appropriate choices for restoring cardiovascular function and maintaining splanchnic circulation during isoflurane-induced hypotension in neonatal foals, based on improvements in MAP, CI, and overall oxygen delivery (Do_2) in the absence of detrimental effects on ΔCO_2. In contrast, VP failed to increase CI and Do_2 and resulted in an increase in ΔCO_2.

Norepinephrine and vasopressin had more favorable risk-benefit profiles than epinephrine in a canine model of septic shock (n = 78)

In a canine study, epinephrine therapy (0.2–2 µg/kg/min) caused a dose-dependent decrease in the survival of septic dogs (induced by intraperitoneal implantation of *E coli*) compared with concurrent controls, whereas NE (0.2–2 µg/kg/min) and VP (0.01–0.04 U/min) therapy improved survival [94]. Epinephrine also caused a significantly greater and dose-dependent decrease in mean CI and increase in SVR compared with NE and VP therapy. Epinephrine and NE significantly increased MAP in septic dogs compared with controls ($P<.01$), however, whereas VP did not. The effects of vasopressors were independent of the severity of infection but depended on the type and dose of vasopressor used [94].

Clinical relevance

The application of VP in critically ill equine patients has gained significant attention over the past years, especially for the treatment of septic neonatal foals. This interest is based on encouraging results from several human studies, which have documented endogenous VP deficiency in established sepsis [66,75] as well as superior management of cardiocirculatory failure using low-dose VP infusion in septic shock that is unresponsive to other vasoactive drugs [70,74]. VP was also reported to improve endotoxin-induced renal dysfunction [78] and to reduce catecholamine requirements (drug-sparing effect) [70]. Nevertheless, high-dose VP infusion, especially as the sole vasopressor, is believed to be limited by a variety of side effects, including reduced CO and oxygen delivery [77], worsened gastrointestinal perfusion [80–82,89], and ISLs in people [83]. Although VP is empirically used in equine practice, current research remains insufficient to verify superior efficacy of VP over catecholamines in neonatal septic foals [89].

In the clinical setting, dobutamine (enhancing CO) and NE (counteracting peripheral vasodilation) are often first-line choices for restoring cardiovascular function in hypotensive neonatal foals unresponsive to fluid therapy. Combined NE and dobutamine infusion in sedated healthy foals has been shown to cause unique hemodynamic improvements without affecting renal function [90]. Some equine clinicians propose that the circulatory effects of dopamine may be more difficult to predict because of its variable effects on arterial BP and SVR, which is supported by the current literature in healthy horses [84,85]. Neither epinephrine nor phenylephrine is generally recommended as a first-line choice in the treatment of septic shock.

References

[1] Sackett D, Strauss S, Richardson W, et al. Evidence-based medicine: how to practice and teach EBM. 2nd edition. New York: Churchill Livingstone; 2000.
[2] WA PTAo. Evidence-based practice and physical therapy. Available at: http://www.ptwa.org/EBP.htm. Accessed November 2006.
[3] What is EBM? In: Oxford Centre for Evidence Based Medicine. Available at: http://www.cebm.net. Accessed November 2006.
[4] Pickering GW. BMJ 1956;2:113–6.
[5] Roy MF. Sepsis in adults and foals. Vet Clin North Am Equine Pract 2004;20:41–61.
[6] Bedenice D, Heuwieser W, Solano M, et al. Risk factors and prognostic variables for survival of foals with radiographic evidence of pulmonary disease. J Vet Intern Med 2003;17:868–75.
[7] Corley KT. Inotropes and vasopressors in adults and foals. Vet Clin North Am Equine Pract 2004;20:77–106.
[8] Rivers E, Nguyen B, Havstad S, et al. Early goal-directed therapy in the treatment of severe sepsis and septic shock. N Engl J Med 2001;345:1368–77.
[9] Beal AL, Cerra FB. Multiple organ failure syndrome in the 1990s. Systemic inflammatory response and organ dysfunction. JAMA 1994;271:226–33.
[10] Trzeciak S, Dellinger RP, Abate NL, et al. Translating research to clinical practice: a 1-year experience with implementing early goal-directed therapy for septic shock in the emergency department. Chest 2006;129:225–32.
[11] Elliott DC. An evaluation of the end points of resuscitation. J Am Coll Surg 1998;187:536–47.
[12] Rhodes A, Bennett ED. Early goal-directed therapy: an evidence-based review. Crit Care Med 2004;32:S448–50.
[13] Gattinoni L, Brazzi L, Pelosi P, et al. A trial of goal-oriented hemodynamic therapy in critically ill patients. SvO2 Collaborative Group. N Engl J Med 1995;333:1025–32.
[14] Kortgen A, Niederprum P, Bauer M. Implementation of an evidence-based "standard operating procedure" and outcome in septic shock. Crit Care Med 2006;34:943–9.
[15] Dellinger RP, Vincent JL. The Surviving Sepsis Campaign sepsis change bundles and clinical practice. Crit Care 2005;9:653–4.
[16] Beale RJ, Hollenberg SM, Vincent JL, et al. Vasopressor and inotropic support in septic shock: an evidence-based review. Crit Care Med 2004;32:S455–65.
[17] Vincent JL, Dufaye P, Berre J, et al. Serial lactate determinations during circulatory shock. Crit Care Med 1983;11:449–51.
[18] Bakker J, Coffernils M, Leon M, et al. Blood lactate levels are superior to oxygen-derived variables in predicting outcome in human septic shock. Chest 1991;99:956–62.

[19] Corley K, Donaldson L, Furr M. Arterial lactate concentration, hospital survival, sepsis and SIRS in critically ill neonatal foals. Equine Vet J 2005;37:53–9.
[20] Hoffman AM, Staempfli HR, Willan A. Prognostic variables for survival of neonatal foals under intensive care. J Vet Intern Med 1992;6:89–95.
[21] Bedenice D, Heuwieser W, Brawer R, et al. Clinical and prognostic significance of radiographic pattern, distribution, and severity of thoracic radiographic changes in neonatal foals. J Vet Intern Med 2003;17:876–86.
[22] Lorenz J, Markarian K, Oliver M, et al. Serum anion gap in the differential diagnosis of metabolic acidosis in critically ill newborn foals. J Pediatr 1999;135:751–5.
[23] Constable P, Hinchcliff K, Muir W. Comparison of anion gap and strong ion gap as predictors of unmeasured strong ion concentration in plasma and serum from horses. Am J Vet Res 1998;59:881–7.
[24] Gossett KA, Cleghorn B, Adams R, et al. Contribution of whole blood L-lactate, pyruvate, D-lactate, acetoacetate, and 3-hydroxybutyrate concentrations to the plasma anion gap in horses with intestinal disorders. Am J Vet Res 1987;48:72–5.
[25] Rackow EC, Mecher C, Asitz M, et al. Unmeasured anion during severe sepsis with metabolic acidosis. Circ Shock 1990;30:107–15.
[26] Furr M, Lessard P, White NA. Development of a colic severity score for predicting the outcome of equine colic. Vet Surg 1995;24:97–101.
[27] Parry B, Anderson G, Gay C. Prognosis in equine colic: a comparative study of variables used to assess individual cases. Equine Vet J 1983;15:211–5.
[28] Kawcak CE, Baxter GM, Getzy DM, et al. Abnormalities in oxygenation, coagulation, and fibrinolysis in colonic blood of horses with experimentally induced strangulation obstruction. Am J Vet Res 1995;56:1642–50.
[29] Wilkins PA, Ducharme NG, Lowe JE, et al. Measurements of blood flow and xanthine oxidase activity during postischemic reperfusion of the large colon of ponies. Am J Vet Res 1994;55:1168–77.
[30] Moore JN, Owen RR, Lumsden JH. Clinical evaluation of blood lactate levels in equine colic. Equine Vet J 1976;8:49–54.
[31] Boluyt N, Bollen CW, Bos AP, et al. Fluid resuscitation in neonatal and pediatric hypovolemic shock: a Dutch Pediatric Society evidence-based clinical practice guideline. Intensive Care Med 2006;32(7):995–1003.
[32] So KW, Fok TF, Ng PC, et al. Randomised controlled trial of colloid or crystalloid in hypotensive preterm infants. Arch Dis Child Fetal Neonatal Ed 1997;76:F43–6.
[33] Bland RD, Clarke TL, Harden LB, et al. Early albumin infusion to infants at risk for respiratory distress. Arch Dis Child 1973;48:800–5.
[34] Group NNNIT. Randomised trial of prophylactic early fresh-frozen plasma or gelatin or glucose in preterm babies: outcome at 2 years. Northern Neonatal Nursing Initiative Trial Group. Lancet 1996;348:229–32.
[35] Group NNNINT. A randomized trial comparing the effect of prophylactic intravenous fresh-frozen plasma, gelatin or glucose on early mortality and morbidity in preterm babies. The Northern Neonatal Nursing Initiative [NNNI] Trial Group. Eur J Pediatr 1996;155:580–8.
[36] Kirpalani H. The use of albumin and/or colloids in newborns: a meta-analysis. Pediatr Crit Care Med 2001;2:S14–9.
[37] Reviewers CIGA. Human albumin administration in critically ill patients: systematic review of randomised controlled trials. BMJ 1998;317:235–40.
[38] Schierhout G, Roberts I. Fluid resuscitation with colloid or crystalloid solutions in critically ill patients: a systematic review of randomised trials. BMJ 1998;316:961–4.
[39] Alderson P, Schierhout G, Roberts I, et al. Colloids versus crystalloids for fluid resuscitation in critically ill patients. Cochrane Database Syst Rev 2000;CD000567.
[40] Alderson P, Bunn F, Lefebvre C, et al. Human albumin solution for resuscitation and volume expansion in critically ill patients. Cochrane Database Syst Rev 2002;CD001208.

[41] Bisonni RS, Holtgrave DR, Lawler F, et al. Colloids versus crystalloids in fluid resuscitation: an analysis of randomized controlled trials. J Fam Pract 1991;32:387–90.
[42] Bunn F, Alderson P, Hawkins V. Colloid solutions for fluid resuscitation. Cochrane Database Syst Rev 2001;CD001319.
[43] Choi PT, Yip G, Quinonez LG, et al. Crystalloids vs. colloids in fluid resuscitation: a systematic review. Crit Care Med 1999;27:200–10.
[44] Velanovich V. Crystalloid versus colloid fluid resuscitation: a meta-analysis of mortality. Surgery 1989;105:65–71.
[45] Wilkes MM, Navickis RJ. Patient survival after human albumin administration. A meta-analysis of randomized, controlled trials. Ann Intern Med 2001;135:149–64.
[46] Finfer S, Bellomo R, Boyce N, et al. A comparison of albumin and saline for fluid resuscitation in the intensive care unit. N Engl J Med 2004;350:2247–56.
[47] Rackow EC, Falk JL, Fein IA, et al. Fluid resuscitation in circulatory shock: a comparison of the cardiorespiratory effects of albumin, hetastarch, and saline solutions in patients with hypovolemic and septic shock. Crit Care Med 1983;11:839–50.
[48] Vincent JL, Gerlach H. Fluid resuscitation in severe sepsis and septic shock: an evidence-based review. Crit Care Med 2004;32:S451–4.
[49] Astiz ME, Rackow EC. Crystalloid-colloid controversy revisited. Crit Care Med 1999;27:34–5.
[50] Rackow EC, Weil MH, Macneil AR, et al. Effects of crystalloid and colloid fluids on extravascular lung water in hypoproteinemic dogs. J Appl Physiol 1987;62:2421–5.
[51] Berger A. Why albumin may not work. BMJ 1998;317:240.
[52] Metildi LA, Shackford SR, Virgilio RW, et al. Crystalloid versus colloid in fluid resuscitation of patients with severe pulmonary insufficiency. Surg Gynecol Obstet 1984;158:207–12.
[53] Meister D, Hermann M, Mathis G. Kinetics of hydroxyethyl starch in horses. Schweiz Arch Tierheilkd 1992;134:329–39.
[54] Bertone JJ, Gossett KA, Shoemaker KE, et al. Effect of hypertonic vs isotonic saline solution on responses to sublethal Escherichia coli endotoxemia in horses. Am J Vet Res 1990;51:999–1007.
[55] Jones PA, Tomasic M, Gentry P. Oncotic, hemodilutional and hemostatic effects of isotonic saline and hydroxyethyl starch infusions in clinically normal ponies. Am J Vet Res 1997;58(5):541–8.
[56] Grocott M, Hamilton M. Resuscitation fluids. Vox Sang 2002;82:1–8.
[57] Traylor R, Pearl R. Crystalloid vs. colloid vs. colloid: all colloids are not created equal. Anesth Analg 1996;83:209–12.
[58] Hallowell GD, Corley KT. Preoperative administration of hydroxyethyl starch or hypertonic saline to horses with colic. J Vet Intern Med 2006;20:980–6.
[59] Schmall LM, Muir WW, Robertson JT. Haemodynamic effects of small volume hypertonic saline in experimentally induced haemorrhagic shock. Equine Vet J 1990;22:273–7.
[60] Jones PA, Bain FT, Byars TD, et al. Effect of hydroxyethyl starch infusion on colloid oncotic pressure in hypoproteinemic horses. J Am Vet Med Assoc 2001;218:1130–5.
[61] Phillips T. Retrospective analysis of the results of 151 exploratory laparotomies in horses with gastro-intestinal disease. Equine Vet J 1993;25:427–31.
[62] Dyson DH, Pascoe PJ. Influence of preinduction methoxamine, lactated Ringer solution, or hypertonic saline solution infusion or postinduction dobutamine infusion on anesthetic-induced hypotension in horses. Am J Vet Res 1990;51:17–21.
[63] Delmas A, Leone M, Rousseau S, et al. Clinical review: vasopressin and terlipressin in septic shock patients. Crit Care 2005;9:212–22.
[64] Landry DW, Oliver JA. The pathogenesis of vasodilatory shock. N Engl J Med 2001;345:588–95.
[65] Mutlu GM, Factor P. Role of vasopressin in the management of septic shock. Intensive Care Med 2004;30:1276–91.

[66] Landry DW, Levin HR, Gallant EM, et al. Vasopressin deficiency contributes to the vasodilation of septic shock. Circulation 1997;95:1122–5.
[67] Landry D, Levin H, Gallant E, et al. Vasopressin pressor hypersensitivity in vasodilatory septic shock. Crit Care Med 1997;25:1279–82.
[68] Dunser MW, Mayr AJ, Ulmer H, et al. The effects of vasopressin on systemic hemodynamics in catecholamine-resistant septic and postcardiotomy shock: a retrospective analysis. Anesth Analg 2001;93:7–13.
[69] Holmes CL, Walley KR, Chittock DR, et al. The effects of vasopressin on hemodynamics and renal function in severe septic shock: a case series. Intensive Care Med 2001;27:1416–21.
[70] Dunser MW, Mayr AJ, Ulmer H, et al. Arginine vasopressin in advanced vasodilatory shock: a prospective, randomized, controlled study. Circulation 2003;107:2313–9.
[71] Tsuneyoshi I, Yamada H, Kakihana Y, et al. Hemodynamic and metabolic effects of low-dose vasopressin infusions in vasodilatory septic shock. Crit Care Med 2001;29:487–93.
[72] Malay MB, Ashton RC Jr, Landry DW, et al. Low-dose vasopressin in the treatment of vasodilatory septic shock. J Trauma 1999;47:699–703 [discussion: 703–5].
[73] Patel BM, Chittock DR, Russell JA, et al. Beneficial effects of short-term vasopressin infusion during severe septic shock. Anesthesiology 2002;96:576–82.
[74] Holmes CL, Walley KR. Vasopressin in the ICU. Curr Opin Crit Care 2004;10:442–8.
[75] Sharshar T, Blanchard A, Paillard M, et al. Circulating vasopressin levels in septic shock. Crit Care Med 2003;31:1752–8.
[76] Sun Q, Dimopoulos G, Nguyen DN, et al. Low-dose vasopressin in the treatment of septic shock in sheep. Am J Respir Crit Care Med 2003;168:481–6.
[77] Westphal M, Stubbe H, Sielenkamper AW, et al. Effects of titrated arginine vasopressin on hemodynamic variables and oxygen transport in healthy and endotoxemic sheep. Crit Care Med 2003;31:1502–8.
[78] Guzman JA, Rosado AE, Kruse JA. Vasopressin vs norepinephrine in endotoxic shock: systemic, renal, and splanchnic hemodynamic and oxygen transport effects. J Appl Physiol 2003;95:803–9.
[79] Levy B, Vallee C, Lauzier F, et al. Comparative effects of vasopressin, norepinephrine, and L-canavanine, a selective inhibitor of inducible nitric oxide synthase, in endotoxic shock. Am J Physiol Heart Circ Physiol 2004;287:H209–15.
[80] van Haren FM, Rozendaal FW, van der Hoeven JG. The effect of vasopressin on gastric perfusion in catecholamine-dependent patients in septic shock. Chest 2003;124:2256–60.
[81] Klinzing S, Simon M, Reinhart K, et al. High-dose vasopressin is not superior to norepinephrine in septic shock. Crit Care Med 2003;31:2646–50.
[82] Martikainen T, Tenhunen J, Uusaro A, et al. The effects of vasopressin on systemic and splanchnic hemodynamics and metabolism in endotoxin shock. Anesth Analg 2003;97:1756–63.
[83] Dünser M, Mayr A, Tur A, et al. Ischemic skin lesions as a complication of continuous vasopressin infusion in catecholamine-resistant vasodilatory shock: incidence and risk factors. Crit Care Med 2003;31:1394–8.
[84] Lee YH, Clarke KW, Alibhai HI, et al. Effects of dopamine, dobutamine, dopexamine, phenylephrine, and saline solution on intramuscular blood flow and other cardiopulmonary variables in halothane-anesthetized ponies. Am J Vet Res 1998;59:1463–72.
[85] Swanson CR, Muir WW 3rd, Bednarski RM, et al. Hemodynamic responses in halothane-anesthetized horses given infusions of dopamine or dobutamine. Am J Vet Res 1985;46:365–70.
[86] Donaldson LL. Retrospective assessment of dobutamine therapy for hypotension in anesthetized horses. Vet Surg 1988;17:53–7.
[87] Wertz E, Dunlop D, Wagner AE, et al. Cardiovascular and oxygen responses to dobutamine and dopamine in halothane anesthetized horses. Vet Surg 1992;21:501–2.
[88] Trim CM, Adams JG, Cowgill LM, et al. A retrospective survey of anaesthesia in horses with colic. Equine Vet J 1989;(Suppl 7):84–90.

[89] Valverde A, Giguere S, Sanchez C, et al. Effects of dobutamine, norepinephrine, and vasopressin on cardiovascular function in anaesthetized neonatal foals with induced hypotension. American Journal of Veterinary Research 2006;67:1730–7.

[90] Hollis AR, Ousey JC, Palmer L, et al. Effects of norepinephrine and a combined norepinephrine and dobutamine infusion on systemic hemodynamics and indices of renal function in normotensive neonatal Thoroughbred foals. Journal of Veterinary Internal Medicine 2006;20(6):1437–42.

[91] Sneddon J, Van der Walt J, Mitchell G, et al. Effects of dehydration and rehydration on plasma vasopressin and aldosterone in horses. Physiol Behav 1993;54:223–8.

[92] Picker O, Schwarte LA, Roth HJ, et al. Comparison of the role of endothelin, vasopressin and angiotensin in arterial pressure regulation during sevoflurane anaesthesia in dogs. Br J Anaesth 2004;92:102–8.

[93] O'Connor SJ, Gardner DS, Ousey JC, et al. Development of baroreflex and endocrine responses to hypotensive stress in newborn foals and lambs. Pflugers Arch 2005;450:298–306.

[94] Minneci PC, Deans KJ, Banks SM, et al. Differing effects of epinephrine, norepinephrine, and vasopressin on survival in a canine model of septic shock. Am J Physiol Heart Circ Physiol 2004;287:H2545–54.

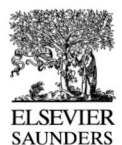

An Evidence-Based Approach to Clinical Questions in the Practice of Equine Neurology

Jérôme Van Biervliet, DVM[a,b,*]

[a]Neuronal Cell Biology and Gene Transfer Laboratory, Department for Molecular and Developmental Genetics, VIB, Leuven, Belgium
[b]Neuronal Cell Biology and Gene Transfer Laboratory, Center for Human Genetics, K.U., Leuven, Herestraat 49-602, 3000 Leuven, Belgium

As the understanding of equine diseases has rapidly grown, studies have been published that enable clinicians to take an evidence-based approach in daily practice, allowing a more accurate diagnosis of cervical vertebral compressive myelopathy (CVCM). The equine clinician should consider all components of the diagnostic process from history taking and clinical examination to advanced imaging as tests, each of which has its own inherent accuracies and limitations. Clinicians should also be aware of the precise prevalence of the disease in question and its differential diagnoses as well as the limitations of each of the diagnostic tests and, more importantly, of the combination of all of them.

Pathogenesis and pathologic findings

CVCM is characterized by the compression of the spinal cord at the level of two adjacent cervical vertebrae. This compression results in chronic or repetitive trauma, nerve conduction block, and, finally, axonal loss causing neurologic signs.

Clinical signs attributable to CVCM are most commonly insidious in onset. Typically, they are also progressive. However, acute exacerbation after what may seem to be a minor trauma is common in the history, and owners frequently report an acute onset of gait deficits. Clinical signs of mild ataxia

* Neuronal Cell Biology and Gene Transfer Laboratory, Center for Human Genetics, K.U., Leuven, Herestraat 49-602, 3000 Leuven, Belgium
 E-mail address: jerome.vanbiervliet@med.kuleuven.be

and paresis may be frequently missed by the owners and, in fact, may be the cause of a falling episode leading up to the exacerbation of clinical signs [1].

CVCM occurs in two broad classes of horses. A first type of CVCM is essentially a developmental disease in which malformation and malarticulation of the cervical vertebrae cause spinal cord compression. The higher incidence of this disease in Thoroughbred horses suggests an inherited basis, but attempts at characterizing the mode of inheritance have failed so far. It is more likely a multifactorial disease to which environmental influences and genetic predisposition contribute [1]. Young male horses, especially rapidly growing individuals, are at higher risk. A high carbohydrate ration and dietary zinc excess and copper deficiency seem to predispose to the development of CVCM [2,3]. Possibly, traumatic events and activity level at a young age can influence the onset of clinical signs as well. In this and other aspects, CVCM is similar to other developmental orthopedic diseases, such as osteochondrosis, epiphysitis, and acquired angular limb deformities, and such disorders do occur in the same patients [4]. Nevertheless, it should be repeated that the exact cause of CVCM in young growing horses has not been determined.

A second class of horses affected by CVCM is generally of old age, although it can occur in young adults. A breed predisposition for this type of CVCM is not readily apparent. These cases are characterized by spinal cord compression attributable to osteoarthritic enlargement of articular processes. To complicate matters, however, such osteoarthritic enlargement is frequently seen in older horses without neurologic signs. This perhaps suggests that only predisposed individuals develop neurologic signs, and such predisposition might include individuals with a relatively narrow vertebral canal.

Describing the pathologic changes found in CVCM before discussing the diagnostic tests used in the live animal is useful and important, because projections of pathologic changes on radiographs are used as diagnostic tests. Postmortem confirmation of the presence and nature of spinal cord compression is the diagnostic "gold standard" that measures the accuracy of these radiographic tests. Multiple pathologic changes can be seen in cases of CVCM. Individuals often have several of these bony and soft tissue changes [5,6].

In the CVCM of younger horses, vertebral malformation results in a disproportionately shorter vertebral body compared with an apparently caudally extended vertebral arch and a narrower vertebral canal, especially in a dorsoventral direction, at the caudal vertebral orifice. This gives the affected vertebrae an overall funnel shape, which may contribute to instability between adjacent vertebrae. This instability then results in secondary changes, such as angular (lordotic or kyphotic) deviations of the vertebrae, dorsal flare of the caudal epiphysis of the vertebral body, and degenerative osteoarthritis of the articular processes with possible osteophyte formation. At this abnormal articulation, the cranial orifice of the vertebral foramen of the more caudal vertebra is also often narrowed dorsoventrally. Importantly, soft tissue changes can also be involved in the compression, including thickening of the ligamentum flavum, thickening of the joint capsules, and extradural synovial cyst formation.

The CVCM seen in older horses is usually attributable to severe osteoarthritis of the articular processes. This type of CVCM is associated with extensive bone proliferation and joint capsule thickening, which compresses the spinal cord in a dorsolateral direction.

Clinical signs and neurologic examination

A careful and complete neurologic examination should be the first step in the diagnostic process. The neurologic examination is solely intended to make an accurate neuroanatomic diagnosis, from which a suitable list of differential diagnoses can be drawn. In other words, the clinician should attempt to locate the lesion to the spinal cord, brain stem, cerebellum, forebrain, or peripheral nerves and to determine whether it is focal, multifocal, or diffuse.

The neurologic examination of a horse with CVCM reveals clinical signs related to the dysfunction of the upper motor neuron (UMN) and general proprioceptive (GP) tracts in all four limbs. These clinical findings place a lesion in the cervical spinal cord [1,7]. The UMN tracts descend from higher centers. They are responsible for the regulation of muscle tone in supporting the body against gravity and in initiating voluntary movement of different muscles and parts of the body. Their dysfunction causes a spastic form of paresis. The GP tracts are ascending. They function to transmit sensory information about position and movement of muscles, tendons, and joints to higher centers. Hence, interruption of these GP tracts results in ataxia because of the loss of control of the position of the limbs in space, and thus the ability to coordinate voluntary movements accurately.

The clinical signs seen with CVCM are always a combination of deficits in both functional systems—spastic paresis and ataxia. Ataxia, or incoordination of movements, spasticity, or inappropriate rigidity, and paresis, or weakness, in all four limbs are the clinical signs caused by cervical spinal cord lesions. It is nearly impossible to attribute specific signs to either system individually, nor is it important to do so. Clinical signs are usually symmetric and are present in the thoracic and pelvic limbs, because the cervical spinal cord contains tracts to and from both. Signs are frequently more obvious in the pelvic limbs; however, because of the more superficial location within the spinal cord of the tracts related to the pelvic limbs.

Evaluating postural reactions (eg, hopping) is difficult in adult horses and can be dangerous in neurologic patients. Therefore, the neurologic examination aimed at detecting evidence of spinal cord disease mostly consists of judicious evaluation of the patient's gait on a nonslippery surface. Several maneuvers can be performed. These maneuvers require finely tuned coordination of UMN and GP functions, and therefore might exacerbate the clinical signs if such coordination is lacking.

Walking the horse in a straight line may show the following gait deficits in different combinations: varying stride lengths, floating or dragging of the hooves, outward or inward swaying of the limbs in motion, and unsteady movement of the pelvis and trunk. Head elevation can worsen these signs, especially the "floating" of the thoracic limbs and buckling of distal limbs, which may also be combined with scuffing the hooves. Care needs to be taken with horses of certain breeds when interpreting floating (eg, Paso Finos, Tennessee Walking Horses), because some mild but consistent floating can be present normally.

Horses with neurologic deficits may also have difficulty in walking on and off a step or a slope and may hit the step or stumble. Walking the horse in tight circles is probably the most sensitive clinical test of normal UMN and GP function. The animal with UMN and GP deficits is slow in protraction of the limbs; commonly pivots on the inside limb; circumducts the outer pelvic limb in a spastic rigid manner; and sometimes scuffs its hooves, steps on itself, or strikes the inside of its own limbs. Repeating this maneuver with the head slightly elevated on a slight slope, on and off a step, or more rapidly can often make subtle abnormalities more noticeable.

Paresis can be subjectively evaluated by pulling the horse's tail or mane firmly to either side (preferably when the horse is in, or just before, the weight-bearing phase of the gait on the ipsilateral limb). Horses with CVCM can be more easily pulled over, and the horse sometimes stumbles in an attempt to correct its posture. Spinal cord disease also commonly results in difficulty in backing the horse; it appears awkward, and the limbs can drag and protract quite slowly. In severe cases, the horse can fall backward.

In clear contrast to young horses with CVCM, manipulation of the head and neck of older horses with CVCM can sometimes appear painful, likely because of painful osteoarthritic disease of the articular processes rather than the spinal cord disease itself. Results of cerebrospinal fluid analyses are normal, although the fluid may rarely be slightly xanthochromic (yellow), the presence of which is good evidence to support a history of an intrathecal bleeding episode.

Imaging

To help confirm the suspicion of CVCM, properly positioned lateral survey radiographs of the occiput, all the cervical vertebrae, and T1 should be taken with the horse standing and the neck in a neutral posture (ie, neither flexed nor extended). This can most easily be performed under light sedation, because long exposure times require the horse to stand still. Several pathologic changes can be recognized, and these characteristic observations can be graded (Fig. 1) as follows [8]:

1. Mild subluxation of the vertebrae, seen as the degree of dorsal angulation between the adjacent vertebrae
2. Physeal enlargement and dorsal projection of the caudal physis of the vertebral body
3. Osteoarthritis and bony proliferation of the articular processes
4. Osteochondrotic changes, including incomplete or delayed postnatal ossification at the articular processes
5. Apparent caudal extension of the dorsal aspect of the vertebral arch over the cranial physis of the next caudal vertebral body

A measurement of the sagittal ratio can help to estimate the relative size of the vertebral foramen. The sagittal ratio is calculated as the ratio of the minimum sagittal diameter of the vertebral foramen to the maximum sagittal diameter of the vertebral body, taken at the cranial aspect of the vertebra and perpendicular to the vertebral canal (Fig. 2) [9]. Because it is taken within the vertebral body, it is also called the "intravertebral" sagittal ratio. Taking two measurements in the same plane of magnification eliminates differences caused by body size and radiographic magnification. A ratio less than 52% for C3-C4, C4-C5, and C5-C6 and less than 56% for C6-C7 is indicative of vertebral foramen narrowing and was suggested as a criterion for the diagnosis of CVCM. The sensitivity and specificity of this test in detecting CVCM-affected horses are approximately 90% [9]. Some care should be taken in the individual case, however, because this measurement likely does not indicate the site of compression accurately. In addition, depending on the prevalence of CVCM and other differential diagnoses in a particular population of horses with signs of cervical spinal cord disease, the chance of classifying the individual horse correctly as affected or not based on sagittal ratios only (so-called "predictive values") may not be the same everywhere. It is thus logical not to rely on sagittal ratios exclusively but to combine several readouts from diagnostic tests (radiographs) to improve the overall accuracy of the diagnosis.

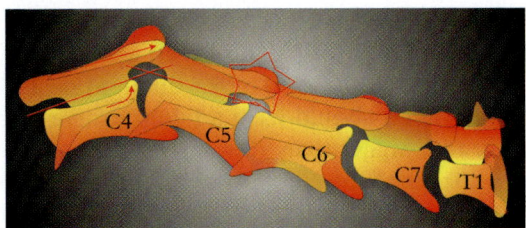

Fig. 1. Schematic drawing of the cervical vertebrae in neutral position illustrating the survey radiographic changes in CVCM: subluxation, apparent extension of the vertebral arch, dorsal projection of the caudal epiphysis, and degenerative changes of the articular processes. Note that C6 can easily be recognized by its broad lateral process in most horses.

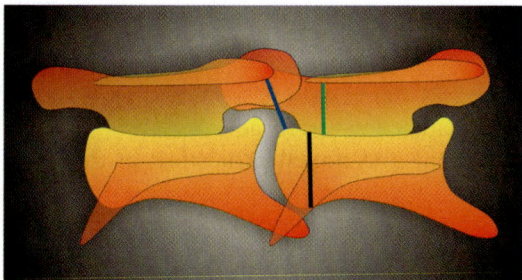

Fig. 2. Schematic drawing of the cervical vertebrae illustrating the sagittal ratios: the intravertebral sagittal ratio is calculated as the ratio of the minimum sagittal diameter of the spinal canal (*green line*) to the maximum sagittal diameter of the vertebral body, taken at the cranial aspect of the vertebra and perpendicular to the spinal canal (*black line*). The intervertebral sagittal ratio is the ratio of the minimal distance taken from the most cranial aspect of the vertebral body to the most caudal aspect of the vertebral arch of the more cranial vertebra (*blue line*) and the maximal sagittal diameter of the vertebral body (*black line*).

Recently, intervertebral sagittal ratios have been proposed as readouts taken from survey radiographs that could possibly assist in the diagnosis of spinal cord compression (J. Mayhew and C. Hahn, personal communication, 2004) [10]. In essence, this is a ratio of the minimal distance taken from the most craniodorsal aspect of the vertebral body to the most caudal aspect of the vertebral arch of the more cranial vertebra and the maximal sagittal diameter of the cranial region of the caudal vertebral body (see Fig. 2). The hypothesis for using this ratio is that it may correlate more closely to the occurrence of spinal cord compression, because, in CVCM, this compression occurs most often at the articulation of two adjacent vertebrae.

This hypothesis was tested in a population of horses with CVCM, with a confirmed site of compression postmortem as a gold standard. The sagittal ratios in horses with CVCM were compared with the ratios of horses affected by spinal cord diseases other than CVCM. The intra- and intervertebral sagittal ratios were statistically lower in CVCM-affected horses.

Adequate decision criteria can be identified to separate CVCM-affected versus nonaffected cases (Fig. 3) based on the receiver operator characteristic (ROC) curves. These curves plot the false-negative rate (or sensitivity) and the false-positive rate (specificity) of the different possible cutoff values. Preferably, decision criteria should have a false-positive rate less than 10% and a false-negative rate higher than 90%, placing adequate cutoff values in the left uppermost corner of the curve. Interestingly, it seems that the intervertebral sagittal ratio is a superior criterion compared with the intravertebral sagittal ratio (larger area under the curve [AUC]).

If an attempt is made to predict the site of compression, however, the ratios of the compressed sites should be compared with those of noncompressed sites in horses with other diseases (controls) and CVCM cases

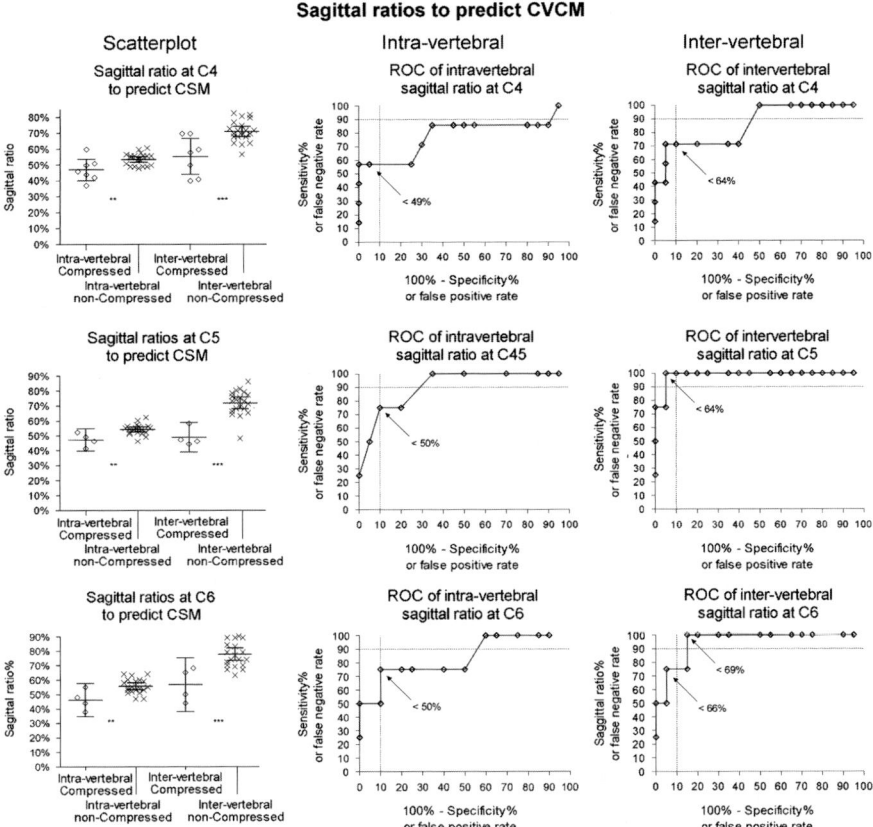

Fig. 3. As control values, the sagittal ratios of corresponding sites are taken in horses with other diseases than CVCM. Receiver operator characteristic curves can be drawn to select actual cutoff values for the intra- and intervertebral sagittal ratios. Cutoff values that result in a lower false-positive rate and the highest possible sensitivity (or false-negative rate) should be selected. The dotted lines indicate the desired 10% and 90% values respectively. The cutoff value with the best combination of sensitivity and false-positive rate is indicated. Possibly, the intervertebral sagittal ratio could be a superior criterion compared with the intravertebral sagittal ratio (area under the curve larger in most instances). In the left column, scatterplots, means, and 95% confidence intervals of the sagittal ratios at the inter- or intravertebral sites of C4, C5, and C6, respectively, are shown with the statistical significance indicated (Student's t test; $*P<0.05$; $**P<0.01$; $***P<0.001$).

(compressed at other sites). Such comparison introduces significant overlap between the values of compressed and control values (Fig. 4); it becomes difficult to identify a cutoff value with an adequate false-positive rate and false-negative rate in an ROC curve [10]. It can therefore be concluded that the intervertebral sagittal ratio, like the intravertebral sagittal ratio, cannot be used to predict the site of compression in CVCM. The intervertebral sagittal ratio seems to be a slightly superior criterion for diagnosis when compared with the intravertebral sagittal ratio.

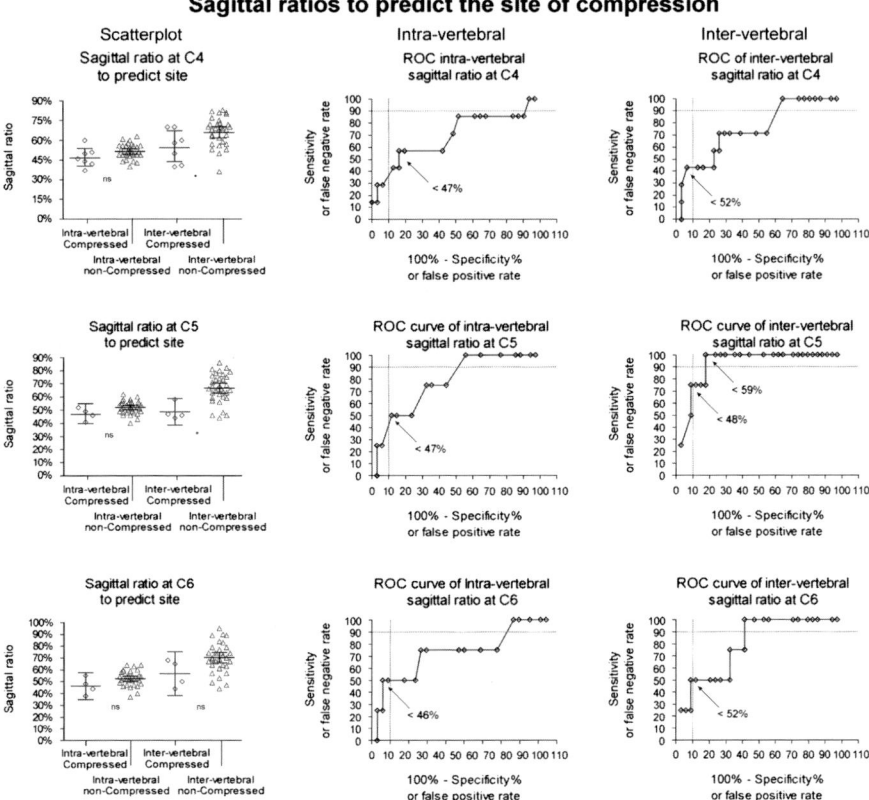

Fig. 4. As control values, the sagittal ratios of all corresponding noncompressed sites are taken in horses with diseases other than CVCM as well as in horses with CVCM but with a different site of compression than the site in question. Again, scatterplots (means and 95% confidence intervals [Student's t test; $*P<0.05$; $**P<0.01$; $***P<0.001$]) and ROC curves can be drawn for the intra- and intervertebral sagittal ratios, with 10% and 90% values indicated by the dotted line. Importantly, the differences seen before between CSM and non-CSM horses are lost to some degree; as a result, the decision criteria that can be defined have a poor accuracy. Therefore, neither the intravertebral nor the intervertebral sagittal ratio should be used to predict the site of compression in CSM.

Cervical myelography can also be a useful asset in helping to confirm a diagnosis of CVCM. In many cases, it remains the only tool available to assist in defining the site of spinal cord compression when the intention is surgical correction. The procedure for this test is fairly straightforward. Under general anesthesia, the horse is placed in lateral recumbency and a spinal needle is placed in the subarachnoid space of the cerebellomedullary cistern (cisterna magna). The preferred contrast medium in the horse is iohexol (iodine, 240 mg/mL), and a volume of 50 to 75 mL is injected slowly into the subarachnoid space. After the injection and removal of the needle, the horse's head and neck are elevated at approximately 30° for 5 to 10 minutes to aid in the caudal flow of the contrast medium. At least three radiographic views are usually necessary for good visualization of all cervical vertebrae. These views should be evaluated in neutral and flexed positions. Adequate flexion of the neck is empiric but has generally been achieved when the horse's nose is placed between the carpi.

It should be noted that from an evidence-based perspective that the diagnostic criteria for compression based on myelographic observations have not been definitively established. Reduction of the dorsal myelographic column (DMC) at the intervertebral junction to a value of 50% or less of that within the vertebra has been traditionally used to predict compression at this site.

Recently, this traditional test was examined in a similar manner as described previously. As a result, it is apparent that the DMC reduction should be interpreted conservatively, because the diagnostic accuracy of this criterion is less than desirable (Table 1) [11]. It is likely that more compression (up to 70% reduction of the DMC) is necessary to avoid false-positive diagnoses. Possibly, reduction of the total height of the dural sac, represented in a ratio of the minimal dural diameter at the intervertebral junction (left green line, Fig. 5) to the maximal dural diameter at the level of the midvertebral body (right green line, see Fig. 5), might reflect spinal cord compression more accurately. Greater than a 20% reduction has been suggested as potentially being useful in diagnosis of CVCM (Table 2) [11].

Table 1
Sensitivity and specificity of the "dorsal myelographic column (DMC) reduction rule" (compression present when the intervertebral DMC is reduced to greater than or equal to the cutoff value compared with the intravertebral DMC) change if the decision criterion is changed

		75%		70%		65%		60%		55%		50%		40%		30%	
Site	Position	Se	Sp	Se	Sp	Se	Sp	Se	Sp	Se	Sp	Se	Sp	Se	Sp	Se	Sp
C3–4	N	0	**100**	0	**100**	0	**100**	0	**100**	0	97	0	97	60	**90**	60	86
	F	0	89	14	89	29	85	57	81	57	78	71	78	86	74	86	67
C4–5	N	0	**100**	0	**100**	20	97	20	97	40	97	40	**90**	60	80	80	63
	F	60	**90**	60	**90**	60	**90**	60	83	80	80	80	73	80	63	80	60
C5–6	N	33	**100**	33	**100**	33	97	33	**94**	33	**90**	33	**90**	33	81	67	52
	F	0	**94**	50	**94**	50	**94**	50	**91**	50	**91**	50	88	100	85	100	73
C6–7	N	100	**93**	100	**90**	100	86	100	83	100	79	100	76	100	55	100	41
	F	50	**100**	50	**100**	50	**100**	50	**100**	50	**96**	50	**96**	50	**96**	100	81

The author suggests choosing a cutoff value based on the Sp because of the severe implications of a false-positive diagnosis and the smaller confidence intervals associated with the Sp. Using a more stringent reduction of the DMC (eg, 65%–70%) instead of the suggested 50% leads to acceptable specificity.

Specificities of 90% or greater have been indicated in bold to ease the selection of decision criteria, because using criteria with a specificity equal to or greater than 90% results in 10% or less false-positive diagnoses.

Abbreviations: F, flexed; N, neutral; Se, sensitivity; Sp, specificity.

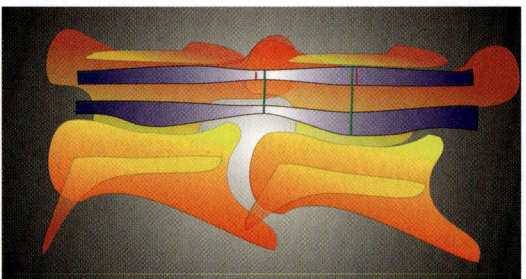

Fig. 5. Schematic drawing of cervical myelogram illustrating the dural diameter reduction (*green lines*) and the dorsal myelographic column reduction (*pink lines*).

It should be stressed that it is especially difficult to diagnose definitively the site of compression correctly in all CVCM cases, because affected horses seem to have a narrowed vertebral canal at several sites and compression could be located at any or several of these. Flexion of the neck can exacerbate the cord compression in CVCM cases, especially in the midcervical region. Nevertheless, flexion may also create reduction of the DMC in normal horses or, more importantly, at functionally nonaffected sites, thus leading to a false-positive diagnosis [11].

Fortunately, myelography is relatively safe, although a proportion of the horses can have complications. Complications range from prolonged

Table 2
Sensitivity and specificity for the accuracy of the "dural diameter (DD) reduction rule" (compression present when the intervertebral DD is reduced to greater than or equal to the cutoff value)

		45%		40%		35%		30%		25%		20%		15%	
Site	Position	Se	Sp	Se	Sp	Se	Sp	Se	Sp	Se	Sp	Se	Sp	Se	Sp
C3–4	N	0	**100**	0	**100**	0	**100**	14	**100**	29	**100**	57	**97**	57	83
	F	0	**96**	43	88	43	77	71	62	86	54	86	27	100	19
C4–5	N	0	**100**	0	**100**	20	**100**	20	**100**	40	**97**	60	**97**	60	**90**
	F	0	**100**	20	**97**	40	87	60	77	80	50	80	37	100	17
C5–6	N	0	**100**	0	**100**	0	**100**	0	**100**	0	**100**	33	**94**	33	87
	F	0	**100**	0	**97**	50	**94**	50	84	50	75	100	59	100	47
C6–7	N	0	**100**	33	**100**	33	**100**	100	**97**	100	**97**	100	**93**	100	87
	F	0	**100**	50	**100**	50	**100**	50	**100**	100	**100**	100	**100**	100	**91**

Using similar logic as for the dorsal myelographic column reduction rule, one can withhold a 20% reduction as a cutoff value to avoid false-positive diagnoses, especially in the neutral view.

Specificities of 90% or greater have been indicated in bold to ease the selection of decision criteria, because using criteria with specificity greater than or equal to 90% results in 10% or less false-positive diagnoses.

Abbreviations: F, flexed; N, neutral; Se, sensitivity; Sp, specificity.

recovery from anesthesia, seizures, and cortical blindness to nonsuppurative meningitis and associated fever. Mostly these complications are self-limiting [12].

CT to diagnose CVCM is of limited value because of size limitations. Most machines can only accommodate the horse's head and neck up to C4. In addition, the horse's neck must remain in extension during the CT procedure, preventing any flexion studies.

Summary

One should consider the process of the clinical evaluation and ancillary diagnostic procedures as tests that are run in series and in parallel, which, together, are capable of improving the overall accuracy of diagnosis of CVCM. Importantly, in all likelihood, there is no diagnostic test that is accurate enough on its own. Even with the available tests, it remains a challenge to find the site of compression, particularly when surgical correction is intended. Hopefully, development in CT and MRI hardware may make these (and other) imaging modalities available for use in the diagnosis of CVCM. Perhaps functional conduction studies may be established to determine the site of conduction block. Interestingly, even though elderly human patients with cervical spondylotic myelopathy have a different pathogenesis than equine patients with CVCM, they also frequently have multilevel vertebral canal narrowing, and a comparison of the MRI imaging with functional conduction testing has revealed that the sites of maximal compression did not always correlate to the site of maximal functional conduction block [13]. The extent to which this is a problem in horses has not yet been determined.

References

[1] Mayhew IG. Problem 10: large animal neurology: a handbook for veterinary clinicians. Philadelphia: Lea & Febiger; 1989. p. 243–66.
[2] Kronfeld DS, Meacham TN, Donoghue S. Dietary aspects of developmental orthopaedic disease. Vet Clin North Am Equine Pract 1990;6:451–65.
[3] Knight DA, Gabel AA, Reed SM. Correlation of dietary mineral to incidence and severity of metabolic bone disease in Ohio and Kentucky. Proceedings of the AAEP 1985;31:445–61.
[4] Stewart RH, Reed SM, Weisbrode SE. Frequency and severity of osteochondrosis in horses with cervical stenotic myelopathy. Am J Vet Res 1991;52:873–9.
[5] Trostle SS, Dubielzig RR, Beck KA. Examination of frozen cross sections of cervical spinal intersegments in nine horses with cervical vertebral malformation: lesions associated with spinal cord compression. J Vet Diagn Invest 1993;5:423–31.
[6] Cummings JF, Summers B, de Lahunta A. Injuries to the central nervous system: vertebral malformations and injuries to the spinal cord. Veterinary Neuropathology. Philadelphia: WB Saunders; 1995. p. 193–8.
[7] de Lahunta A. Veterinary neuroanatomy and clinical neurology. Philadelphia: WB Saunders; 1989.

[8] Mayhew IG, Donawick WJ, Green SL, et al. Diagnosis and prediction of cervical vertebral malformation in Thoroughbred foals based on semi-quantitative radiographic indicators. Equine Vet J 1993;25:435–40.
[9] Moore BR, Reed SM, Biller DS, et al. Assessment of vertebral canal diameter and bony malformations of the cervical part of the spine in horses with cervical stenotic myelopathy. Am J Vet Res 1994;55:5–13.
[10] Van Biervliet J. Survey radiographs of the cervical spine in the horse. Presented at the BEVA annual meeting. Birmingham, September 3, 2004. p. 134–5.
[11] van Biervliet J, Scrivani PV, Divers TJ, et al. Evaluation of decision criteria for detection of spinal cord compression based on cervical myelography in horses: 38 cases (1981–2001). Equine Vet J 2004;36:14–20.
[12] Van Biervliet J, J.F, Divers TJ, et al. The febrile response after cervical myelography in the horse: a retrospective analysis and experimental study [abstract 35]. Presented at the ACVIM annual meeting. Minneapolis (MN), June 6, 2004.
[13] Tani T, Kawasaki M, Taniguchi S, et al. Functional importance of degenerative spondylolisthesis in cervical spondylotic myelopathy in the elderly. Spine 2003;28:1128–34.

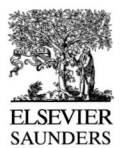

Evidence-Based Literature Pertaining to Thyroid Dysfunction and Cushing's Syndrome in the Horse

Nat T. Messer IV, DVM*, Philip J. Johnson, BVSc (Hons), MS, MRCVS

Department of Veterinary Medicine and Surgery, Veterinary Medical Teaching Hospital at Clydesdale Hall, College of Veterinary Medicine, University of Missouri, Columbia, MO 65211, USA

Thyroid dysfunction

Does primary hypothyroidism occur in horses?

Primary hypothyroidism has been reported in specific instances in horses. Goitrous autoimmune thyroiditis (Hashimoto's disease) and atrophic autoimmune thyroiditis are two recognized causes of primary hypothyroidism in human beings [1]. Atrophic autoimmune thyroiditis seems to be closely related to canine lymphocytic thyroiditis [2]. A recent report describing a Hashimoto's thyroiditis-like disease in horses from Eastern Europe indicates that up to 25% of slaughtered horses had abnormal thyroid glands, with microscopic alterations consistent with immune-mediated thyroiditis [3]. A subpopulation of those horses also had increased levels of thyroglobulin, of antithyroglobulin, and of antithyroid peroxidase autoantibodies compared with controls, helping to confirm the histopathologic diagnosis. Unfortunately, insofar as a diagnosis of primary hypothyroidism is concerned, there was no description of any abnormal clinical signs associated with this group of horses or any antemortem analysis of thyroid hormone (TH) levels. As a result, it is not known if this is an incidental finding or one that is isolated to a specific geographic region. There have been no similar reports from other parts of the world.

A congenital syndrome consisting of thyroid gland hyperplasia and TH-musculoskeletal deformity (TH-MSD) has been reported in the Pacific Northwest region of the North American continent [4–9]. It most often

* Corresponding author.
E-mail address: messern@missouri.edu (N.T. Messer).

occurs in the western provinces of Canada, but other cases have been described from Wisconsin, Washington, Oregon, and New York as well. Affected foals have variable clinical signs, but enough similarities exist between most foals to be able to identify a distinct syndrome [7].

There is no breed or gender predilection. Most affected foals are delivered after prolonged gestation (340–400 days). Despite the prolonged gestation, foals are dysmature with a short silky hair coat, pliable ears, muscle weakness, and incomplete skeletal development. In some instances, multiple cases occur on one farm. Dams have normal thyroid function at the time of parturition and are asymptomatic [8].

Serum thyroid hormone concentrations in foals with TH-MSD are usually low normal or lower than normal [6,9], and the thyroid glands do not respond to stimulation by thyroid-stimulating hormone (TSH). Histopathologic examination of the thyroid gland reveals colloid goiter with a large variation in follicular size or thyroid hyperplasia with small, crowded, irregular follicles.

The clinical signs most often reported are musculoskeletal abnormalities, especially failure of the cuboidal bones of the carpus and tarsus to ossify and mandibular prognathism. Less commonly reported signs are goiter, muscle weakness, rupture of the common digital extensor tendons, angular limb deformities, subnormal temperature, anemia, persistent lipemia, and listlessness. Most foals die or are euthanized in the first week of life. Those that survive display persistent musculoskeletal disease that is not reversed by thyroxine (T_4) supplementation. Even in foals first seen when several months old, a history reveals that the problems were present at birth [5].

The exact cause of TH-MSD is still not determined. An epidemiologic study of foals with this syndrome revealed that pregnant mares that were fed green feed, did not receive supplemental minerals, or grazed irrigated pastures had an increased risk of producing foals with the syndrome [9]. It was concluded that a combination of nitrate ingestion and low iodine levels in the feed may be responsible for the condition. If this is the case, iodine supplementation during gestation may help to prevent the syndrome.

What constitutes thyroid dysfunction in horses?

There are no studies that evaluate the incidence of thyroid dysfunction in horses in the general equine population. Controversial associations between hypothyroidism and obesity, abnormal accumulation of fat, and laminitis have arisen out of anecdotal reports. These associations must be viewed critically and carefully, however, because none of the latter clinical signs have ever been observed in thyroidectomized horses. Indeed, in one study of horses with obesity and chronic laminitis, triiodothyronine (T_3) levels were actually higher than in control animals and there was no difference in T_4 levels between affected animals and normal controls [10].

Much of the information about thyroid dysfunction has been derived from experimental models. These models give a much different constellation of clinical signs than do clinical cases, reported anecdotally or in case studies, which have had signs that have historically been attributed to low serum levels of THs. For example, in adult horses, low serum levels of THs have been associated with alopecia [11], anhidrosis [12], episodic rhabdomyolysis [13], and agalactia [14]. In foals, low serum levels of thyroid hormones have been associated with developmental orthopedic disease [4–7,9], respiratory distress [15], and stress and gastric ulcers [16]. When adult horses are made hypothyroid by surgical thyroidectomy [17–19], however, they demonstrate different clinical signs than those described in clinical reports, in which the diagnosis of hypothyroidism is based primarily on the measurement of serum TH levels. In thyroidectomized foals, clinical signs of developmental orthopedic disease and dysmaturity more closely resemble the signs observed clinically in foals with low serum levels of THs [20]. When adult horses are made hypothyroid by the administration of propylthiouracil (PTU), however, they show no clinical signs [21,22].

Surgical thyroidectomy has been performed in horses and ponies ranging in age from a 202-day-old fetus to an 18-year-old mare [17–20,23–25]. Thyroidectomized adult horses exhibit cold intolerance with shivering observed during cool weather, lethargy, reduced feed consumption, static growth rates, diminished sexual activity, thickening of the face, nonpainful swelling of the eyelids, rear limb edema, a coarse hair coat, mild alopecia, and delayed shedding of hair [17,18,23,25]. Of these clinical signs, only cold intolerance and hair coat abnormalities have been consistently observed. In fact, thyroidectomized horses are often clinically indistinguishable from normal healthy horses. Hypothyroidism might even go unnoticed because it is not life threatening and seems to be compensated for by other body processes [17].

Hypothyroid horses have been followed for as long as 3 years after thyroidectomy [17,24]. Thyroidectomized mares have experienced normal estrous cycles, and these mares have been successfully bred and subsequently delivered normal foals [23–25]. Thyroidectomized stallions demonstrated reduced libido; however, normal blood androgen concentrations have been detected, and mares have been successfully impregnated by these stallions (Figs. 1 and 2) [24,26].

Physical examination and laboratory findings for thyroidectomized horses include lower heart rates and rectal temperatures, reduced packed cell volume with normochromic normocytic anemia, and hypophosphatemia [18,19,23–25]. Blood lipoproteins are also affected by thyroidectomy. Hypothyroidism significantly alters blood lipid concentrations, resulting in elevated levels of very-low-density lipoproteins (VLDLs), the appearance of triglyceride-rich VLDLs in serum, increased levels of triglycerides and total cholesterol, and decreased blood levels of nonesterified fatty acids [18]. Alterations in cardiovascular function and exercise tolerance have been described in thyroidectomized horses [19]. It was proposed that hypothyroidism results in a reduction in the number or function of β-adrenergic receptors within cardiac tissues. Younger horses that have not yet reached

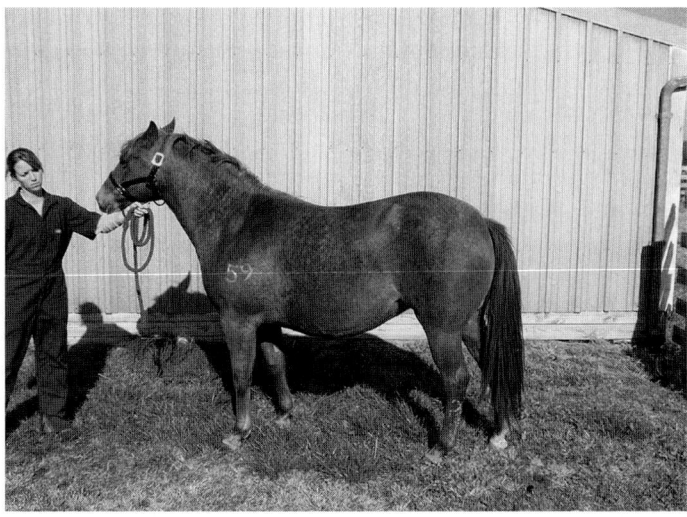

Fig. 1. "Sugar" (marked with a 59 freeze brand) before thyroidectomy at the time of acquisition in the autumn of 2003 and before thyroidectomy. The mare was thyroidectomized in the autumn of 2004.

maturity are more affected by thyroidectomy [17,20,23]. Compared with euthyroid controls, thyroidectomized yearlings and 2-year-olds were significantly shorter [17]. Body weight gains were 30% to 60% lower in three thyroidectomized mares compared with two controls. Delayed physeal closure and retention of deciduous teeth also occurred [17]. Severe stunting was observed in a thyroidectomized 1-month-old pony foal [23]. In utero partial thyroidectomy at approximately 8 months of gestation resulted in profound skeletal immaturity and abnormal mentation when the foals were born [20].

Hypothyroidism has been induced in horses through the oral administration of PTU at a dose of 4 mg/kg/d for 6 weeks [21,22]. PTU interferes with iodine binding to thyroglobulin within the thyroid gland and inhibits 5′-monodeiodinase activity in other tissues [22]. In the reports describing this model, laboratory test results for treated horses were consistent with primary hypothyroidism [21,22]. Serum T_3 and T_4 concentrations declined and TSH concentrations rose during the treatment period. After 6 weeks, a thyrotropin-releasing hormone (TRH) challenge resulted in a delayed and blunted response for T_3 and T_4 and an exaggerated rise in TSH. Results were suggestive of increased secretory activity of pituitary thyrotropes. Clinical signs of hypothyroidism were not observed in any of the treated animals.

In sum, based on experimental evidence and as opposed to clinical suggestions, when criteria established from studies of thyroidectomized animals are applied, adult-onset primary hypothyroidism seems to be a rare disease in horses [27].

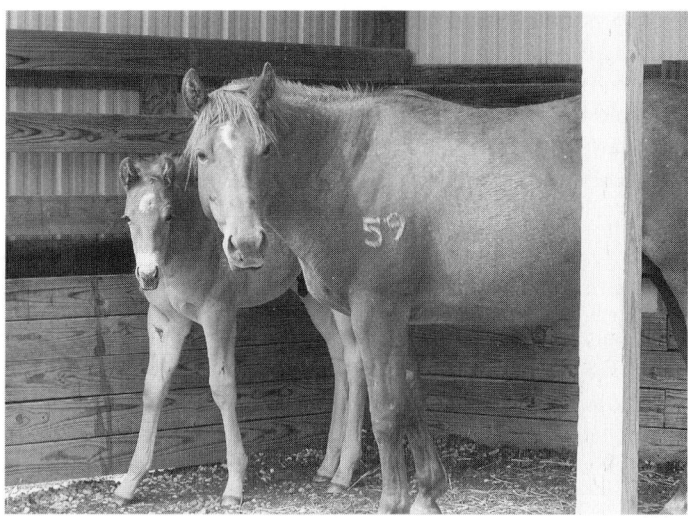

Fig. 2. "Sugar" with her 1-month-old normal foal born on March 6, 2007, nearly 2.5 years after thyroidectomy. The only thyroid hormone supplement the mare received after being thyroidectomized was in the spring of 2005 for a period of 4 weeks as part of a study on the effects of supplementation. The mare has had no supplementation of thyroid hormone since that time, even during pregnancy.

What is the best way to diagnosis hypothyroidism?

Serum total T_3 and T_4 measurements are readily obtained from diagnostic laboratories, but results are often misleading [27–31]. To diagnose hypothyroidism correctly, additional tests must be performed to determine if the hypothalamic-pituitary-thyroid axis is functioning normally. Animals should not be referred to as hypothyroid if the hormonal axis is normal [27]. Low TH concentrations detected in such cases are more likely to be a result of factors outside the thyroid gland.

To distinguish primary hypothyroidism from other disturbances of the hypothalamic-pituitary-thyroid axis, TSH concentrations must be measured. Subnormal serum concentrations of total T_3, total T_4, free (f) T_3, or fT_4 are accompanied by elevated TSH concentrations [21,22]. Pituitary secretion of TSH increases in an attempt to stimulate TH synthesis within the diseased thyroid gland. The use of fT_4 by equilibrium dialysis has recently been shown to be helpful in distinguishing nonthyroidal illness syndrome from other types of hypothyroidism [32].

Diagnostic testing for primary hypothyroidism is therefore limited to the measurement of serum TH concentrations and TRH response tests. To perform the TRH response test, a dose of TRH (1 mg) is administered intravenously and blood samples are collected after 2 and 4 hours [33,34]. In normal healthy horses, blood concentrations of T_3 and T_4 are twice that of baseline after 2 and 4 hours, respectively. This test should be used to confirm a diagnosis of hypothyroidism by documenting abnormal hypothalamic-pituitary-thyroid axis function. It cannot be used to distinguish primary disease from other types of hypothyroidism unless TSH concentrations are measured concurrently.

Does secondary (central, pituitary-dependent, idiopathic) hypothyroidism occur in horses?

Low TH levels also occur as a result of suppression of TSH formation or TRH-induced TSH release. Several nonthyroidal factors potentially affect the hypothalamic-pituitary-thyroid axis in horses, resulting in low levels of circulating TH, including phenylbutazone administration [35–37], high-energy diets [38], high-protein diets [39], diets high in zinc and copper [39], diets with a high carbohydrate/roughage ratio [40], glucocorticoid administration [41], food deprivation [42], level of training [43], stage of pregnancy [44–47], and ingestion of endophyte-infected fescue grass [48]. All have been shown to be associated with or to cause low levels of TH in euthyroid horses. In another study, the pituitary-thyroid axis was not affected in adult horses fed endophyte-infected fescue seed [49].

In patients with secondary hypothyroidism, the thyroid gland itself is normal and capable of responding to stimulation with TSH or TRH. The well-described effects of phenylbutazone therapy serve as a good example. Serum total T_4 concentrations were significantly lower on day 4 of phenylbutazone therapy (4.4 mg/kg administered intravenously for 5 days) and remained at lower than baseline values for 10 days [37]. Free T_4 concentrations also decreased significantly on day 4 but returned to normal 1 day after completion of therapy. Phenylbutazone is a highly protein-bound drug capable of displacing TH from carrier proteins. Increased availability of free hormone exerts a negative effect on the TH feedback pathway and inhibits the hypothalamic-pituitary-thyroid axis. Thyroid hormone secretion by the thyroid gland is thereby inhibited, resulting in reduced serum total T_3 and T_4 levels.

Most cases of apparent thyroid dysfunction in horses are diagnosed on the basis of clinical signs or on the basis of detecting low resting levels of TH in serum. Using these criteria alone, it is impossible to distinguish primary from secondary hypothyroidism [50]. Therefore, the use of TSH or TRH stimulation tests and measurements of TSH are necessary to differentiate primary from secondary hypothyroidism [51]. Unfortunately, these tests are used infrequently in horses because of expense, limited availability, safety issues, and the potential for spurious results. For example, depending on the underlying cause of secondary hypothyroidism, lack of response to TRH stimulation may, in fact, result in the misdiagnosis of primary hypothyroidism, because some causes of secondary hypothyroidism (ie, states of glucocorticoid excess) suppress TRH-induced TSH release [41]. Because validated assays for equine TSH are not yet readily available for routine testing, naturally occurring thyroid dysfunction in adult horses remains difficult to characterize; however, it seems that secondary forms of hypothyroidism are potentially more common causes of low TH levels in horses than disorders of the thyroid gland itself.

Many horses receive TH supplementation once low TH levels are detected in serum without regard for the type of hypothyroidism present and despite what seems to be an extremely low incidence of primary hypothyroidism in horses. The effects of TH supplementation in euthyroid horses or in horses with secondary hypothyroidism have yet to be determined, and TH supplementation should therefore be used with caution. Such supplementation may actually further suppress pituitary function in horses with low TH levels because of secondary hypothyroidism [52].

How should horses with secondary hypothyroidism be treated?

Identification and treatment of the underlying problem that has caused secondary hypothyroidism to occur should be the first priority. TH supplementation is of unknown benefit in cases of secondary hypothyroidism and could, at least theoretically, be detrimental in horses with low serum TH caused by certain nonthyroidal factors. That said, there are other endocrine disorders not related to thyroid disease that have historically been associated with thyroid dysfunction in which thyroid hormone supplementation seems to be beneficial [53].

Do horses get thyroid tumors?

Benign adenomas comprise most thyroid gland tumors. These tumors are not uncommon in older horses [54]. A sign associated with these adenomas is usually enlargement of the gland; rarely, if ever, does this result in hypothyroidism or hyperthyroidism. In addition, a few cases of C-cell tumors have been reported in horses. These horses have also been relatively free of abnormal clinical signs, with the exception of enlargement of the thyroid gland and continual gulping [55]. There are two reports of aged horses with hyperthyroidism and thyroid neoplasia. In one case [56], an aged Quarter Horse gelding with unilateral enlargement of the thyroid gland, there were clinical signs similar to those seen in other species with hyperthyroidism, including weight loss, hyperexcitability, polyphagia, and tachycardia. A hemithyroidectomy resulted in resolution of clinical signs and a return to normal of TH levels, which were persistently elevated before surgery. A histologic diagnosis of adenomatous hypertrophy or thyroid adenoma was made on the excised portion of the thyroid gland. In the other case [57], an aged half-Arabian gelding, there was also gross enlargement of the thyroid gland, weight loss, tachycardia, tachypnea, and behavioral abnormalities characterized by constant pacing in the paddock and difficulty in handling. Measurement of T_4 levels was within the normal range, but levels of fT_4 were markedly elevated. After surgical thyroidectomy, clinical signs disappeared and TH levels eventually returned to normal.

Summary

Occasional diagnoses of primary thyroid dysfunction are supported by a "gold standard" of postmortem evidence in a few instances. The currently available evidence would suggest that primary hypothyroidism is a rarely occurring disease in horses, however. A clinically relevant experimental model has been developed (thyroidectomized horses), and such animals do not fit the clinical picture typically described in many suspected clinical cases. There is a need for a reliable diagnostic test for hypothyroidism in horses. Although TH supplementation may have some clinical benefit in selected cases, such benefit has largely not been established in a solid foundation of evidence.

Equine Cushing's syndrome

Is there any evidence that the incidence of equine Cushing's syndrome is increasing?

The frequency with which veterinarians make a diagnosis of equine pituitary Cushing's syndrome (pituitary pars intermedia dysfunction [PPID]) seems to have increased during the past several years. This trend has likely been fueled by horse owners wishing to optimize the health of their older horses, substantial improvements in many aspects of the veterinary care of the older horse, enhanced interest in and awareness of the disease resulting from extensive new information published in the veterinary scientific literature, and the availability of new diagnostic tests [58]. Estimates of the prevalence of PPID have varied from 0.075% to 0.5% of the equine population, based largely on data published from veterinary teaching hospitals [59,60]. Newer publications have emphasized that PPID clearly arises in a younger population of horses than that previously believed and that subclinical PPID may be more widespread than generally recognized [61]. Therefore, these estimates of the prevalence of PPID should be regarded as conservative. There is no scientific evidence that the true incidence of the condition has changed, however.

What is equine Cushing's syndrome, and how long has it been recognized?

By definition, the term *Cushing's syndrome* describes the clinical consequence of glucocorticoids acting in excess of physiologic requirements.

Harvey Cushing originally described the clinical features of hypercortisolism ("Cushing's disease") in human patients experiencing the effects of a corticotropin-secreting corticotrope tumor in the pars distalis (PD), the most common form of Cushing's syndrome in people [62]. An equine form of the disease was recorded shortly afterward [63].

In contrast to the human condition, equine Cushing's syndrome is almost invariably attributable to clonal expansion of the melanotrope cell population in the pars intermedia (PI) of the pituitary gland. The resulting changes in the PI of affected horses have been variously referred to as pituitary hypertrophy, pituitary hyperplasia, or pituitary adenoma. The condition is currently widely referred to as PPID and represents one of the most common endocrinopathic conditions of older horses [64–66]. Evidence that Cushing's syndrome attributable to corticotropin-secreting adenohypophyseal tumors in the PD (corticotropinomas) ever arises in horses is virtually nonexistent [67]. Hypercortisolism resulting from primary adrenal gland tumors is also evidently rare in horses (Fig. 3) [68–70].

What is the primary underlying cause of pituitary pars intermedia dysfunction in horses?

Mounting evidence suggests that PPID arises as a consequence of a primary hypothalamic abnormality [71]. The secretion of proopiomelanocortin (POMC)-derived peptides from melanotropes in the PI is normally under the primary control of dopaminergic neurons originating in the hypothalamus [72,73]. Moreover, unlike corticotropin secretion by corticotropes in the

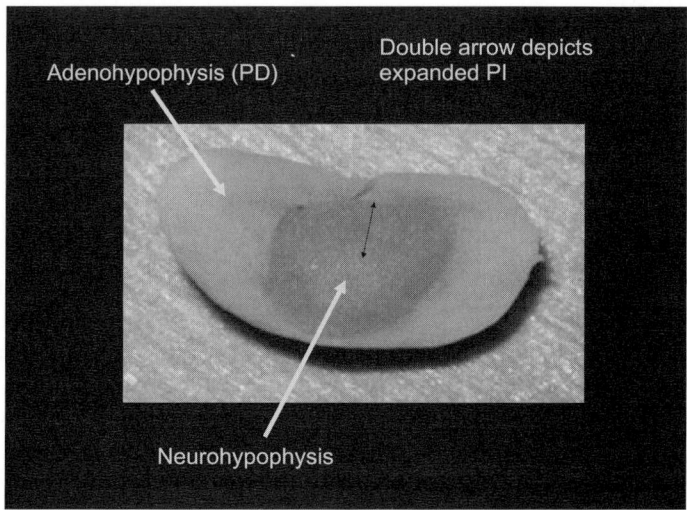

Fig. 3. Image of PPID-derived pituitary in cross section.

PD, the secretion of corticotropin (and other POMC-derived peptides) by melanotropes in the PI does not undergo circadian variance and is not under the influence of negative feedback associated with high circulating levels of glucocorticoids [74–76].

Strong evidence now points to the fact that PPID occurs as a result of a loss of this (inhibitory) dopaminergic influence from the hypothalamus. There exists little evidence to support the concept that melanotropic hyperplasia (neoplasia) in the PI arises as a spontaneous primary disease (as is thought to be the case in human patients with Cushing's syndrome with corticotrope adenomas in the PD) [60]. Specifically, there exists a reduced number of dopaminergic neurons in the periventricular nuclei (cell bodies) of the hypothalamus and in the PI (nerve terminals) of PPID-affected equids. This loss of inhibitory neurons has been attributed to the effects of oxidative stress (dopaminergic neurons are especially susceptible to oxidative stress) [71]. In one other study, horses with PPID also had increased circulating markers of oxidative stress, strengthening the hypothesis that PPID results from oxidative stress-associated neurodegenerative changes in dopaminergic nerves [77].

In further support of this hypothesis, the histologic appearance of the PI obtained from PPID-affected equids is similar to that seen in rats after PI denervation [78]. The concentration of dopamine (and its metabolites) in the PI of affected horses is markedly reduced, and the expression of type-2 dopamine receptors in affected melanotropes is increased (consistent with a response to dopaminergic denervation) [79,80]. Furthermore, the clinical signs of PPID and the circulating concentration of POMC peptides (products of PI melanotrope secretion) are significantly reduced after treatment using dopamine or dopaminergic agonists in affected horses [75,81,82].

How is the pituitary gland affected by loss of dopaminergic inhibition?

Biochemical studies of equine pituitary PI tumors have demonstrated that the hormonal profile of the abnormal state (PPID) resembles that of the normal PI [75,80,83,84]. Immunocytochemical studies have also confirmed that the POMC-derived peptides in equine pituitary adenomas resemble those of the normal PI [80,85,86]. Specifically, in equine PPID, the plasma concentrations of b-endorphin (b-END), a-melanocyte-stimulating hormone (a-MSH), b-MSH, g-MSH, and corticotropin-like intermediate peptide (CLIP) are increased [75,80,87]. In contrast to the situation in human patients affected with corticotrope tumors of the PD, the plasma concentration of corticotropin in many PPID-affected horses is relatively less elevated.

Macroscopic (gross) enlargement of the pituitary gland (macroadenoma) is not evident in all cases of PPID. Microscopic examination is necessary to demonstrate small adenoma formation (microadenoma) in the PI of a few affected pituitary glands [85]. It should be noted that nonfunctional pituitary adenomas represent incidental findings in approximately 25% of human autopsies [88]. It is being increasingly reported that PI adenomas are identified in young horses in which there are no clinical signs of Cushing's disease [89].

Although the major pathologic disturbance affects the intermediate lobe of the pituitary gland, abnormalities in the PD and the neurohypophysis may play a role in the clinical expression of PPID in some instances. For example, multinodular corticotrope hyperplasia has been described in the PD of some PPID-affected horses [85]. It has been suggested that, as is the case in other species, the presence of multinodular corticotrope hyperplasia in PPID-affected horses may result from inappropriate release of corticotropin-releasing factor (CRF) from the hypothalamus. This observation is relevant, because recent work has strongly implicated a role for perturbed hypothalamic function as the primary underlying basis for PPID in horses [71]. In some cases, clonal expansion of melanotropes leads to infiltration and destructive compression of the neurohypophysis [67,85,90].

Several publications have documented the cell population characteristics of the PI and the PD based on histologic and immunohistochemical staining techniques. A large precursor peptide, POMC, is the earliest product of the biosynthetic pathway in corticotropes in the PD and melanotropes in the PI. The posttranslational processing of POMC differs between corticotropes and melanotropes, however. In corticotropes, POMC is primarily processed to corticotropin, b-lipotropin, and lesser quantities of g-lipotropin and b-END. In melanotropes, corticotropin is further processed into a-MSH and CLIP [76,83,85]. This difference in the manner by which POMC is processed in corticotropes and melanotropes is attributable to the fact that corticotropes lack specific prohormone convertases I and II, the enzymes responsible for cleaving corticotropin (eg, to a-MSH) [91]. Therefore, corticotropin is the major product of POMC processing by corticotropes, whereas a-MSH is produced by melanotropes [80,91].

Immunohistochemical studies have demonstrated that most cells in the PI (melanotropes) stain strongly for POMC and a-MSH but are only weakly positive for corticotropin [85,89]. The population of cells within the PI is not homogeneous, however, and there exist small islands of cells close to the boundary with the neurohypophysis that stain positively for b-END [85,92]. Moreover, there exists a population of cells within the PI that lie in close proximity to the PD and are characterized by relatively higher immunoreactivity to corticotropin (compared with most cells in the PI) [89]. Some have suggested that it is an increase in this population of cells that explains the elevated circulating corticotropin concentrations and hypercortisolism seen in some PPID-affected horses [89]. Positive immunostaining for corticotropin has been reported to be greater in the PI of PPID-affected horses than in the PI of unaffected horses [67,86,89,93].

Although pathologic changes (adrenocortical hyperplasia) are also reported in the adrenal glands from some PPID-affected equids, this finding is relatively uncommon and is clearly only evident in a few (approximately 20%) cases [67,85,89]. Nodular or diffuse adrenocortical hyperplasia was demonstrated in only 4 of 19 PPID-affected horses in one report, underscoring the fact that excessive cortisol production is not a clinical feature in most affected horses [85]. That hypercortisolism is not common in PPID is likely explained by the observation that biochemically demonstrable corticotropin and corticotropin immunostaining in the normal PI and in PI adenomas is relatively weak and that the circulating corticotropin concentration is often not highly elevated [75,84–87]. Although corticotropin is secreted in relatively smaller quantities compared with other melanotrope-derived POMC peptides, excessive secretion of the other POMC peptides acts to potentiate the effectiveness of corticotropin at the adrenal glands (the steroidogenic action of corticotropin is increased sixfold by the other melanotrope-derived POMC peptides) [94,95].

The clinical consequences of PPID result from a constellation of various different pathologic processes. The old-fashioned concept that equine Cushing's syndrome results simply from excessive corticotropin production by a functional PI adenoma and resulting hypercortisolism (as is the case in many human and canine cases) has been replaced by a more complex and diverse pathophysiologic picture. Primary attenuation of hypothalamus-derived dopaminergic inhibition of melanotropes in the PI leads to hypersecretion of multiple POMC-derived peptides. Loss of normal physiologic inhibition results in melanotrope hypersecretion or clonal expansion (or both). If clonal expansion occurs to a sufficient extent, enlargement of the PI may occur, causing a macroscopically evident pituitary "adenoma." In those cases in which physical expansion of the PI occurs, adjacent structures, such as the PD, neurohypophysis, optic chiasm, and overlying hypothalamus, might be compressed. In a few cases, macroscopically evident PI expansion does not occur and the clinical results of melanotrope hypersecretion might be more simply attributable to the consequences of POMC-peptide excess. The extent to which the adrenal cortices are affected by PPID is also variable. Structurally evident adrenocortical hypertrophy has been reported in only approximately 20% of PPID-affected horses.

Is there a breed or gender predilection for pituitary pars intermedia dysfunction, and is it more likely at specific times of the year?

Morgan horses and pony breeds seem to be at greater risk for the development of PPID, but it can affect any breed [60,82,96–98]. In one study in which the association between laminitis and PPID was examined, PPID-affected ponies represented 40% of the study population compared with only 7.5% of ponies in the general equine hospital population over the same period [99].

There does not seem to be a gender predilection for PPID in horses based on more recent publications [60,67,82,85,96,100]. Earlier published reports suggested that female horses might be predisposed (as is the case for human beings with PD tumors), but those observations might have been attributable to the greater tendency to allow broodmares to live longer [67,85,101]. Some earlier reports suggested that male horses might be predisposed to PPID [96].

The age of most horses that are presented to veterinarians for PPID tends to exceed 18 years [60,82,100,101]. The mean age of horses with PPID reported in one literature analysis ranged from 18 to 23 years [82]. The minimum age at which PPID has been recorded in the literature is 7 years [75,85]. More recent publications have suggested that PPID may be under-recognized in younger horses [61]. Moreover, there is growing recognition that PPID is present in younger horses in the absence of the classic clinical signs, such as hirsutism and weight loss (Fig. 4).

In one study, the time of onset of laminitis in PPID-affected horses was reported to occur predominantly during the month of September [99]. Although a full explanation for the seasonal onset of laminitis in affected equids has not been ascertained, plausible explanations that have been proposed include the following: the pasture grass content of hydrolysable carbohydrates (a risk factor for laminitis) is increased at that time [102]; the risk of laminitis associated with ingestion of endophyte-affected tall fescue is greater at this time, possibly associated with higher plant content of endophytic alkaloids [103,104]; and the secretory output of the normal and PPID-affected equine pituitary gland seems to be increased during the autumn (September) [105].

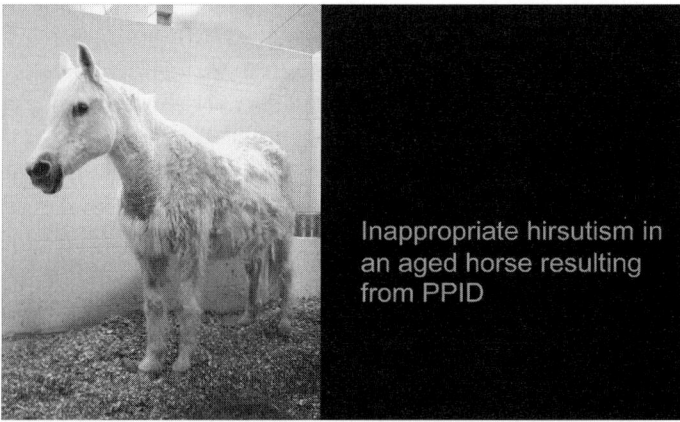

Fig. 4. Inappropriate hirsutism in an aged horse resulting from PPID.

Corroborating the clinical diagnosis of pituitary pars intermedia dysfunction

The diagnosis of PPID in older horses that have developed inappropriate hirsutism is often presumptively made without resort to further corroborative endocrinologic characterization. Inappropriate hirsutism has been described as a pathognomonic sign of PPID in affected horses [106]. Nevertheless, in light of the fact that the cost of (and lifelong commitment to) treatment for PPID using pergolide is not inconsequential, endocrinologic corroboration should be considered. Moreover, it is becoming evident that PPID occurs more commonly in younger horses than previously believed and that the clinical expression of the disease in these younger horses may not be so pathognomonic. Diagnosis of PPID in the absence of inappropriate hirsutism is challenging [106]. Several aspects of the clinical appearance of PPID-affected horses could just as likely be attributed to other primary diseases (eg, laminitis) or the effects of advancing age. Corroboration of the PPID diagnosis requires specific endocrinologic testing.

Is the determination of plasma cortisol concentration helpful for diagnosis of pituitary pars intermedia dysfunction?

It is not possible to differentiate normal from abnormal horses satisfactorily by simply measuring the plasma cortisol concentration, because hypercortisolemia is not evident in many PPID-affected horses [96,101]. Moreover, numerous other conditions and circumstances may be associated with elevated cortisol secretion, such as management, stress, effects of hospitalization, pain, and concurrent disease [66]. When the plasma cortisol was measured on a frequent basis (every 4 hours) during a 24-hour period, PPID-affected horses could be differentiated based on a loss of diurnal rhythmicity in one study [67]. Those authors concluded that substantial variation between individual horses would preclude the practical use of any single time point measurements of cortisol for purposes of making a diagnosis, however. Another author suggested that loss of diurnal rhythmicity, as demonstrated by simply comparing the plasma cortisol concentration measured in the morning with that in the afternoon, could be useful for the diagnosis of PPID. That concept has not been validated, however, and it should only be regarded as a screening tool at best [107].

Based on a small number of horses, the urinary concentration of cortisol, expressed as a ratio with the concentration of urinary creatinine, has been suggested as a potentially useful test for PPID in horses [108,109]. Supporting data are needed for validation before this diagnostic test can be recommended, however. Preliminary data pertaining to the measurement of cortisol in saliva suggest that the determination of salivary cortisol concentration may lack sufficient sensitivity and specificity for clinical application as a diagnostic test for PPID [110].

Should the low-dose dexamethasone suppression test be regarded as the gold standard for antemortem diagnosis of pituitary pars intermedia dysfunction?

The overnight low-dose dexamethasone (DEX) suppression test (DST) is often advocated as the classic gold standard antemortem test for PPID. This contention is supported by excellent research that entailed a series of endocrinologic testing protocols employing 66 PPID-affected horses (all confirmed at autopsy) and 55 normal controls (most of which were confirmed at autopsy) [67]. It has been advocated as the most practical and most reliable test for PPID in horses [67]. Failure of DEX to suppress the plasma cortisol concentration has been attributed to uninhibited production of corticotropin by melanotropes in the PI that is not under the influence of negative feedback.

In this test, DEX is administered as an intramuscular injection (0.04 mg/kg of body weight), and its effect on the circulating plasma (or serum) concentration of cortisol is evaluated after 19 hours [66]. In healthy horses, DEX inhibits the release of corticotropin from the PD (negative feedback) and the cortisol concentration decreases to less than 1 mg/dL [67]. In horses affected with PPID, the cortisol concentration is not reduced to this extent after treatment with DEX. As with most diagnostic tests (but with less frequency than many), false-positive [111] and false-negative [87] results have been reported for the DST. Although initial reports suggested that the DST had a sensitivity and specificity of 100% [67], more recent observations suggest that it may be a somewhat less reliable test than previously suggested [112].

Other potentially confounding effects on the DST have been reported, including the effect of seasonality. Specifically, DEX evidently fails to cause suppression of corticotropin release in many normal equids in September [113]. It has been suggested that the failure of DEX to suppress corticotropin release may arise in the later stages of the disease and that the high sensitivity of the DST reported previously [67] could be attributable to the fact that the horses in that study were relatively old (ie, the disease was relatively advanced) [114].

The most commonly cited objection to the DST pertains to the fact that administration of DEX has been associated with the risk for inducing or exacerbating laminitis, one of the commonly reported presenting clinical signs of PPID [66]. In one study in which 66 horses with PPID were treated with DEX, however, laminitis was not observed [67]. It has been suggested that if specific concern exists regarding the risk of laminitis after administration of the DST, a lower dose of DEX (0.02 mg/kg of body weight) might be just as useful as that originally published [66]. Although some clinicians have suggested that the presence of stress or pain might interfere with the veracity of the DST, one author has reported that the DST correctly demonstrated (using the lower dose of DEX) absence of PPID in 3 horses affected with painful acute laminitis [66]. Nevertheless, it seems that the risk of inciting or aggravating laminitis as a result of the DST is small.

Is the administration of thyrotropin-releasing hormone useful for the diagnosis of pituitary pars intermedia dysfunction?

TRH causes elevations in the plasma concentration of corticotropin, cortisol, and a-MSH in PPID-affected equids. This response has been attributed to relatively greater expression of TRH receptors in melanotropes (cf, corticotropes) [33,114]. Subsequently, the use of TRH in diagnostic tests has been advocated because it eliminates the necessity of administering DEX to patients affected with PPID.

In one study, the administration of TRH to PPID-affected horses (n = 7) and ponies (n = 4) caused an increase in the circulating concentration of cortisol after 15 to 90 minutes [33]. The circulating concentration of cortisol did not change when TRH was administered to healthy horses (n = 12) [33]. These observations formed the basis of the TRH stimulation test that has been used for the diagnosis of PPID in horses. TRH has also been reported to stimulate cortisol release in some normal horses, however [114]. In another study, the TRH stimulation test proved to be superior to a single-sample plasma corticotropin determination (4 horses) and the DST (1 horse) for identification of PPID (confirmed at necropsy) [61].

In one study, resting plasma concentrations of a-MSH (representing PI-derived POMC peptide secretion) and corticotropin (representing primarily PD-derived POMC peptide secretion) were increased in PPID-affected equids compared with normal horses. This study also showed that the plasma concentrations of α-MSH and corticotropin were increased after treatment with TRH in healthy horses (n = 16) and PPID-affected equids (n = 7) [114]. The extent to which corticotropin increased after treatment with TRH was much less than the extent to which α-MSH increased in normal horses.

In that report, the increased concentrations of α-MSH and corticotropin after TRH treatment were greater in the PPID-affected equids. It should be noted, however, that although the absolute plasma α-MSH concentration was greater in horses with PPID before and at 30 minutes after TRH administration, the magnitude of the plasma TRH-induced response did not differ between horses with PPID compared with the normal controls (618% ± 149% versus 1046% ± 492% of control [$P = .43$], healthy and PPID-affected horses, respectively) [114]. Treatment of the same horses with TRH also led to an increased plasma cortisol concentration, but the extent to which cortisol increased was not significantly different between normal and abnormal horses [114].

The authors of this study went on to confirm that increases in plasma α-MSH were a direct consequence of the action of TRH on melanotropes by treating PI and PD tissue explants with TRH for 24 hours ex vitro.

Treatment of PI tissue with TRH produced an increase in the α-MSH concentration in the supernatant, but α-MSH was not produced by the PD explants. All PD explants showed an increase in supernatant corticotropin concentration after treatment with TRH, but corticotropin was not produced by PI explants [114]. Using polymerase chain reaction (PCR) technology, evidence was also obtained to demonstrate that melanotropes (in the PI) and corticotropes (in the PD) express TRH receptors [114].

Although earlier reports suggested that an increase in cortisol after treatment with TRH could be useful for the diagnosis of PPID [33], more recent reports have suggested that significantly elevated cortisol secretion may also be provoked by TRH in many normal horses [114]. Differences in the results of these two studies could be attributable to seasonal variation in pituitary function (seasonality was not tested in these reports). Season certainly affects pituitary secretion of corticotropin and α-MSH as well as pituitary responsiveness to DEX [105,113]. It remains an untested possibility that the TRH response test could be clinically useful when performed at certain times of the year.

In conclusion, the TRH stimulation test, when based on cortisol response, is not reliable for discrimination between normal horses and those affected with PPID. Moreover, the unavailability of medical-grade TRH has caused some to shy away from using this test, which presently requires that TRH be purchased as a chemical-grade product. Although it has been shown that TRH acts to stimulate the release of POMC-derived peptides in healthy and PPID-affected horses, further work is needed to explore its utility for the diagnosis of PPID [114]. Unfortunately, measurement of plasma α-MSH concentration is not currently offered by veterinary diagnostic laboratories.

What is the combined dexamethasone suppression test/thyrotropin-releasing hormone stimulation test?

As originally described, the TRH stimulation test, which measures the extent to which the plasma cortisol concentration is increased after injection of TRH, has also been criticized because there is so much variability in the baseline cortisol concentration, regardless of the effectiveness of TRH. To overcome this problem of variability in the baseline cortisol concentration, the TRH stimulation test has been modified by performing it in conjunction with a DST (the combined DST/TRH stimulation test) [111–116]. In this test protocol, PPID suspects are first treated with DEX, such that any potential corticotropin release by corticotropes in the PD is theoretically inhibited. TRH is administered 3 hours after DEX has been administered. If TRH treatment (after administration of DEX) leads to elevation in the plasma cortisol concentration, it is concluded that TRH effected significant corticotropin release by melanotropes (implying the presence of PPID) [111,115,116].

The combined DST/TRH stimulation test entails injecting the patient first with DEX (0.04 mg/kg administered intramuscularly) and second with TRH (0.5–1.0 mg administered intravenously) 3 hours later. Four blood samples are collected for cortisol determination. The first sample is acquired just before the administration of DEX, the second sample is acquired just before the administration of TRH, the third sample is acquired 30 minutes after the TRH treatment, and the fourth sample is acquired 24 hours after the DEX treatment. Diagnosis of PPID is supported by two possible outcomes: an increase of at least 66% in the plasma cortisol concentration at 30 minutes after administration of TRH (compared with the measurement obtained just before TRH is administered) or plasma cortisol concentration greater than 1.0 μ/dL at 24 hours after administration of DEX (compared with the measurement obtained just before DEX is administered) [115].

Results of combined DST/TRH stimulation tests performed on 42 equids were recently reported and shown to be more predictive of a correct diagnosis of PPID (based on autopsy confirmation) than the simple TRH stimulation test or the DST. The combined DST/TRH stimulation test had sensitivity, specificity, positive predictive value, and negative predictive values of 88%, 76%, 71%, and 90%, respectively [116]. Interestingly, in that study, the best predictor of a correct PPID diagnosis was simply the presence of inappropriate hirsutism.

Needless to say, use of the combined DST/TRH stimulation test fails to eliminate the need for administering DEX to patients potentially affected with PPID. Moreover, this test is not easily accomplished by veterinary practitioners in the field because it requires four different time points for veterinary attention. As noted previously, medical-grade TRH is not currently available; although it has been used safely in large numbers of horses, some veterinarians have avoided using the chemical-grade product. The extent to which seasonal factors affect the outcome of this test protocol has not been ascertained.

Is measurement of resting plasma corticotropin concentration useful for the diagnosis of pituitary pars intermedia dysfunction?

The demonstration of an elevated plasma corticotropin concentration is a convenient diagnostic test commonly used for the diagnosis of PPID in horses and ponies, with reportedly good sensitivity (84%) and specificity (78%) [106]. Others have reported even higher values [100,109]. That plasma corticotropin and cortisol levels are not suppressed by DEX in PPID-affected horses suggests that increased and unfettered corticotropin secretion is derived from melanotropes. There has been substantial discussion regarding how corticotropin is secreted from melanotropes in PPID-affected horses, however, in light of the fact that, as noted previously, melanotropes have been characterized by the presence of relatively small quantities of corticotropin based on biochemical and immunohistochemical studies.

A satisfactory explanation for the derivation of increased corticotropin release from the PI in PPID has not been established. Several explanations have been proposed, including the following: although melanotropes only produce small quantities of corticotropin, clonal expansion or hypersecretion could be sufficient to release pathologic quantities of corticotropin into the circulation; when affected by PPID, melanotropes process corticotropin differently, yielding greater quantities of corticotropin (and relatively reduced quantities of α-MSH) [83,86]; the bioactivity of corticotropin derived from melanotropes may be different (less) than that of corticotropin derived from corticotropes (leading to relatively less cortisol production) [86]; some melanotropes at the border region of the PI (with the PD) are more immunoreactive for corticotropin than others and could contribute relatively greater corticotropin if stimulated [117].

Metabolic and endocrinologic differences between horses and ponies [118,119] are also reflected in differences in the reference range for corticotropin between the two groups. Specifically, the reference range for corticotropin in ponies has been reported to be less than that for horses [100]. The plasma corticotropin concentration tends to increase with age [113]. As is the case for other species, the plasma corticotropin concentration also varies with the season in healthy horses and ponies [113]. Specifically, the plasma corticotropin concentration is significantly higher in the month of September when compared with the months of January and May. The extent to which seasonal variance might affect corticotropin release in other months has not been reported. It is important to consider the (September) seasonal factor when interpreting plasma corticotropin results for diagnosis of PPID, because plasma corticotropin values often exceed the reference range in September in normal horses [113]. The fact that younger evidently healthy horses may have elevated plasma corticotropin levels has been observed in small numbers of horses, although necropsy confirmation of the absence of PPID in those horses was not available [106,120,121].

Although it has been suggested that false-positive elevated plasma corticotropin measurements could be attributable to other stressful circumstances (eg, pain, especially severe laminitis), some studies have shown that plasma corticotropin is not elevated by pain or other illnesses. Specifically, plasma corticotropin levels were normal in one study in which experimentally induced, short-term, moderate hoof pain was induced [122]. In another study, plasma corticotropin levels were normal in four horses that were affected by illness unrelated to PPID [100]. General anesthesia is stressful and may be associated with elevated plasma corticotropin levels [123,124]. Other conditions that may lead to increased corticotropin secretion by the equine pituitary gland include vigorous exercise, colic, and dysautonomia (grass disease) [125–128].

The rate of release of corticotropin by the pituitary gland fluctuates throughout the day as a result of pulsatile release [121,129,130]. These fluctuations can significantly affect the significance of a single plasma corticotropin determination. Veterinarians should therefore be cautious when interpreting single-sample determinations of plasma corticotropin concentration for purposes of diagnosis of PPID, especially if their clinical index of suspicion is high and the plasma corticotropin concentration is not elevated (false-negative result).

Does the corticotropin stimulation test have a place in the diagnosis of pituitary pars intermedia dysfunction?

The administration of corticotropin to normal and PPID-affected horses causes an increase in the plasma cortisol concentration. Conceptually, for the purpose of diagnosing PPID, the resulting increase in cortisol concentration would be greater in the face of PPID (assuming that adrenocortical hyperplasia had developed). As noted previously, however, adrenocortical hyperplasia is only identified in a few (approximately 20%) PPID-affected horses. Two independent studies failed to discriminate between healthy and PPID-affected horses on the basis of this test protocol [65,100]. Furthermore, specific criteria by which the corticotropin stimulation test should be performed in horses have not been defined (eg, dose of corticotropin, route of administration, time of day, timing of measurements of cortisol after corticotropin administration) [131]. The corticotropin stimulation test may be useful for the purpose of identifying those PPID-affected horses in which adrenocortical hyperplasia has arisen [66].

What is the combined dexamethasone suppression test/corticotropin stimulation test?

The corticotropin stimulation test was modified by combining it with a precedent DEX treatment (combined DST/corticotropin stimulation test) [132]. The rationale for developing a combined test has been that an exaggerated cortisol response to corticotropin would be more clearly evident in PPID-affected horses if endogenous cortisol production has been inhibited before administration of corticotropin. In one study, application of the combined DST/corticotropin stimulation test failed to differentiate between six PPID-affected horses and six normal horses [67]. The combined DST/corticotropin stimulation test is not commonly performed.

What is the value of measuring plasma insulin concentration or insulin sensitivity in the diagnosis of pituitary pars intermedia dysfunction?

Hyperinsulinemia (potentially implicative for insulin resistance [IR]) is commonly identified in equids diagnosed with PPID [96,109,133,134]. Hyperinsulinemia might also occur from stimulated pancreatic β-cell secretion resulting from elevated release of CLIP, a potent β-cell secretagogue, from melanotropes in PPID-affected equids [135].

There are multiple other potential explanations for the development of hyperinsulinemia and IR in older horses, however. For example, the accretion of new adipose tissue, physical inactivity, and the presence of chronic inflammation, all features of PPID, could contribute to the development of hyperinsulinemia and IR [118]. Although excessive glucocorticoids represent a powerful cause of IR [136], it should be noted that hypercortisolism (adrenocortical hyperplasia) is only evident in a few PPID-affected equids. In one study based on examination of 12 necropsy-confirmed cases of PPID, measurement of fasting serum insulin concentration had a sensitivity of 92% for diagnosis of PPID using a cutoff point of 57 µ/mL [109]. The serum concentration of insulin fluctuates substantially when repeated within a short space of time, casting further doubt on the validity of spot test single-sample measurements of this hormone for diagnostic purposes (Fig. 5) [133].

In conclusion, the use of tests to demonstrate the presence of IR or simple hyperinsulinemia should probably be regarded as lacking sufficient sensitivity or specificity for the diagnosis of PPID. Furthermore, assigning clinical significance to single-sample insulin determinations should be avoided, because the circulating plasma concentration of insulin is highly variable throughout a given 24-hour period [137].

What is the most practical way to demonstrate insulin resistance?

The demonstration of IR in PPID-affected equids may provide specific guidance to veterinary practitioners regarding type of treatment (dietary adjustments) and response to treatment. Long-term survival was reduced in those cases of PPID in which hyperinsulinemia was identified at the outset of treatment [137]. Moreover, it is possible that the presence of IR could predispose PPID-affected equids to laminitis [138].

The best tests for IR include the frequently sampled intravenous glucose tolerance test (FSIGT) and the euglycemic hyperinsulinemic clamp technique. Unfortunately, these tests are impractical for practicing veterinarians, and less specific alternative diagnostic approaches are recommended. The

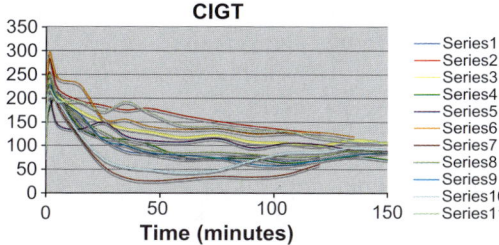

Fig. 5. Results of CGITs from 11 horses (see the report by Eiler and colleagues [139] for method). Horse 2 (*red line*) represents poor insulin sensitivity; horse 7 (*brown line*) exhibits higher insulin sensitivity.

easiest diagnostic test for IR is to determine the serum insulin concentration. Compensatory hyperinsulinemia is a common finding in IR-affected equids. Veterinarians should be extremely cautious when interpreting the results of single-sample insulin determinations without due consideration of possible confounding factors.

In addition to insulin sensitivity of the individual, serum insulin concentration is also influenced by other factors, including time since the animal was last fed, circulating cortisol concentration (diurnal variance, excitement, pain and stress, and PPID), type of food on which the ration is based, reproductive status, and physiologic status (fitness or illness). Fasting concentrations of insulin and glucose tend to be relatively constant, however, and may be used to provide insight into the patient's insulin sensitivity. Horses and ponies affected with IR tend to be characterized by a high normal or slightly elevated plasma glucose concentration (reference range: 80–115 mg/dL) and hyperinsulinemia (reference range: <42 μ/mL [<300 pmol/L]). There may be some value in comparing the plasma glucose concentration (mg/dL) with the serum insulin concentration (μ/mL) as a ratio.

In light of the fact that fasting could represent a stressor, it has been recommended that the samples should be obtained after a period of several days; during that time, the patient is fed an ad libitum grass hay ration. As a matter of standardization, it is generally recommended that samples should always be obtained at the same time of day (we strive to obtain endocrine test samples between 7:00 and 10:00 AM). It should be further noted that in early cases of IR, use of serum insulin concentration may yield a significant number of false-negative results.

Although somewhat more complicated, a better diagnostic test for IR in clinical patients is the combined intravenous glucose-insulin test (CGIT) [139]. Horses are tested by administering glucose and insulin (glucose, 150 mg/kg; insulin, 0.1 U/kg) and measuring the blood glucose concentration for 2 hours (12 blood glucose determinations). Results of a CGIT are characterized by a two-phase curve with positive (hyperglycemic) and negative (hypoglycemic) portions. The CGIT represents a potentially practical clinical measurement of insulin sensitivity because it provides integrated information and more information than the singular glucose tolerance test or an insulin sensitivity test [139]. Investigators compared the results of the CGIT between six healthy mares and one mare affected with a pituitary adenoma [139]. The CGIT results from the PPID-affected mare were, in this case, supportive of the presence of IR.

Could the diagnosis of pituitary pars intermedia dysfunction be made from single blood samples using other proopiomelanocortin peptide assays?

Although plasma corticotropin concentration is commonly used for the diagnosis of PPID, several problems with this assay have been outlined previously. The plasma concentration of α-MSH and β-END could be useful for the diagnostic corroboration of PPID, especially from the perspective of simplifying the diagnosis in the field using a single-sample test. In one study, plasma concentrations of corticotropin, α-MSH, and β-END were elevated in 25 PPID-affected equids when compared with 38 age-matched controls (all diagnoses based on results of a DST) [140]. In another study, plasma α-MSH concentration was increased in 7 PPID-affected equids (diagnosis based on results of a DST or autopsy) when compared with 16 age-matched normal controls (confirmed at autopsy) [114].

Commercially available assays for α-MSH and β-END are not presently available, however. It is likely that, as is the case for corticotropin, plasma concentrations of α-MSH and β-END may be elevated in the autumn in such a manner as to lead to false-positive results for diagnosis of PPID at that time of the year. Seasonal elevation of α-MSH has been demonstrated in healthy equids in September [105].

Can the effect of domperidone on the pituitary gland be helpful for the diagnosis of pituitary pars intermedia dysfunction?

Domperidone is commonly used for the management of fescue agalactia in pregnant mares. Domperidone is an orally administered dopamine receptor antagonist. It is useful in fescue agalactia because it antagonizes the dopaminergic effects of endophyte alkaloids to promote the secretion of prolactin by lactotropes in the PD. In normal horses, the administration of domperidone does not affect the plasma corticotropin concentration. In PPID-affected equids, treatment with domperidone causes a significant elevation of the plasma corticotropin concentration [141]. This effect has been attributed to the concept that hypertrophied melanotropes in the PI of PPID-affected equids continue to be under some degree of dopaminergic inhibition and that treatment with domperidone would effectively neutralize residual inhibition, leading to an elevation in the plasma corticotropin concentration.

In one study, an oral dose of domperidone (2.5 mg/kg) caused the plasma corticotropin concentration to be elevated (2.9 ± 0.68 times over baseline) in PPID-affected equids 4 hours after treatment (n = 8); a similar increase was not observed in normal horses (n = 8) [141]. Diagnosis of PPID was based on clinical signs (inappropriate hirsutism, lack of shedding, and abnormal fat deposition), results of a DST, or necropsy findings (the specific method for each horse was not provided); normal controls were defined by the absence of inappropriate hirsutism, normal shedding, and normal DST results (the specific method for each horse was not provided). Interestingly, in that study, five of the eight PPID-affected equids were characterized by a normal resting plasma corticotropin concentration at the beginning of the study, further pointing to the fact that care should be taken when simply measuring the plasma corticotropin concentration for purposes of making a diagnosis of PPID. Although preliminary results regarding the domperidone challenge test indicate that is practical and safe and promises high diagnostic accuracy, further work on a larger number of normal and PPID-affected equids must yet be undertaken to determine its sensitivity and specificity. Similarly, it remains to be seen whether the test might yield a relatively higher number of false-positive test results in the autumn.

Is imaging of the pituitary gland a useful diagnostic tool?

Physical enlargement of the pituitary gland can be demonstrated using CT and radiography [142–144]. As noted previously, however, physical enlargement of the pituitary gland is only evident in approximately two thirds of PPID-affected equids at necropsy [97]. The frequency with which pituitary gland enlargement occurs for reasons unrelated to PPID in horses has not been extensively reported. For example, in one recent study, the size and microscopic anatomy of the pituitary gland were found to vary with age and gestational status in mares [145]. Interestingly, in that study, microscopic lesions could be identified in the PI of almost 50% of horses that were not exhibiting any clinical signs of PPID.

Are there times of the year when diagnostic testing for pituitary pars intermedia dysfunction is especially unreliable?

In recent years, several publications have addressed the observation that secretion of some POMC-derived peptides from the healthy pituitary gland is increased during the autumn (specifically, September). These observations are important when considering a diagnosis of PPID in equids in the Northern Hemisphere, based on elevated plasma corticotropin and α-MSH [105,113]. Therefore, testing normal horses at this time of the year is associated with an increased risk of a false-positive test result. As noted previously, results of the DST were also falsely positive at this same time of the year (September) in 10 of 39 healthy horses [113].

Seasonal elevation in the pituitary secretion of POMC-derived peptides has been attributed to physiologic processes intended to "gear up" the horse in readiness for winter. The extent to which this phenomenon affects equids during other months of the year is incompletely understood.

How is pituitary pars intermedia dysfunction best managed?

The treatment of PPID generally falls into two categories: nonspecific management of the older horse and pharmacologic strategies aimed specifically at the hormonal manifestations of PPID. Unfortunately, pharmacokinetic studies to investigate the appropriate dose for the most commonly used drugs to treat PPID (pergolide, cyproheptadine, and trilostane) have not been reported in horses and are based on extrapolations from human studies. The two most commonly prescribed drugs for the management of PPID, cyproheptadine and pergolide, were originally recommended in 1983 [146].

Nonspecific health management strategies should be carefully individualized to the needs of the patient. As with all older horses, PPID-affected equids require special attention regarding the health of their teeth, nutrition, and feet. Morbidity associated with age-dependent dental attrition is often more severe in PPID-affected equids because of the combined effects of immune compromise and osteoporosis. PPID-affected equids are commonly affected with laminitis, requiring special attention by the veterinarian and farrier. The nutritional requirements of PPID-affected equids should take into account the likelihood of complicating dental attrition and the observation that many of these horses are concomitantly affected with IR. Hirsute horses are customarily clipped to help with thermoregulation in the warmer months of the year. Affected horses may be treated with long-term antimicrobials to control the morbidity associated with low-grade subclinical infections (especially affecting the lower urinary and respiratory tracts) [66].

On the basis of the fact that serotonin stimulates the release of corticotropin from the PI of rats, the serotonin antagonist cyproheptadine has been advocated for the management of PPID in horses [147]. Cyproheptadine treatment of three PPID-affected horses over the course of 4 to 8 weeks was initially reported to cause remarkable improvement in clinical appearance as well as normalization of blood glucose concentrations, cortisol levels, and results of DEX suppression tests [146]. More recently, however, cyproheptadine treatment failed to cause further clinical improvement in a group of PPID-affected horses in which clinical improvement had already been established through management adjustments (deworming, dental work, and improved nutrition) [148]. Other more recent reports also suggest that cyproheptadine often might not be effective for the management of PPID. In one study, treatment using cyproheptadine resulted in clinical improvement in only 25% of treated PPID-affected ponies [98].

Only 2 of 7 owners of PPID-affected equids reported clinical improvement after treatment using cyproheptadine in one recent study in which cyproheptadine treatment (7 horses) was compared with pergolide treatment (20 horses) [81]. In that same study, 17 of 20 owners reported that pergolide treatment resulted in clinical improvement. Treatment with pergolide was also more effective in terms of reducing the plasma corticotropin concentration compared with cyproheptadine [81]. In another study, the administration of cyproheptadine was judged to be effective for the management of PPID in terms of the clinical response [149]. In that same study, the plasma corticotropin concentration was reduced by the treatment in all the clinically improved horses.

The current widespread use of pergolide, a dopaminergic agonist, for treatment of PPID is based on the original observation that intravenous infusion of dopamine inhibited the pituitary release of POMC peptides in a PPID-affected mare [75]. The dose of pergolide (5 mg) used in that study was quite high by current standards. The currently recommended "low-dose" pergolide treatment (0.0017 mg/kg every 24 hours) for horses and ponies affected with PPID was originally published in 1995 [150].

Pergolide was also shown to decrease circulating POMC peptide concentrations in PPID-affected mares and was reported to be clinically effective for the management of PPID in a large case series [151,152]. As noted previously, pergolide was reported to cause clinical improvement in 17 of 20 treated PPID-affected equids (compared with clinical improvement seen in only 2 of 7 horses treated using cyproheptadine) [81]. Moreover, reported reductions in plasma corticotropin concentrations after initiation of treatment with pergolide were correlated with the duration of treatment and the dose of pergolide administered [81].

Pergolide has been reported to be a more effective treatment for PPID than cyproheptadine in terms of clinical response (85% favorable outcome for pergolide versus 43% for cyproheptadine) and normalizing the results of a DST (35% versus 15%, respectively) [82]. Pergolide was also reported to be superior to cyproheptadine for the management of PPID by another author [153]. There have been several other reports in which pergolide treatment was introduced to good effect after a failed period (several months) of cyproheptadine treatment [146,148]. It has been suggested that administration of a combination of pergolide and cyproheptadine might increase the likelihood of a favorable treatment response in refractory cases of PPID, but there have been no published studies that served to review this combined treatment approach to date [66].

Unfortunately, although it has been shown to be effective, pergolide is likely to become unavailable to equine practitioners. On March 29, 2007, the US Food and Drug Administration (FDA) announced that manufacturers of pergolide drug products, which are used to treat Parkinson's disease, are voluntarily removing these drugs from the market because of the risk of serious damage to patients' heart valves [154]. The products being withdrawn are Permax, the trade name for pergolide marketed by Valeant Pharmaceuticals, and two generic versions of pergolide manufactured by Par and Teva Pharmaceuticals. Thus, to continue to use the drug, equine practitioners have to use compounded sources of the drug, which may themselves become unavailable, because the equine market for pharmaceuticals is so much smaller than the human market. Other dopamine agonists available on the human market, including cabergoline, are likely to be evaluated for suitability for the management of equine PPID in the near future.

Another dopaminergic agonist, bromocriptine, had been advocated for the management of PPID in earlier literature, but its efficacy is limited by poor oral bioavailability in horses [148,155]. Bromocriptine is not currently recommended for the treatment of PPID in horses.

Trilostane is another drug that has been recently introduced for the management of PPID in horses. Trilostane is a competitive inhibitor of adrenal steroidogenesis (specifically, it inhibits the enzyme 3β-hydroxysteroid dehydrogenase). In support of its place for the management of PPID, the authors reported that treatment with trilostane caused improvement in signs of laminitis, PU/PD ratio, and lethargy [156]. In that study, the diagnosis of PPID in 16 ponies and four horses was based on results of physical examination and a combined TRH/DEX test. Although results of the TRH/DEX tests were improved by 30 days of treatment with trilostane (reduced cortisol response to administered TRH), treatment did not cause the endocrinologic abnormalities to become normal.

Trilostane is not readily available to veterinarians in the United States. In light of the fact that, as noted previously, adrenocortical hyperplasia is identified in only 20% of PPID-affected equids, inhibition of adrenal biosynthesis of cortisol may not be particularly effective in most treated patients. Nevertheless, if available, trilostane might be considered as an adjunct to the treatment of PPID in those cases for which pergolide seems to be relatively ineffective.

Prompted by lay interest in the treatment, another study reported the results of treating 14 PPID-affected horses using *Vitex agnus castus* (chaste berry) extract (Hormonize) [157]. Diagnosis of PPID was based on clinical signs and an elevated plasma corticotropin concentration ($n = 12$) or an abnormal DST result ($n = 2$). The dose of chaste berry extract followed the manufacturer's recommendation. Clinical and endocrinologic criteria worsened in all but 1 of the treated horses. Although it had been planned that treatment (based on the manufacturer's recommendations) would be undertaken for 6 months, deterioration in clinical signs and endocrine test results necessitated that the treatment be curtailed prematurely in 8 of the horses [157]. The authors concluded that chaste berry extract did not cause clinical improvement or improve the endocrinologic test results in PPID-affected horses.

If pituitary pars intermedia dysfunction is a result of oxidative stress, should dietary supplementation with antioxidants be a part of the treatment?

As noted previously, there is good evidence that PPID results from oxidative damage to dopaminergic nerves derived from the hypothalamus that normally inhibit melanotropes in the PI. Oxidative damage could be attributed to an increase in the production of oxidants, a reduction in the availability of antioxidants, or a combination of both factors. In one study in which 20 unaffected older horses were compared with 20 PPID-affected equids, there was no evidence of systemic accumulation of oxidative stress markers or deficiencies in antioxidant capacity in horses with PPID, suggesting that these are unlikely to be major predisposing factors in the development of PPID [158]. Oxidative-stress associated pathologic findings in PPID seem to be a localized tissue-specific phenomenon, occurring specifically in dopaminergic nerve terminals of the PI, in the face of adequate antioxidative capacity [159]. Therefore, at this time, there seems to be no evidence to suggest that dietary supplementation with antioxidants would necessarily affect the clinical course of PPID.

After diagnosis, how is response to treatment best evaluated?

It has been stressed that any clinical improvement that might be evident after initiation of treatment of PPID using cyproheptadine or pergolide could be simply attributable to management adjustments that are invariably adopted at the same time [66]. The extent to which any treatment for PPID-affected equids is effective in terms of clinical signs or restoration of normal endocrinologic parameters has not been reported extensively [149,155,159]. For many treated horses, it is further evident that there is clinical improvement but that the endocrinologic test results remain abnormal. In one study, owners reported that clinical improvement was evident in greater than 80% of pergolide-treated horses but evidence of improvement based on results of endocrinologic tests was only evident in approximately one third of those horses [82]. Results of the DST returned to normal in only 7 of 20 PPID-affected horses after treatment using 2 mg per dose of pergolide [82].

Plasma corticotropin concentration has been advocated as a useful test for determining whether endocrinologic normalization is being achieved during the management of PPID [106]. Pharmacologic treatment of PPID may not necessarily result in reductions of the plasma corticotropin concentration into the reference range, but a reduction of the measured level of corticotropin has been interpreted as a sign of response to treatment [106]. In that study, treatment with pergolide or cyproheptadine was associated with improvement in hirsutism and reductions in plasma corticotropin concentration, but the effectiveness of pergolide seemed to be more significant (interpretation of results was limited by the small sample size). These authors concluded that plasma corticotropin levels may be helpful for monitoring response to treatment but that improvement in clinical signs was the most important index of treatment effectiveness. The same authors did not identify any difference between pergolide and cyproheptadine in terms of clinical improvement during treatment of PPID. As had been reported previously, there did not seem to be any association between changes in corticotropin and improvement in clinical signs resulting from treatment of PPID using cyproheptadine.

Interestingly, in one report, the clinical signs of PPID in 3 horses treated with cyproheptadine improved but their plasma corticotropin levels increased [149]. The plasma corticotropin concentration was reduced in 9 of 20 horses treated with cyproheptadine. Reported signs of clinical improvement included changes in hair coat characteristics (65%), reduced laminitic pain (60%), and improved behavior (50%) in 20 of 29 PPID-affected equids that were treated with cyproheptadine [149]. In another study that investigated the clinical response to pergolide and cyproheptadine treatments for PPID, the authors were unable to distinguish between the two drugs based on surveys sent to veterinarians [106]. In that study, treatment with pergolide or cyproheptadine tended to cause a reduction in the plasma corticotropin concentration when blood was retested. In another study, the extent to which the plasma corticotropin concentration was decreased after initiation of treatment using pergolide was correlated with the period of treatment and the dose of pergolide used for treatment [81]. In that study, the authors recognized a correlation between improvement in clinical signs and decreasing plasma corticotropin levels.

There presently exists a lack of evidentiary support for the application of any diagnostic endocrinologic test for purposes of demonstrating clinical resolution or control during the pharmacologic management of PPID. At best, veterinary clinicians may elect to monitor the resting plasma corticotropin concentration as an indicator of improvement (reduction in corticotropin), but plasma corticotropin concentrations may remain elevated in the face of improvement in clinical signs. As noted previously, some workers have suggested that clinical observation remains the best method to evaluate response to treatment.

Acknowledgment

The authors thank Kate Anderson for excellent and expert assistance with the management of library resources.

References

[1] Greenspan FS. The thyroid gland. In: Greenspan FS, Strewler GJ, editors. Basic and clinical endocrinology. 5th edition. Connecticut: Appleton & Lange; 1997. p. 192–262.
[2] Graham PA, Nachreiner RF, Refsal KR, et al. Lymphocytic thyroiditis. Vet Clin North Am Small Anim Pract 2001;31(5):915–33.
[3] Perillo A, Passantino G, Passantino L, et al. First observation of an Hashimoto thyroiditis-like disease in horses from Eastern Europe: histopathological and immunological findings. Immunopharmacol Immunotoxicol 2005;27(2):241–53.
[4] Shaver JR, Fretz PB, Doige CE, et al. Skeletal manifestations of suspected hypothyroidism in two foals. J Equine Med Surg 1979;3:269–75.
[5] Vivrette SL, Reimers TJ, Krook L. Skeletal disease in a hypothyroid foal. Cornell Vet 1884; 74(4):373–86.
[6] McLaughlin BG, Doige CE, McLaughlin PS. Thyroid hormone levels in foals with congenital musculoskeletal lesions. Can Vet J 1986;27(7):264–7.
[7] Allen AL, Doige CE, Fretz PB, et al. Hyperplasia of the thyroid gland and concurrent musculoskeletal deformities in western Canadian foals: reexamination of a previously described syndrome. Can Vet J 1994;35(1):31–8.
[8] Fretz PB. Congenital hypothyroidism-dysmaturity syndrome in western Canadian foals: clinical manifestations, management, treatment, prognosis, and follow-up. In: Proceedings of the 40th Convention of the American Association of Equine Practitioners. Vancouver; 1994. p. 63.
[9] Allen AL, Townsend HGG, Doige CE, et al. A case-control study of congenital hypothyroidism and dysmaturity syndrome of foals. Can Vet J 1996;37:349–58.
[10] Hood DM. Thyroid function in horses affected with laminitis. Southwest Vet 1987;38: 85–91.

[11] Stanley O, Hillidge CJ. Alopecia associated with hypothyroidism in a horse. Equine Vet J 1982;14(2):165–7.
[12] Correa JE, Calderin GG. Anhidrosis, dry coat syndrome in the Thoroughbred. J Am Vet Med Assoc 1966;149:1556–60.
[13] Waldron-Mease E. Hypothyroidism and myopathy in racing Thoroughbreds and Standardbreds. J Equine Med Surg 1979;3(3):124–8.
[14] Thompson FN, Caudle AB, Kemppainen RJ, et al. Thyroidal and prolactin secretion in agalactic mares. Theriogenology 1986;25(4):575–80.
[15] Murray MJ. Hypothyroidism and respiratory insufficiency in a neonatal foal. J Am Vet Med Assoc 1990;197(12):1635–8.
[16] Furr MO, Murray MJ, Ferguson DC. The effects of stress on gastric ulceration, T3, T4, reverse T3, and cortisol in neonatal foals. Equine Vet J 1992;24:37–9.
[17] Lowe JE, Baldwin BH, Foote RH, et al. Equine hypothyroidism: the long term effects of thyroidectomy on metabolism and growth in mares and stallions. Cornell Vet 1974;64(2):276–95.
[18] Frank N, Sojka JE, Latour MA, et al. Effect of hypothyroidism on blood lipid concentrations in horses. Am J Vet Res 1999;60:730–3.
[19] Vischer CM, Foreman JH, Constable PD, et al. Hemodynamic effects of thyroidectomy in sedentary horses. Am J Vet Res 1999;60:14–21.
[20] Allen AL, Fretz PB, Card CE, et al. The effects of partial thyroidectomy on the development of the equine fetus. Equine Vet J 1998;30:53–9.
[21] Breuhaus BA. Thyroid-stimulating hormone in adult euthyroid and hypothyroid horses. J Vet Intern Med 2002;16:109–15.
[22] Johnson PJ, Messer NT, Ganjam VK, et al. Effects of propylthiouracil and bromocriptine on serum concentrations of thyrotrophin and thyroid hormones in normal female horses. Equine Vet J 2003;35:296–301.
[23] Lowe JE, Kallfelz FA. Thyroidectomy and the T-4 test to assess thyroid dysfunction in the horse and pony. Proceedings of the 16th American Association of Equine Practitioners. 1970. p. 135–54.
[24] Lowe JE, Baldwin BH, Foote RH, et al. Semen characteristics in thyroidectomized stallions. J Reprod Fertil Suppl 1975;23:81–6.
[25] Lowe JE, Foote RH, Baldwin BH, et al. Reproductive patterns in cyclic and pregnant thyroidectomized mares. J Reprod Fertil Suppl 1987;35:281–8.
[26] Ganjam VK, Kenney RM. Androgens and oestrogens in normal and cryptorchid stallions. J Reprod Fertil Suppl 1975;23:67–73.
[27] Frank N, Sojka J, Messer NT. Equine thyroid dysfunction. Vet Clin North Am Equine Pract 2002;18:305–19.
[28] Beech J. Evaluation of thyroid, adrenal, and pituitary function. Vet Clin North Am Equine Pract 1987;3(3):649–60.
[29] Harris P, Marlin D, Gray J. Equine thyroid function tests: a preliminary investigation. Br Vet J 1992;148(1):71–80.
[30] Mooney CT, Murphy D. Equine hypothyroidism: the difficulties of diagnosis. Equine Veterinary Education 1995;7:242–5.
[31] Sojka JE, Levy M. Evaluation of endocrine function. Vet Clin North Am Equine Pract 1995;11(3):415–35.
[32] Breuhaus BA, Refsal KR, Beyerlein SL. Measurement of free thyroxine concentration in horses by equilibrium dialysis. J Vet Intern Med 2006;20:371–6.
[33] Beech J, Garcia M. Hormonal response to thyrotropin-releasing hormone in healthy horses and in horses with pituitary adenoma. Am J Vet Res 1985;46(9):1941–3.
[34] Chen CL, Li OW. Effect of thyrotropin releasing hormone (TRH) on serum levels of thyroid hormones in Thoroughbred mares. Equine Vet Sci 1986;6:58–61.
[35] Morris DD, Garcia M. Thyroid-stimulating hormone response test in healthy horses, and effect of phenylbutazone on equine thyroid hormones. Am J Vet Res 1983;44(3):503–7.

[36] Morris DD, Garcia M. Effects of phenylbutazone and anabolic steroids on adrenal and thyroid gland function tests in healthy horses. Am J Vet Res 1985;46:359–64.
[37] Ramirez S, Wolfsheimer KJ, Moore RM, et al. Duration of effects of phenylbutazone on serum total thyroxine and free thyroxine concentrations in horses. J Vet Intern Med 1997;11:371–4.
[38] Glade MJ, Reimers TJ. Effects of dietary energy supply on serum thyroxine, triiodothyronine, and insulin concentrations in young horses. J Endocrinol 1985;104:93–8.
[39] Swinker AM, McCurley JR, Jordan ER, et al. Effects of dietary excesses on equine serum thyroid hormone levels. J Anim Sci 1989;65(Suppl 1):255–6.
[40] Powell DM, Lawrence LM, Fitzgerald BP, et al. Effect of short-term feed restriction and calorie source on hormonal and metabolic responses in geldings receiving a small meal. J Anim Sci 2000;78:3107–13.
[41] Messer NT, Ganjam VK, Nachreiner RF, et al. Effect of dexamethasone administration on serum thyroid hormone concentrations in clinically normal horses. J Am Vet Med Assoc 1995;206(1):63–6.
[42] Messer NT, Johnson PJ, Refsal KR, et al. Effect of food deprivation on baseline iodothyronine and cortisol concentrations in healthy, adult horses. Am J Vet Res 1995;56(1):116–21.
[43] Bayly W, Andrea R, Smith B, et al. Thyroid hormone concentrations in racing Thoroughbreds. Pferdeheilkunde 1996;12:534–8.
[44] Symonds ME. Thyroid hormones and nutrient supplementation during pregnancy. Equine Veterinary Education 1995;7(5):246–8.
[45] Flisinska-Bojanowska A, Komosa M, Gill J. Influence of pregnancy on diurnal and seasonal changes in cortisol, T_3 and T_4 levels in the mare blood serum. Comp Biochem Physiol 1991;98A(1):23–30.
[46] Messer NT, Riddle WT, Traub-Dargatz JL. Thyroid hormone levels in Thoroughbred mares and their foals at parturition. In: Proceedings of the 44th Convention of the American Association of Equine Practitioners. Baltimore; 1998. p. 248–51.
[47] Meredith TB, Dobrinski I. Thyroid function and pregnancy status in broodmares. J Am Vet Med Assoc 2004;224:892–4.
[48] Boosinger TR, Brendemuehl JP, Bransby DL, et al. Prolonged gestation, decreased triiodothyronine concentration, and thyroid gland histomorphologic features in newborn foals of mares grazing *Acremonium coenophialum*-infected fescue. Am J Vet Res 1995;56(1):66–9.
[49] Breuhaus BA. Thyroid function in mature horses ingesting endophyte-infected fescue seed. J Am Vet Med Assoc 2003;223:340–5.
[50] Sojka JE. Factors which affect serum T_3 and T_4 levels in the horse. Equine Practice 1993; 15(10):15–9.
[51] Sojka JE, Johnson MA, Bottoms GD. Serum triiodothyronine, total thyroxine, and free thyroxine concentrations in horses. Am J Vet Res 1993;54(1):52–5.
[52] Sommardahl CS, Frank N, Elliott SB, et al. Effects of oral administration of levothyroxine sodium on serum concentrations of thyroid gland hormones and responses to injections of thyrotropin-releasing hormone in healthy adult mares. Am J Vet Res 2005;66:1025–31.
[53] Frank N, Sommardahl CS, Eiler H, et al. Effects of oral administration of levothyroxine sodium on concentrations of plasma lipids, concentration and composition of very-low density lipoproteins, and glucose dynamics in healthy adult mares. Am J Vet Res 2005; 66:1032–8.
[54] Beech J. Disorders of thyroid gland function. In: Watson T, editor. Metabolic and endocrine problems of the horse. Philadelphia: WB Saunders; 1998. p. 69–74.
[55] Lucke VM, Lane JG. C-cell tumours of the thyroid in the horse. Equine Vet J 1984;16(1): 28–30.
[56] Alberts MK, McCann JP, Woods PR. Hemithyroidectomy in a horse with confirmed hyperthyroidism. J Am Vet Med Assoc 2000;217:1051–4.
[57] Ramirez S, McClure JJ, Moore RM, et al. Hyperthyroidism associated with a thyroid adenocarcinoma in a 21-year-old gelding. J Vet Intern Med 1998;12:475–7.

[58] Mellor D, Love S, Gettinby G, et al. Demographic characteristics of the equine population of northern Britain. Vet Rec 1999;145:299–304.
[59] Evans DR. The recognition and diagnosis of a pituitary tumor in the horse. American Association of Equine Practitioners 1973.
[60] van der Kolk JH, Kalsbeek HC, Vangarderen E, et al. Equine pituitary neoplasia—a clinical report of 21 cases (1990–1992). Vet Rec 1993;133(24):594–7.
[61] Donaldson MT, Jorgensen AJR, Beech J. Evaluation of suspected pituitary pars intermedia dysfunction in horses with laminitis. J Am Vet Med Assoc 2004;224(7):1123–7.
[62] Cushing H. The basophil adenomas of the pituitary body and their clinical manifestations (pituitary basophilism). Bull Johns Hopkins Hosp 1932;50:137–95.
[63] Pallaske G. Zur kasuistik seltnere Geschwülste bei den Haustieren. Z Krebsforsch 1932;36: 342 [in German].
[64] Brosnahan M, Paradis M. Demographic and clinical characteristics of geriatric horses: 467 cases (1989–1999). J Am Vet Med Assoc 2003;223:93–8.
[65] Dybdal NO, Hargreaves KM, Madigan JE, et al. Diagnostic testing for pituitary pars intermedia dysfunction in horses. J Am Vet Med Assoc 1994;204(4):627–32.
[66] Schott HC II. Pituitary pars intermedia dysfunction: equine Cushing's disease. Vet Clin North Am Equine Pract 2002;18(2):237–70.
[67] Boujon CE, Bestetti GE, Meier HP, et al. Equine pituitary adenoma: a functional and morphological study. J Comp Pathol 1993;109(2):163–78.
[68] Sokkar S, Mahmoud A. Adrenocortical carcinoma in a donkey. Dtsch Tierarztl Wochenschr 2003;110(4):176–7.
[69] van der Kolk JH, Ijzer J, Overgaauw PA, et al. Pituitary-independent Cushing's syndrome in a horse. Equine Vet J 2001;33(1):110–2.
[70] van der Kolk JH, Mars M, van der Gaag I. Adrenocortical carcinoma in a 12-year-old mare. Vet Rec 1994;134(5):113–5.
[71] McFarlane D, Dybdal N, Donaldson MT, et al. Nitration and increased alpha-synuclein expression associated with dopaminergic neurodegeneration in equine pituitary pars intermedia dysfunction. J Neuroendocrinol 2005;17(2):73–80.
[72] Kemppainen R, Zerbe C, Sartin J. Regulation and secretion of proopiomelanocortin peptides from isolated perfused dog pituitary pars intermedia cells. Endocrinology 1989;124: 2208–17.
[73] Kemppainen RJ, Peterson ME. Regulation of alpha-melanocyte-stimulating hormone secretion from the pars intermedia of domestic cats. Am J Vet Res 1999;60(2):245–9.
[74] Moore JN, Steiss J, Nicholson WE, et al. A case of pituitary adrenocorticotropin-dependent Cushing's syndrome in the horse. Endocrinology 1979;104(3):576–82.
[75] Orth DN, Holscher MA, Wilson MG, et al. Equine Cushing's disease: plasma immunoreactive proopiolipomelanocortin peptide and cortisol levels basally and in response to diagnostic tests. Endocrinology 1982;110(4):1430–41.
[76] Malven P. Pituitary gland neuroendocrinology. Presented at the 15th Annual Forum of the American College of Veterinary Internal Medicine, Lake Buena Vista, Florida, 1997.
[77] Keen JA, McLaren M, Chandler KJ, et al. Biochemical indices of vascular function, glucose metabolism and oxidative stress in horses with equine Cushing's disease [see comment]. Equine Vet J 2004;36(3):226–9.
[78] Ooki T, Kotsu T, Kinutani M. Pars intermedia of the hypophysis of rats after early postnatal lesions of the basal hypothalamus. Quantitative and qualitative observations. Neuroendocrinology 1973;11:22–45.
[79] Levy M, Dybdal N. Pituitary pars intermedia dysfunction in the horse. Part 1: clinical signs and pathophysiology. Presented at the 15th Annual Forum of the American College of Veterinary Internal Medicine, Lake Buena Vista, Florida, 1997.
[80] Millington WR, Dybdal NO, Dawson R Jr, et al. Equine Cushing's disease: differential regulation of beta-endorphin processing in tumors of the intermediate pituitary. Endocrinology 1988;123(3):1598–604.

[81] Donaldson MT, LaMonte BH, Morresey P, et al. Treatment with pergolide or cyproheptadine of pituitary pars intermedia dysfunction (equine Cushing's disease). J Vet Intern Med 2002;16(6):742–6.
[82] Schott H, Coursen C, Eberhart S. The Michigan Cushing's Project. Presented at the 47th Annual Convention of the American Association of Equine Practitioners. San Diego, California, November 24–28, 2001.
[83] Wilson MG, Nicholson WE, Holscher MA, et al. Proopiolipomelanocortin peptides in normal pituitary, pituitary tumor, and plasma of normal and Cushing's horses. Endocrinology 1982;110(3):941–54.
[84] Pauli BU, Rossi Straub R. [Interstitial cell adenoma of the hypophysis with Cushing-like symptomatology in the horse]. Vet Pathol 1974;11(5):417–29 [in German].
[85] Heinrichs M, Baumgartner W, Capen C. Immunocytochemical demonstration of proopiomelanocortin-derived peptides in pituitary adenomas of the pars intermedia in horses. Vet Pathol 1990;27:419–25.
[86] Orth DN, Nicholson WE. Bioactive and immunoreactive adrenocorticotropin in normal equine pituitary and in pituitary tumors of horses with Cushing's disease. Endocrinology 1982;111(2):559–63.
[87] Wallace MA, Crisman MV, Pickett JP, et al. Central blindness associated with a pituitary adenoma in a horse. Equine Practice 1996;18(8):8–13.
[88] Cotran R, Kumar V, Collins T. The endocrine system. 6th edition. Philadelphia: WB Saunders; 1999.
[89] Okada T, Shimomuro T, Oikawa M, et al. Immunocytochemical localization of adrenocorticotropic hormone-immunoreactive cells of the pars intermedia in Thoroughbreds. Am J Vet Res 1997;58(8):920–4.
[90] Horvath CJ, Ames TR, Metz AL, et al. Adrenocorticotropin-containing neoplastic cells in a pars intermedia adenoma in a horse. J Am Vet Med Assoc 1988;192(3):367–71.
[91] Raffin-Sanson M, de Keyzer Y, Bertangna X. Proopiomelanocortin, a polypeptide precursor with multiple functions: from physiology to pathological conditions. Eur J Endocrinol 2003;149:79–90.
[92] Amann J, Smith R, Ganjam V. Distribution and implications of b-endorphin and ACTH-immunoreactive cells in the intermediate lobe of the hypophysis in healthy equids. Am J Vet Res 1987;48:323–7.
[93] Yoshikawa H, Oishi H, Sumi A, et al. Spontaneous pituitary adenomas of the pars intermedia in 5 aged horses: histopathological, immunohistochemical and ultrastructural studies. SO - Journal of Equine Science 2001;12(4):119–26.
[94] Shanker G, Sharma RK. Beta-endorphin stimulates corticosterone synthesis in isolated rat adrenal cells. Biochem Biophys Res Commun 1979;86(1):1–5.
[95] Seger M, Bennett H. Structure and bioactivity of the amine terminal of proopiomelanocortin. J Steroid Biochem 1986;25:703–10.
[96] Hillyer M, Taylor F, Mair T. Diagnosis of hyperadrenocorticism in the horse. Equine Veterinary Education 1992;4:131–4.
[97] van der Kolk JH. Equine Cushing's disease. Equine Veterinary Education 1997;9:209–14.
[98] Love S. Equine Cushing's disease. Br Vet J 1993;149(2):139–53.
[99] Donaldson MT. Equine Cushing's disease and laminitis. Large animal. Presented at the Proceedings of the North American Veterinary Conference, vol. 18. Orlando, Florida, USA, January 17–21, 2004.
[100] Couëtil L, Paradis MR, Knoll J. Plasma adrenocorticotropin concentration in healthy horses and in horses with clinical signs of hyperadrenocorticism. J Vet Intern Med 1996; 10(1):1–6.
[101] van der Kolk JH. Diseases of the pituitary gland, including hyperadrenocorticism. London: Saunders, WB; 1998.
[102] Hoffman R, Wilson J, Kronfeld D. Hydrolyzable carbohydrates in pasture, hay, and horse feeds: direct assay and seasonal variation. J Anim Sci 2001;79:500–6.

[103] Rohrbach B, Green E, Oliver J. Aggregate risk study of exposure to endophyte-infected (Acremonium coenophialum) tall fescue as a risk factor for laminitis in horses. Am J Vet Res 1995;56:22–6.
[104] Rottinghaus G, Garner G, Cornell C. HPLC method for quantitating ergovaline in endophyte-infected tall fescue: seasonal variation of ergovaline levels in stems with leaf sheaths, leaf blades, and seed heads. J Agric Food Chem 1991;39:112–5.
[105] McFarlane D, Donaldson MT, McDonnell SM, et al. Effects of season and sample handling on measurement of plasma alpha-melanocyte-stimulating hormone concentrations in horses and ponies. Am J Vet Res 2004;65(11):1463–8.
[106] Perkins GA, Lamb S, Erb HN, et al. Plasma adrenocorticotropin (ACTH) concentrations and clinical response in horses treated for equine Cushing's disease with cyproheptadine or pergolide. Equine Vet J 2002;34(7):679–85.
[107] Douglas R. Circadian cortisol rhythmicity and equine Cushing's-like disease. J Equine Vet Sci 1999;19(11):684–753.
[108] van der Kolk JH, Kalsbeek HC, Wensing T, et al. Urinary concentration of corticoid in normal horses and horses with hyperadrenocorticism. Res Vet Sci 1994;56(1):126–8.
[109] van der Kolk JH, Wensing T, Kalsbeek HC, et al. Laboratory diagnosis of equine pituitary pars intermedia adenoma. Domest Anim Endocrinol 1995;12(1):35–9.
[110] van der Kolk JH, Nachreiner RF, Schott HC, et al. Salivary and plasma concentration of cortisol in normal horses and horses with Cushing's disease. Equine Vet J 2001;33(2): 211–3.
[111] Eiler H, Oliver JW, Andrews FM, et al. Results of a combined dexamethasone suppression/thyrotropin-releasing hormone stimulation test in healthy horses and horses suspected to have a pars intermedia pituitary adenoma. J Am Vet Med Assoc 1997;211(1):79–81.
[112] Miesner T, Beard L, Schmall S, et al. Results of overnight dexamethasone suppression test repeated over time in horses suspected of having equine Cushing's disease [abstract]. J Vet Intern Med 2003;7:420.
[113] Donaldson MT, McDonnell SM, Schanbacher BJ, et al. Variation in plasma adrenocorticotropic hormone concentration and dexamethasone suppression test results with season, age, and sex in healthy ponies and horses [see comment]. J Vet Intern Med 2005;19(2): 217–22.
[114] McFarlane D, Beech J, Cribb A. Alpha-melanocyte stimulating hormone release in response to thyrotropin releasing hormone in healthy horses, horses with pituitary pars intermedia dysfunction and equine pars intermedia explants. Domest Anim Endocrinol 2006; 30(4):276–88.
[115] Andrews FM, Frank N, Sommardahl CS, et al. Diagnostic value of a combined dexamethasone suppression/thyrotropin-releasing hormone stimulation test in equine Cushing's disease. Presented at the Proceedings of the 50th Annual Convention of the American Association of Equine Practitioners. Denver, Colorado, USA, December 4–8, 2004.
[116] Frank N, Andrews FM, Sommardahl CS, et al. Evaluation of the combined dexamethasone suppression/thyrotropin-releasing hormone stimulation test for detection of pars intermedia pituitary adenomas in horses. J Vet Intern Med 2006;20(4):987–93.
[117] Okada T, Yuguchi K, Kiso Y, et al. A case of a pony with Cushing's disease. J Vet Med Sci 1997;59(8):707–10.
[118] Freestone J, Beadle R, Shoemaker K. Improved insulin sensitivity in hyperinsulinaemic ponies through physical conditioning and controlled feed intake. Equine Vet J 1992;24: 187–90.
[119] Jeffcott L, Field J, McLean J. Glucose tolerance and insulin sensitivity in ponies and Standardbred horses. Equine Vet J 1986;18:97–101.
[120] McFarlane D, Sellon D, Gaffney D, et al. Hematologic and serum biochemical variables and plasma corticotropin concentration in healthy, aged horses. Am J Vet Res 1998;59: 1247–51.

[121] Redekopp C, Irvine C, Donald R, et al. Spontaneous and stimulated adrenocorticotropin and vasopressin pulsatile secretion in the pituitary venous effluent of the horse. Endocrinology 1986;118:1410–6.
[122] Xie H, Ott E, Colahan P. Influence of acupuncture on experimental lameness in horses. Proceedings of the 47th Annual Convention of the American Association of Equine Practitioners 2001:347–57.
[123] Luna S, Taylor P. Pituitary-adrenal activity and opioid release in ponies during thiopentone/halothane anaesthesia. Res Vet Sci 1995;58(1):35–41.
[124] Taylor P. Equine stress responses to anaesthesia. Br J Anaesth 1989;63(6):702–9.
[125] Alexander S, Irvine C, Ellis M, et al. The effect of acute exercise on the secretion of corticotropin-releasing factor, arginine vasopressin, and adrenocorticotropin as measured in pituitary venous blood from the horse. Endocrinology 1991;128(1):65–72.
[126] McCarthy R, Jeffcott L, Funder J, et al. Plasma beta-endorphin and adrenocorticotrophin in young horses in training. Aust Vet J 1991;68:359–61.
[127] Nagata S, Takeda F, Kurosawa M, et al. Plasma adrenocorticotropin, cortisol and catecholamine response to various exercises. Equine Vet J Suppl 1999;30:570–4.
[128] Hodson N, Wright J, Hunt J. The sympathoadrenal system and plasma levels of adrenocorticotropic hormone, cortisol and catecholamines in equine grass sickness. Vet Rec 1986;118: 148–50.
[129] Cudd T, Leblanc M, Silver M, et al. Ontogeny and ultradian rhythms of adrenocorticotropin and cortisol in the late-gestation fetal horse. J Endocrinol 1995;45:271–83.
[130] Toutain P, Oukessou M, Autefage A. Diurnal and episodic variations of plasma hydrocortisone concentrations in horses. Domest Anim Endocrinol 1988;5:55–9.
[131] Eiler H, Goble D, Oliver J. Adrenal gland function in the horse: effects of cosyntropin (synthetic) and corticotropin (natural) stimulation. Am J Vet Res 1979;40:724–8.
[132] Eiler H, Oliver J, Goble D. Combined dexamethasone-suppression cosyntropin (synthetic ACTH-) stimulation test in the horse: a new approach to testing of adrenal gland function. Am J Vet Res 1980;41:430–4.
[133] Reeves HJ, Lees R, McGowan CM. Measurement of basal serum insulin concentration in the diagnosis of Cushing's disease in ponies. Vet Rec 2001;149(15):449–52.
[134] Garcia MC, Beech J. Equine intravenous glucose tolerance test: glucose and insulin responses of healthy horses fed grain or hay and of horses with pituitary adenoma. Am J Vet Res 1986;47(3):570–2.
[135] Beevor S, Beloff-Chain A, Donaldson A. Pituitary intermediate lobe function in generically obese (ob/ob) and lean mice. J Physiol 1978;275:55P.
[136] Qi D, Rodrigues B. Glucocorticoids produce whole body insulin resistance with changes in cardiac metabolism. Am J Physiol Endocrinol Metab 2007;292(3):E654–7.
[137] McGowan CM, Frost R, Pfeiffer DU, et al. Serum insulin concentrations in horses with equine Cushing's syndrome: response to a cortisol inhibitor and prognostic value [see comment]. Equine Vet J 2004;36(3):295–8.
[138] Treiber K, Kronfeld D, Hess T, et al. Evaluation of genetic and metabolic predispositions and nutritional risk factors for pasture-associated laminitis in ponies. J Am Vet Med Assoc 2006;228(10):1538–45.
[139] Eiler H, Frank N, Andrews FM, et al. Physiologic assessment of blood glucose homeostasis via combined intravenous glucose and insulin testing in horses. Am J Vet Res 2005;66(9): 1598–604.
[140] Horowitz M, Neal L, Watson J. Characteristics of plasma adrenocorticotropin, beta-endorphin and alpha-melanocyte stimulating hormone as diagnostic tests for pituitary pars intermedia dysfunction in the horse [abstract]. J Vet Intern Med 2003;17(3):386.
[141] Sojka J, Jackson L, Moore G, et al. Domperidone causes an increase in endogenous ACTH concentration in horses with pituitary pars intermedia dysfunction (equine Cushing's disease). In: Proceedings of the 52nd Annual Convention of the American Association of Equine Practitioners 2006. p. 320–3.

[142] Allen JR, Barbee DD, Crisman MV. Diagnosis of equine pituitary tumors by computed tomography—part I. Compendium on Continuing Education for the Practicing Veterinarian 1988;10(9):1103–6.
[143] Allen JR, Crisman MV, Barbee DD. Diagnosis of equine pituitary tumors by computed tomography—part II. Compendium on Continuing Education for the Practicing Veterinarian 1988;10(10):1196–200.
[144] Levy M, Blevins W, Janovitz E. Radiological diagnosis of pituitary adenoma in the horse. Presented at the Third Congress of the World Equine Veterinary Association, 1993.
[145] van der Kolk JH, Heinrichs M, van Amerongen JD, et al. Evaluation of pituitary gland anatomy and histopathologic findings in clinically normal horses and horses and ponies with pituitary pars intermedia adenoma. Am J Vet Res 2004;65(12):1701–7.
[146] Beech J. Tumors of the pituitary gland (pars intermedia). 1st edition. Philadelphia: WB Saunders; 1983.
[147] Fischer J, Moriarty M. Control of bioactive corticotropin release from the neurointermediate lobe of the rat pituitary in vitro. Endocrinology 1977;100:1047–54.
[148] Dybdal N, Levy M. Pituitary pars intermedia dysfunction in the horse. Part II: diagnosis and treatment. Presented at the 15th Annual Forum of the College of Veterinary Internal Medicine. Lake Buena Vista, Florida, 1997.
[149] Couëtil LL. Clinical response and plasma adrenocorticotropin concentration in horses with equine Cushing's disease treated with cyproheptadine. Presented at the 42nd Annual Conference of the American Association of Equine Practitioners. Denver (CO), December 8–11, 1996, p. 297–8.
[150] Peters D, Erfle J, Slobojan G. Low-dose pergolide mesylate treatment for equine hypophyseal adenomas (Cushing's syndrome). Presented at the 41st Annual Conference of the American Association of Equine Practitioners. Lexington (KY), December 3–6, 1995. p. 154–5.
[151] Nicholson W, Wilson M, Holscher M, et al. Tissue and plasma levels of proopiolipomelanocortin (POLMC) peptides in the normal and Cushing's horse [abstract]. 62nd Annual Meeting of the Endocrinology Society 1981;403:183.
[152] Beech J. Treatment of hypophysial adenomas. Compendium of Continuing Education for the Practicing Veterinarian 1994;16:921–3.
[153] Williams P. Equine Cushing's syndrome—retrospective study of twenty four cases and response to medication [abstract]. Presented at the Proceedings of the 34th Congress of the British Equine Veterinary Association, 1995.
[154] FDA announces voluntary withdrawal of pergolide products. FDA News March 29, 2007. Available at: http://www.fda.gov/bbs/topics/NEWS/2007/NEW01596.html. Accessed April 7, 2007.
[155] Beck D. Effective long-term treatment of a suspected pituitary adenoma with bromocriptine mesylate in a pony. Equine Veterinary Education Journal 1992;4:119–22.
[156] McGowan CM, Neiger R. Efficacy of trilostane for the treatment of equine Cushing's syndrome. Equine Vet J 2003;35(4):414–8.
[157] Beech J, Donaldson MT, Lindborg S. Comparison of Vitex agnus castus extract and pergolide in treatment of equine Cushing's syndrome. Presented at the Proceedings of the 48th Annual Convention of the American Association of Equine Practitioners. Orlando, Florida, USA, December 4–8, 2002. p. 175–7.
[158] McFarlane D, Cribb AE. Systemic and pituitary pars intermedia antioxidant capacity associated with pars intermedia oxidative stress and dysfunction in horses. Am J Vet Res 2005;66(12):2065–72.
[159] Watson J, Dybdal N, Herrgesell E, et al. Equine Cushing's disease and the long-term treatment with oral pergolide mesylate. Presented at the Annual Forum of the American College of Veterinary Internal Medicine. San Diego, California, 1998.

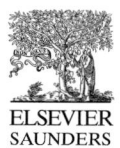

Evidence-Based Equine Nutrition

Sarah L. Ralston, VMD, PhD

Department of Animal Science, School of Environmental and Biological Sciences, Rutgers, The State University of New Jersey, 84 Lipman Drive, New Brunswick, NJ 08901, USA

It is well accepted that horses evolved as grazing animals, with gastrointestinal tracts that are capable of digesting starch, protein, and fat efficiently in the small intestine, also deriving significant nutrition from the fermentation of fiber and other carbohydrates in the cecum and large colon. All vitamin and mineral needs are adequately met with mixtures of forages with the exception of salt, which feral horses obtained from natural salt licks in the wild. Accordingly, most domestic horses that are not subjected to "unnatural" stresses, such as high-level performance or competition, do well on a ration mirroring that of their feral environment, comprised predominantly of free access to good-quality forage, water, and salt.

One of the most difficult problems in equine nutrition research is often the lack of objective and clinically relevant end points. Unlike food animals, in which the only desired nutritional "benefits" can be objectively measured in pounds per day and dollars and cents, the end points in horses often are more subjective and hard to evaluate. For example, it is difficult to quantitate "better quality coat or hooves" or "more manageable behavior" or to assess the relevance of parameters, such as "time to fatigue" and maximum oxygen consumption as measured in treadmill studies, to a real world wherein many other variables come into play in the determination of actual performance.

Nevertheless, this article attempts to present the best evidence (or lack thereof) for some of the most common clinical questions pertaining to such topics as the evaluation of glucose and insulin tolerance and factors that may confound results, dietary management of horses prone to laminitis and rhabdomyolysis, nutritional prevention of gastric ulcers and developmental orthopedic disease (DOD), the efficacy of commonly used herbal products, and feeding geriatric horses.

E-mail address: ralston@aesop.rutgers.edu

The sixth edition of the National Research Council (NRC) *Nutrient Requirements of Horses* contains evidence-based recommendations for some of these clinical topics that were not included in the 1989 edition [1,2]. The exhaustive analyses in the new edition were not available to the author in writing this article, but the recommendations here are based on the same base of literature as well as on some newer studies not available to the 2007 NRC committee members at the time of their deliberations.

Evaluation of glucose and insulin metabolism in horses

There have recently been several in-depth reviews of blood glucose and insulin regulation and evaluation in horses [3–7]. These reviews were stimulated, in part, by a dramatic increase in level 1 and 2 studies that have implicated "hyperinsulinemia" secondary to "high glycemic index feeds" (high nonstructural carbohydrate [NSC] intakes) or abnormal insulin sensitivity to increased risks of laminitis [8–10], DOD [11–14], or rhabdomyolysis [15–18]. Unfortunately, factors that could result in false-"positive" or -"negative" results are often disregarded in the utilization of the results of these studies, such as exactly what constitutes a high glycemic index feed and consideration of other factors that may affect plasma glucose and insulin concentrations.

Question 1: how do feeds affect blood glucose and insulin concentrations in horses?

Glycemic index

The simple definition of the "glycemic index" of a feed is the plasma glucose response (peak values or area under the curve) to ingestion of a measured amount of that feed compared with a standard reference challenge. In human beings the "gold standard" used is always white bread. In the equine literature, however, the standards have varied. Some researchers have used an equivalent weight of oats [19,20], whereas others have used an oral dose of glucose [21] or the responses of adult horses to standardized amounts of NSCs in the feeds [14]. Insulin responses to the feeds usually have not been considered, but when they have been included, higher glycemic index feeds have usually resulted in higher insulin response curves [14,19,22].

In virtually all studies, regardless of the standards used, the mixtures of corn, oats, and barley combined with molasses ("sweet feeds") fed to clinically normal horses cause increases in blood glucose and insulin within as little as 15 minutes of ingestion, with peak values of between 130 and 200 mg/dL at 60 to 90 minutes after feeding, returning to baseline concentrations within 3 to 4 hours after feeding [3,4,14,19–22]. The reported glycemic index of hulled oats and corn is roughly equivalent, but "naked," or hull-less, oats cause more rapid and higher glucose responses after feeding

[19,20], probably because of the higher digestibility of oat starch in comparison to corn starch [22,23]. Barley has consistently been reported to have the lowest glycemic index of the grains commonly used [19–21]. Peak insulin concentrations in "normal" adult horses to meals composed of a variety of grains and grain mixes have ranged between 20 and 60 microIU/mL [14,22].

Pelleting and extrusion also seem to affect the availability of carbohydrates. The pelleted and extruded concentrates tend to result in lower plasma glucose and insulin responses than do textured feeds with the same basic formulation [3,4,24]. This could be attributable to heat-induced changes in the carbohydrates in the feeds during the pelleting and extrusion process that result in lower digestibility [23,25]. Mixed-concentrate feeds containing restricted amounts of sugars and starch (<12% NSCs) and higher fiber (12%–20% NSCs) and fat (5%–12% NSCs) have significantly reduced postprandial glucose and insulin responses relative to feeds with high starch or sugar content (>30% NSCs) and no added fat [26,27].

Traditionally, the glycemic indices of hays and most forages were assumed to be relatively low, and therefore of no consequence if a horse had access to them before drawing a blood sample to evaluate blood glucose and insulin. Grass hays can contain more than 20% NSCs composed of fructans, starches, and sugars) and can cause significant (>10%) increases in plasma glucose and insulin on ingestion, however [28]. The predominant components of NSCs in grass forages are the water-soluble fructans and sugars, whereas legumes, such as alfalfa and clover, accumulate more of the water-insoluble starches [29,30]. Soluble sugars and starches are rapidly digested and absorbed in the small intestine, causing rapid glycemic responses [3,4]. Fructans, conversely, are not amenable to enzymatic digestion but are rapidly fermentable, potentially contributing to the accumulation of endotoxins and monoamines associated with laminitis [30].

In late fall pastures after freezing overnight temperatures, grasses may accumulate even higher concentrations of NSCs than during their rapid growth in spring [29,31]. Pasture water-soluble content can go from 8% to 17% in the course of a day in certain species of grasses on a warm sunny day in the fall [31]. Sunny warm days, followed by freezing temperatures overnight, result in the highest NSC accumulations [29–31]. It is important to note, however, that despite these large fluctuations, most non–insulin-resistant ponies grazing on even spring and late fall pastures on a regular basis are not adversely affected [32].

Ration adaptation

Horses adapted to high glycemic index (high starch and sugar) concentrate rations have reduced insulin sensitivity and higher insulin responses to carbohydrate challenges relative to horses fed higher fiber (>20%) and fat (5%–7%) rations with low glycemic indices [3,4,7,26,27]. This has led to speculation that feeding horses low glycemic index feeds, with or without added fat, may reduce the incidence of laminitis in insulin-resistant horses

[5–8] as well as the incidence of DOD in susceptible growing horses [3,4,13,14]. Such speculation has yet to be confirmed by clinical trials or controlled studies, however. Interestingly, although horses with polysaccharide storage myopathy have increased insulin sensitivity relative to nonaffected horses [15–17], they also seem to respond to restricted starch intakes, purportedly because of the lower availability of glucose for abnormal glycogen synthesis [16,18].

Feeding supplemental fat has been touted by some as a way to improve insulin sensitivity and reduce hyperinsulinemia [18,33,34]. There is no documentation that supplementing fat to horses alters glucose metabolism, however. To date, most studies investigating fat supplementation have substituted carbohydrate calories with fat; thus, the reported effects on insulin sensitivity [18,26,27] may be a result of the reduction of starch or sugar rather than the fat per se. Nevertheless, it is well documented that high-fat rations ($>7\%$ in the total ration) reduce glucose and glycogen utilization in exercising horses because of higher fat utilization in aerobic efforts [33–35], thereby "sparing" plasma glucose and muscle glycogen for anaerobic efforts. This then results in higher concentrations of glucose and muscle glycogen concentration in fat-supplemented horses during and after standardized exercise tests.

Quality of evidence

The evidence for the relative glycemic index of common grains and sweet feeds is strong, despite disparities in methodology. Unfortunately, at this time, there is no strong evidence for the relative glycemic or insulinemic effects of individual commercial pelleted or extruded products. The long-term effects of feeding high starch or sugar rations versus lower starch and higher fiber and fat have repeatedly been well documented. The effect of supplemental fat alone on glucose and insulin metabolism, and on subsequent plasma glucose and insulin concentrations, needs clarification.

Clinical implications

Feeding "low glycemic index" rations to horses results in lower plasma glucose and insulin responses and increased insulin sensitivity. At this time, a low glycemic index would be a mixed feed with restricted or no molasses, corn or oats, fiber ($>12\%$), and fat ($>5\%$). Clinically normal horses that have adapted to predominantly forage rations differ from those accustomed to consuming large meals of grain-based feeds in their responses to standardized challenges, showing lower and more prolonged responses to a dose of dextrose or meal of grain. If evaluating plasma glucose and insulin concentrations in a clinical case, the relative glycemic index ration to which the horse was adapted needs to be taken into consideration as well as the time since the last meal. Horses that have had access to grass hay or pasture within an hour of sampling also may not have "fasting" or "basal" concentrations of glucose and insulin.

Question 2: what other factors should be taken into account when evaluating glucose and insulin responses?

Exercise

Exercise has been documented to improve insulin sensitivity in obese mature ponies [36] and horses [37]. Mild forced exercise (30 minutes at a walk or trot on a treadmill three times per week) also enhanced insulin sensitivity and glucose clearance in yearling Standardbreds [38].

Obesity

It is well documented that healthy obese horses and ponies tend to be insulin resistant, with abnormally high insulin responses to carbohydrate challenges and high basal insulin concentrations [3,4,27,39]. Weight reduction in obese ponies resulted in significant improvement in insulin sensitivity [36] but was accomplished by increasing exercise in addition to feed restriction. It is not known if only caloric restriction resulting in weight loss would have had the same effect.

Age

Standardbred [11], Thoroughbred [40], and Lippizaner [41] horses 3 to 12 months of age have been reported to have lower insulin sensitivity during standardized glucose challenges than when they are 16 to 24 months of age. Similarly, in a study of Quarter Horse foals [42], one weanling was hyperinsulinemic at 5 to 7 months of age but did not differ from others in its treatment group in subsequent tests. This coincides with the period of highest growth hormone release [42]; it has been shown that exogenously administered somatotropins reduce insulin sensitivity [43,44].

Genetic traits

In a relatively large study of Welsh and Dartmoor ponies (n = 257) maintained on pasture [32], there was strong evidence that susceptibility to laminitis was a dominant genetic trait, partially suppressed in male ponies, later proven be associated with compensated insulin resistance [8]. Differences in insulin sensitivity between Standardbred horses and Shetland ponies have also been documented [39].

Diurnal variation and stress

Diurnal or stress-induced elevations in plasma cortisol also reduce insulin sensitivity [4]. This results in higher insulin responses to carbohydrate challenges, although plasma glucose concentration responses may not be altered [3,4,19]. Plasma cortisol has a well-defined diurnal variation, with peak concentrations in the morning hours (7:00–10:00 AM) that gradually decline until 7:00 to 8:00 PM [19,45]. Glucose and insulin responses to a standardized challenge are higher in unstressed horses in the morning than in the early afternoon, but if the horse is stressed by unaccustomed confinement, stressed glucose and insulin concentrations are elevated [3,4].

Quality of evidence

The evidence for obesity, age, and exercise influencing basal and response curves in plasma glucose and insulin is strong. The somewhat weaker evidence for diurnal and stress-induced variations in insulin sensitivity is, however, shored up by strong evidence in the human literature.

Clinical implications

If taking a single or multiple samples of blood to assess glucose and insulin metabolism (see chapter XX for diagnostic protocols), it is important to consider, in addition to feeding history, the age and body condition of the horse. Stressed horses (eg, acute pain) have elevated plasma glucose and insulin concentrations, especially in the morning, that could lead to false conclusions regarding their real insulin sensitivity. Clinically normal horses younger than 1 year of age may have higher fasting plasma glucose and insulin levels than older animals. Therefore "normal ranges" for glucose and insulin established in mature horses should be applied with caution, especially in weanlings and obese animals. To test maximal responses, it is best to run challenges in the morning hours, whereas if an animal is tested in the afternoon, a "within normal range" glucose and insulin response could be misleading.

Feeding insulin-resistant and glucose-intolerant horses

Question 1: what are the best feeds for a horse documented to have insulin resistance or glucose intolerance?

Provision of feeds with restricted starch and sugar content (<12% NSCs) has been well documented to increase insulin sensitivity and glucose tolerance in normal and obese Thoroughbred horses and ponies. That said, the "threshold" for NSCs has not been well established, and efficacy has not been documented in other breeds. Most grass hays would be appropriate as the main component of the ration, but they should be tested for NSC content, especially if the horse has chronic laminitis. If the NSC content of available hays is high (>12%), soaking the hay in warm water for 30 to 60 minutes before feeding leaches out some of the NSCs (and also 30%–50% of the potassium) [10]. High-fat (>7%) and high-fiber concentrate formulas based primarily on beet pulp and barley would be appropriate supplements if additional calories are needed.

The effect of supplementary fat on insulin sensitivity is equivocal. Fat helps to maintain body weight because of its high calorie density but may not be desirable in obese animals for which weight loss is desirable. Because of the high caloric density, if fat is used as a major source of calories in a ration in which the desire is to restrict calories, the amount of feed the horse would be permitted to consume would be drastically reduced. Severe restriction of dry matter intake may predispose the horse to gastric ulceration. Whole grains, especially oats and corn, should be avoided because of their higher glycemic indices.

Feeding young horses

Question 1: what are the critical nutrient concerns in the prevention of developmental orthopedic disease in young horses?

The NRC (1989) recommends that weanlings receive rations containing 70% concentrates to meet their energy, protein, and mineral needs and that yearlings receive 45% to 60% of their total ration in the form of grain-based concentrates, with the rest provided as good-quality forage. No rationale for this recommendation is given, however, and there seems to be no good evidence for it. In a recent survey of feeding practices on 58 Thoroughbred and Quarter Horse breeding farms, it was found that 62% of the farms fed 50% or less of the rations provided to weanlings in the form of grain-based concentrates [46]. Standardbred [38] and draft-cross weanlings and yearlings [47] fed only 40% to 50% of their total caloric intake in the form of grain-based concentrate feeds had growth rates that met or exceeded NRC [2] recommendations. Similarly, draft-cross yearlings fed only 40% of their calories as a concentrate had growth rates that exceeded NRC predictions [47]. As little as 40% of the total caloric intake in the form of concentrates has supported normal to high growth rates in Belgian/Quarter Horse-cross weanlings fed hays of varying quality and nutrient content (S.L. Ralston, unpublished data, 1999–2006). This translates to approximately 0.75% to 1.0% of the foal or weanling body weight per day divided into two or three feedings. Similarly, growth rates and bone densities of Thoroughbred and Quarter Horse weanlings fed a high-fat concentrate at only 50% of the total ration with free access to grass hay did not differ from those offered 65% of their recommended intake in the form of a high-starch ration [48].

In a large study (42 light horse weanlings) in Canada, there were no differences in growth or development between those fed 73% to 77% alfalfa and those fed 63% to 65% grain or grain byproduct concentrates [2,49]. Based on this evidence, it seems that the NRC [1] recommendations for the proportion of concentrates in weanling and yearling rations are excessive.

Feeding high amounts of high starch or sugar (also called "high-energy" feeds in some of the older studies or high glycemic index in more recent reports) concentrates to young horses has now been documented not only to cause insulin resistance [40] but to affect bone mineral content adversely [13]. Feeding high amounts of these feeds was also correlated with a higher incidence of osteochondrosis dissecans (OCD) requiring surgical correction in Thoroughbred yearlings [14]. Rations providing more than 130% of the NRC's recommended amounts of energy for rapid growth in foals cause an increased incidence of DOD, especially if the ration has only 100% or less of the calcium and phosphorus recommended for growth [50–52]. Based on extensive research at several institutions (Virginia Polytech Institute, Rutgers University, and Kentucky Equine Research), it seems that using higher fiber ($>12\%$) and fat (7%–10%) rations that have relatively low glycemic indices for young horses [14] would be preferable to feeding large quantities of high starch or sugar grain based on such indices as growth responses, bone mineral content, and insulin sensitivity.

Protein content of feeds, if in excess of NRC [2] requirements, has no real impact on DOD if mineral requirements are balanced and met [52–54]. Restricting energy and protein intakes to amounts that result in less than 80% of NRC-predicted average daily gain [2] for 4 months, followed by ad libitum access to balanced rations, resulted in four of six Standardbred weanlings developing flexural deformities, however. This outcome was presumably attributable to the rapid compensatory growth rates the animals experienced; similar results were obtained in a parallel experiment in Thoroughbred weanlings [54]. When Arabian foals from a single breeding farm were restricted to 9% protein feeds that resulted in severe stunting for 140 days and were then offered 20% protein rations, similar compensatory growth rates were seen, but no DOD was observed [55].

Mineral imbalances have been well documented to cause DOD. There seems to be a fairly large range of intakes tolerated, however. In addition, factors like growth rates and mineral interactions should be taken into account. Deficiencies of calcium (intakes greater than 15% less than the 1989 NRC-recommended amounts) or phosphorus intakes in excess of calcium (calcium/phosphorus ratio <1.0) have reliably resulted in defective bone maturation in controlled studies in growing horses [2]. In controlled studies [2,53], however, calcium intakes in gross excess of the NRC recommendations ($>1.0\%$ and as high as 2.0%) did not result in an increased incidence of growth abnormalities, however. Similarly "marginally low" phosphorus intake in weanlings (0.24%–0.35% versus the 0.45% recommended in growth rations) did not result in an increase in growth abnormalities in light horse weanlings [56]. Therefore, it can be safely concluded that, to date, "optimal" intakes of calcium and phosphorus have not been well established.

Dry matter intakes of zinc in excess of 1000 mg/kg of body weight have resulted in DOD lesions; however, intakes up to 700 mg/kg failed to create problems [2]. Although the effects of zinc deficiency alone were documented in foals fed only 5 mg/kg [2], minimum requirements are not well defined. Mare's milk, for example, provides zinc at a rate of only 17 to 30 mg/kg DM intake [2], and based on the relatively low incidence of DOD in suckling foals less than 3 months of age (before they start to consume significant amounts of dry feed), this would seem to be in an adequate range. In the author's experience based on nutritional consultations on breeding farms in the northeast region of the United States, total ration dry matter zinc concentrations of 30 to 35 mg/kg are not associated with DOD if the other mineral concentrations in the rations are at or greater than recommended concentrations. The NRC [2] recommendation for growth of dry matter intake of zinc at a rate of 40 mg/kg of body weight is based on limited studies. The minimum required intake of magnesium, another mineral of importance for bone growth, has not been determined.

Quality of evidence

The evidence that severe deficits or excesses of calcium, phosphorus, copper, and zinc can adversely affect growth and development in young horses is strong. The evidence for precise minimum and maximum concentrations in rations, or even optimal intakes, for virtually all the minerals that are well documented to be of importance to growing animals in other species is weak or nonexistent in horses.

Clinical significance

Based on the best evidence available, to avoid compensatory accelerated growth rates that may be associated with an increased incidence of DOD at weaning [56], nursing foals should be introduced to mineral-fortified concentrates when they are 1 to 2 months of age. The concentrates offered should contain 14% to 18% protein. A higher percentage of protein (16%–18%) should be used if only grass hay is available because of its lower protein content (6%–12% on average [2]) relative to mixed pastures and legume or legume mix hays (usually >14% protein dry matter). Weanlings fed rations deficient in protein (less than 12% in total ration dry matter) have reduced growth rates and poor bone mineralization; if they are suddenly placed on adequate rations, they may experience compensatory growth and DOD. Total ration protein intakes of 14% or higher support good growth and development in weanlings of any breed tested to date. Restricting total ration protein to less than 14% in a rapidly growing foal's ration does not result in improved bone growth and may actually be detrimental.

Concentrates should be fed at the rate of 0.25% to 1.0% of body weight, with the emphasis on maintaining lean body condition (ribs not visible but can be felt with mild pressure over the flank; loin, croup, and neck have smooth outlines without creases or visible bony structures). If low amounts of concentrates are fed (less than 0.5% body weight), the addition of a balanced calcium, phosphorus, and trace mineral supplement may be necessary to maintain proper mineral intake. Because pelleted and extruded feeds cause lower glucose and insulin responses than do sweet feeds (see section on evaluation of glucose and insulin metabolism), the former two types of concentrate would be preferable to textured sweet feed mixes, especially in foals from bloodlines or breeds predisposed to DOD.

Ideally, foals should be fed regulated amounts of concentrates that are inaccessible to their dams or other foals at least once, and preferably twice, a day. The dams should be fed the same concentrate if the foal has access to the mare's feed to prevent ingestion of inappropriately balanced concentrates by the growing horse.

Recommendations for mineral content of rations for foals less than 1 year of age cannot be for precise amounts because of the lack of strong evidence for exact requirements and difficulty in achieving a precise "balance" of minerals when formulating rations. Acceptable ranges of total ration mineral intake that, based on the best evidence, support good-quality bone development and growth are more practical and realistic as targets for formulation. These ranges are presented in Table 1.

The total ration intake of the major minerals includes all sources: available forages, concentrates, and other supplements. Weanlings should be fed the same type of concentrate as when they were nursing, and at the same rate as discussed previously, and monitored carefully for signs of excessive weight gain or loss and DOD. Between 0.25% and 1.0% body weight of concentrates used before weaning, divided into two or three meals a day, with free-choice access to good-quality mixed legume or grass hay or pasture, maintains optimal growth rates of most light horse breeds and reduces the risk of DOD. The goal is to maintain steady growth, avoiding sudden increases or decreases, and to maintain body condition. Plain white or trace mineral salt and a good clean source of water should be available free choice at all times.

Based on strong data (S. L. Ralston, unpublished data, 1999–2006) [2], weanling horses voluntarily ingest a maximum of 2.0% to 3.5% of their body weight in dry matter per day. Yearlings can consume 2.0% to 3.0% of their body weight in dry matter per day (S. L. Ralston, unpublished data, 1999–2006) [2]. The recommendations for protein and mineral intakes are based on the assumption that the animals are consuming an average of 2.5% of their body weight per day. Therefore, if intakes are restricted to less than 2.5% of body weight because of high energy density of feeds or other factors, the protein and mineral content of the ration should be increased

Table 1
Recommended nutrient concentrations minerals in total rations fed to rapidly growing young horses

	Range
Calcium	0.8%–1.5%
Phosphorus	0.4%–0.6%[a]
Copper	Feed, 10–20 mg/kg
Zinc	Feed, 40–60 mg/kg[a]

Other minerals, such as manganese, magnesium, selenium, and iron, are important, but there are no reliable data available on requirements of young horses for these nutrients. Also see references in the discussion section.

[a] Minimum amounts, based on type 2 and 3 evidence, may be lower.

Data from National Research Council. Nutrient requirements of horses. 5th edition. Washington (DC): National Academies Press; 1989.

proportionately to provide adequate amounts of the nutrients. Similarly, if trying to determine adequate nutrient concentrations in concentrates to be fed with free access to forage, it is safe to assume that the young horses would consume 2.5% of their body weight minus the amount of concentrate to be fed in the form of the forage per day.

Nutritional prevention of gastric ulcers

Question 1: what is the best feeding regimen to prevent gastric ulceration?

It has been well established that strenuous exercise or training results in gastric ulceration [57] and that intermittent feed deprivation (24 hours of fasting) and confinement also increase the rate and severity of lesions [58]. Even horses fed free-choice grass hay have a greater incidence of gastric ulcers when confined to stalls than when they are maintained on pasture [58].

The role that diet plays in the prevention and treatment of ulcers has only recently been explored [59–61]. In a controlled crossover design study, feeding horses orchard grass hay at a rate of 1.9% of their body weight resulted in more gastric lesions than when the horses were fed 1.9% of their body weight as a mixture of 14% protein sweet feed and alfalfa hay (40%–45% total weight fed as sweet feed divided into two feedings) [59]. Stomach pH and volatile fatty acid production were measured for 24 hours after the morning feeding on test days. The horses fed alfalfa and grain had higher gastric pH but also higher volatile fatty acid production for up to 4 hours after feeding than when adapted to only grass hay. It was hypothesized that the higher calcium and protein content of the alfalfa hay buffered the gastric contents and may have served as a protectant against the adverse effects of the volatile fatty acids generated from fermentation of the grain portion of the ration. Valeric acid, which is produced in greatest quantities during gastric fermentation of carbohydrates (V. Julliand, personal communication, 2006) [59], has been shown to be especially detrimental to gastric mucosal tissues and may be a significant cause of ulceration in horses fed large meals of grains [61]. In controlled studies, feeding corn oil or rice bran oil was not protective against ulceration induced by confinement and exercise [6].

Quality of evidence

It is well documented that feed restriction and strenuous exercise can induce gastric ulceration. Gastric ulcers do not always cause gastric pain [62], however, and the clinical significance of the extremely high rates of ulceration documented in field studies (80%–100% of competitive performance horses) is questionable. The efficacy of feeding regimens, other than the benefits of feeding alfalfa and maximizing pasture access in the prevention of gastric ulceration, has yet to be adequately documented. The correlation between feeding large meals of grain and ulceration is strong but needs to be fully verified in carefully controlled studies.

Clinical significance

Provision of free access to good-quality pasture and offering alfalfa or other high-calcium or high-protein forages may help to prevent gastric ulceration. Sweet feeds (high carbohydrate and high volatile fatty acid production in the stomach if greater than 1 to 2 kg is fed per meal; V. Julliand, personal communication, 2006) should be avoided in horses that are at risk of ulceration (horses subjected to such conditions as high-level performance, confinement to stalls without pasture access, and limited hay). Prolonged fasts (>12 hours) should be avoided if at all possible.

Herbal supplements in horses

Question 1: is there evidence that any of the herbs or nutraceutic agents commonly used in feed supplements are clinically effective?

A 1997 survey of US horse owners found that 70% of horse operations fed at least one nutritional supplement and that nearly 5% fed herbal or nutraceutic supplements [63]. Since then, sales in the herbal market targeting horses have grown exponentially, as evidenced by the number of such products on the market. Most supplements are mixtures of various herbs and "natural" ingredients, with claims ranging from calming effects to immune stimulation. There have been few well-controlled crossover studies testing efficacy of these products. Only herbs and natural ingredients that have at least one controlled study specifically targeting horses and efficacy of claims are discussed.

Bee pollen and propolis

Bee pollen and propolis are resinous substances collected from plants by honey bees and harvested from the hives by the supplement manufacturers. The anecdotal benefits of supplemented bee pollen in horses include improved oxygen utilization, lower heart rate, increased appetite, and firmer muscle tone.

The only controlled study [64] (10 Arabians in endurance training: 5 supplemented and 5 controls) using a "bee pollen" supplement actually tested a product that contained, in addition to bee pollen (37.3 g) and propolis (75 mg), glucosamine hydrogen chloride (HCl), vitamins E and A, five different enzymes and 11 other herbs per 118-g dose. Therefore, the results cannot be attributable solely to the bee pollen or propolis. After supplementation for 18 to 21 days, hay intake and apparent digestion and retention of phosphorus nitrogen, as measured in a 3-day total fecal collection digestion trial, were significantly increased in 3 supplemented horses relative to the 3 pair-matched controls that had been receiving only a placebo. After 42 days of supplementation, physical fitness (based on standardized exercise tests on a treadmill) and immunologic status (leukocyte counts and plasma IgG, IgM, or IgA) did not differ between supplemented horses (n = 5) relative to controls (n = 5), however.

Echinacea

Echinacea (*Echinacea sp*) is commonly touted to have anti-inflammatory and antioxidant properties [65]. Eight horses that were given echinacea for 42 days at a level equivalent to standardized extract at a dose of 1000 mg [65] showed increases in lymphocyte count and decreases in neutrophil count at only day 35 of the 42-day supplementation period, however, and no effect on neutrophil phagocytosis, which does not support the conclusion that there was significant immune stimulation.

Flaxseed

Flaxseed (*Linum usitatissimum*) contains high levels of ω-3 fatty acids and is often reported to enhance a horse's hair coat and hoof quality. In horses, this supplement is marketed for its high ω-3 fatty acid content and is used in coat, skin, and hoof conditioners.

One clinical study tested flaxseed as a treatment for allergic skin diseases in horses and found a significant reduction in the skin test response to *Culicoides*, or "sweet itch," as compared to placebo-treated horses [66]. To the author's knowledge, there have been no other controlled tests of flaxseed in any form on any of the parameters it is advertised to benefit in horses.

Flaxseed is commonly boiled or otherwise processed before feeding to break down the lignified outer layer and to remove cyanogenic compounds [67]. That said, there have been no documented cases of cyanide toxicosis attributed to feeding raw unprocessed flaxseed.

Garlic

Garlic (*Allium sativum*) is purported to have antibacterial, antiviral, antifungal, and antiparasitic properties. Thiosulfinate allicin is supposedly the most active component [68]. There have been no controlled trials demonstrating the efficacy of garlic supplements to repel flies or prevent infections. Toxicity, however, is a possibility. Freeze-dried garlic fed at a rate of greater than 0.4 g/kg of body weight per day resulted in Heinz body anemia in the two horses receiving the supplement [69].

Ginger

Ginger (*Zingiber officinale*) is thought to have antithrombotic, antioxidant, anti-inflammatory, and antibacterial properties. A limited study in horses tested a single oral dose of ginger on anti-inflammatory and cardiovascular responses after exercise [70]. In an uncontrolled study, six horses were administered ginger extract by means of a nasogastric tube 1 hour before exercise and then run on a high-speed treadmill to fatigue. Treated horses had a reduced oxygen consumption per unit time (V_{O_2}) recovery time relative to their performance on the treadmill 1 to 2 weeks before supplementation. Conversely, ginger had a tendency ($P < 0.1$) to increase proinflammatory cytokines tumor necrosis factor (TNF)-α and interferon (IFN)-γ in the blood of supplemented horses. It was speculated that the ginger extract solution irritated the gastrointestinal tract after ingestion, which could be confounded by the increased creatine kinase levels seen after administration as well [70].

Ginseng

Ginseng (*Panax sp*) is commonly used for its reported immunostimulant properties. Ginseng is marketed and sold for use in horses to stimulate the immune system, decrease indices of stress, and increase performance. No controlled research supporting these claims was found in horses, however.

Valerian

Valerian (*Valeriana sp*) is purported to have tranquilizing and sedative properties. No controlled studies have been done in horses to date, but many "calming aids" or "stress relief" supplements include valerian as one of the major active ingredients. The International Federation for Equestrian Sports (FEI) bans this product from use during competition. The basis for the ban, however, is unsubstantiated by clinical trials.

Quality of clinical evidence

Virtually no good evidence exists for significant beneficial effects of supplementation of the various herbal or natural products being marketed. Extensive reviews on the toxicology of herbs in equine medicine reveal that most of the type 1 and 2 evidence is for adverse effects of oversupplementation [71,72].

Clinical significance

Despite manufacturer claims and anecdotal reports of efficacy, to the author's knowledge, none of the herbal supplements have been proven safe or effective for use in horses in well-controlled trials that showed clear benefits. Supplementation with these products cannot be viewed as an evidence-based practice.

Feeding geriatric horses

Question 1: how and when should the ration of an aged horse be changed to meet "geriatric" needs?

Despite controlled studies conducted in the 1980s that showed a reduction in phosphorus, protein, and fiber digestion and lower plasma ascorbic acid in horses older than 20 years of age relative to younger horses fed the same rations [73], horses older than 20 years of age do not necessarily have altered nutritional needs [74,75]. If a horse older than 20 years of age is in good body condition and overall health, no benefits have been found to switching it to a more digestible "senior" feed formulated with higher protein and phosphorus [74]. Horses older than 20 years of age that were unable to maintain Henneke [76] body condition scores greater than 3 on standard hay and grain rations despite good dental care and overall health did gain weight and condition when fed a feed that had increased digestibility and higher quality protein [74].

If old horses start to lose weight, their feed should certainly be evaluated; however, other causes of weight loss need to be ruled out, such as irreparable dental abnormalities (eg, tooth loss); pituitary, renal, or hepatic dysfunction; chronic pain associated with arthritic changes; chronic infections; or neoplasia. Altered nutrition alone may or may not correct all these problems. Although not supported by evidence gained from clinical trials, it is the author's impression that some of the "older horse" feeds on the market may actually be detrimental to horses that have advanced hepatic or pituitary dysfunction.

Reduced digestion of fiber, protein, and phosphorus was reported in horses older than 20 years of age in the 1980s [73]. Based on other studies by the investigators [77,78], it is now hypothesized that chronic parasitic scarring of the large intestine may have been responsible for some of the apparent malabsorption or maldigestion observed in these horses. The digestive alterations observed were virtually identical to those reported for horses after extensive large colon resection, in which the same protocols were utilized to evaluate nutrient digestion as were used in the aged horse studies [77,78], and the aged horses included in the study in the 1980s had not had the lifelong benefit of modern intestinal parasite control [75]. Similar deficits were not found in aged Standardbred horses studied in the 1990s that had had good gastrointestinal parasite control all their lives [75]. The reduction in fiber digestion observed in the original study may also have been attributable to abnormal dentition, although it has been documented that points and hooks less than 3 mm in size do not adversely affect digestion [79] and definitive studies of the effects of gross abnormalities on digestion have not been performed.

The standard indices for renal and hepatic function can be applied to the geriatric horse [80,81]. Further information about indices for pituitary dysfunction can be found in the article on evidence-based endocrinology elsewhere in this issue.

Strength of evidence

The controlled data available on nutritional requirements of old horses are limited and somewhat contradictory, even though conducted by the same researchers.

Clinical significance

Because digestive alterations have not been documented to be present in all older horses and it has been documented that old horses in good body condition do not benefit from dietary change, there is no reason to change a horse's ration on the basis of age alone. Before instituting dietary changes, blood should be drawn for complete blood chemistry to rule out medical causes of weight loss, such as chronic infection, neoplasia, renal dysfunction, or hepatic failure.

If no other medical abnormalities are found, failing older horses may benefit from feeds formulated specifically for geriatric horses. Most major feed companies now offer feeds designed "specifically" for old horses that contain 12% to 16% protein, restricted calcium (<1.0%), and increased phosphorus (0.45%–0.6%), based on the original study in the 1980s. These feeds are "predigested" or extruded, purportedly to increase digestibility by reduction in particle size and heat effects [22,23]. These senior feeds are usually not "high calorie," because most are "complete" feeds designed to be fed at the rate of 1.0% to 2.0% of body weight and as the sole source of nutrition, and are therefore formulated to provide only approximately 9.2 MJ/kg.

Senior feeds are not a panacea for aged horses, and it may be best to avoid them under certain circumstances. For example, if the horse has insulin resistance or pituitary dysfunction, a product that has little or no added molasses should be selected so as to restrict intake of NSCs. If the horse cannot maintain good body condition on 1.0% to 2.0% of body weight of the feed divided into three or four feedings, it may be necessary to supplement with products with a higher caloric density, or a high-calorie supplement, such as edible oils or rice bran products.

Calcium intakes in excess of need result in high urinary calcium excretion in horses (S. L. Ralston, unpublished data, 1999–2006). In the author's experience, there is a high incidence of renal and bladder calculi in old horses fed straight alfalfa. Therefore, alfalfa or other high-calcium feeds should be used with caution in failing older horses.

Aged horses with pituitary adenomas were documented to have lower plasma ascorbic acid than did younger healthy horses [80]. Vitamin C supplementation (0.02 g/kg of body weight given twice a day) has been observed to increase antibody response to vaccines in aged horses with pituitary dysfunction (S. L. Ralston, unpublished data, 1999–2006) and may be tried if chronic infections are a problem, although efficacy has not been proven.

Summary

From an evidence-based perspective, there have been many level 1 and 2 studies published on a wide variety of topics in equine nutrition. The numbers of animals used in controlled studies are usually fairly small (<10 per treatment group), however, and relevant details needed for critical interpretation of the data are often inadequately described or lacking, especially in some of the older reports that are frequently cited as "evidence" for a nutritional recommendation. In field studies involving larger numbers of animals, there are even more confounding factors (eg, season of data collection and details of locally available feeds, climatic conditions, and management) that are often missing. Furthermore, the results from many of the studies are overinterpreted by veterinarians and the public. Accordingly, veterinarians should pay attention to the quality of available evidence when making nutritional recommendations for horses.

References

[1] National Research Council (NRC). Nutrient requirements of horses. 6th revised edition. Washington (DC): National Academies Press; 2007.
[2] National Research Council (NRC). Nutrient requirements of horses. 5th revised edition. Washington, DC: National Academies Press; 1989.
[3] Ralston SL. Insulin and glucose regulation. Vet Clin North Am Equine Pract 2002;18: 295–304.
[4] Ralston SL. Hyperinsulinemia and glucose intolerance. In: Reed S, Bayly W, Sellon D, editors. Equine internal medicine. 2nd edition. St. Louis (MO): Elsevier; 2004. p. 1599–603.
[5] Kronfeld D, Treiber K, Hess T, et al. Insulin resistance in the horse: definition, detection and dietetics. J Anim Sci 2005;83:E22–31.
[6] Kronfeld DS, Treiber KH, Geor RJ. Comparison of nonspecific and quantitative methods for the assessment of insulin resistance in horses and ponies. J Am Vet Med Assoc 2005; 226(5):712–9.
[7] Treiber KH, Kronfeld DS, Geor RJ. Insulin resistance in equids: possible role in laminitis. J Nutr 2006;136(7 Suppl):2094S–8S.
[8] Treiber KH, Kronfeld DS, Hess TM, et al. Evaluation of genetic and metabolic predispositions and nutritional risk factors for pasture-associated laminitis in ponies. J Am Vet Med Assoc 2006;228(10):1538–45.
[9] French KR, Pollitt CC. Equine laminitis: glucose derivation and MMP activation induce dermo- epidermal separation in vitro. Equine Vet J 2004;36:261–6.
[10] Treiber K, Hess T, Kronfeld D, et al. Insulin resistance and compensation in laminitis-predisposed ponies characterised by the minimal model. Proceedings of the Equine Nutrition Conference. Hanover, Germany. Pferdeheilkunde 2005;21:91–2.
[11] Ralston SL. Hyperglycemia/hyperinsulinemia after feeding a meal of grain to young horses with osteochondritis dissecans (OCD) lesions. Pferdeheilkunde 1996;12(3):320–2.
[12] Ralston SL, Black A, Suslak-Brown L, et al. Postprandial insulin resistance associated with osteochondrosis in weanling fillies. J Anim Sci 1998;76(Suppl 1):176.
[13] Hoffman RM, Lawrence LA, Kronfeld DS, et al. Dietary carbohydrates and fat influence radiographic bone mineral content of growing foals. J Anim Sci 1999;77(12):3330–8.
[14] Pagan JD, Geor RJ, Caddel SE, et al. The relationship between glycemic response and the incidence of OCD in Thoroughbred weanlings: a field study. Proc 47th Ann AAEP 2001;323–5.
[15] Annandale EJ, Valberg SJ, Mikelson JR, et al. Insulin sensitivity and skeletal muscle glucose transport horses with polysaccharide storage myopathy. Neuromusc Disord 2004;14: 666–74.
[16] De La Corte FD, Valberg SJ, Mickelson JR, et al. Blood glucose clearance after feeding and exercise in polysaccharide storage myopathy horses. Equine Vet J Suppl 1999;30:324–8.

[17] De La Corte FD, Valberg SJ, Macleay SJ, et al. Glucose uptake in horses with polysaccharide storage myopathy. Am J Vet Res 1999;60:458–562.
[18] Valentine BA, Van Saun RJ, Thompson KN, et al. Role of dietary carbohydrate and fat in horses with equine polysaccharide storage myopathy. J Am Vet Med Assoc 2001;219:1537–44.
[19] Stull CL, Rodiek AV. Responses of blood glucose, insulin, and cortisol concentrations to common equine diets. J Nutr 1988;118:206–13.
[20] Rodiek A, Stull C. Glycemic index of common horse feeds. Proceedings of the 19th Equine Science Society Symposium Tucson (AZ); June, 2005. p. 153.
[21] Jose-Cunilleras E, Taylor LE, Hinchcliff KW. Glycemic index of cracked corn, oat groats and rolled barley in horses. J Anim Sci 2004;82(9):2623–9.
[22] Vervuert I, Coenen M, Bothe C. Glycaemic and insulinaemic indexes of different mechanical and thermal processed grains for horses. Proceedings of the 19th Equine Science Society Symposium Tucson (AZ); June, 2005. p. 154–55.
[23] A de Fombelle AG, Goachet M, Varloud P, et al. Effects of the diet on prececal digestion of different starches in the horse measured with the mobile bag technique. Proc Eq Nutr Physiol Symp 2003;18:113–5.
[24] Ralston SL. Effect of soluble carbohydrate content of pelleted diets on postprandial glucose and insulin profiles in horses. Pferdeheilkunde 1992;3:112–5.
[25] Vervuert I, Coenen M, Bothe C. Effects of oat processing on the glycaemic and insulin responses in horses. J Anim Physiol Anim Nutr (Berl) 2003;87(3–4):96–104.
[26] Williams CA, Kronfeld DS, Staniar WB, et al. Plasma glucose and insulin responses of Thoroughbred mares fed a meal high in starch and sugar or fat and fiber. J Anim Sci 2001;79(8):2196–201.
[27] Hoffman RM, Boston RC, Stefanovski D, et al. Obesity and diet affect glucose dynamics and insulin sensitivity in Thoroughbred geldings. J Anim Sci 2003;81(9):23–8.
[28] Cottrell E, Watts KA, Ralston SL. Soluble sugar content and glucose/insulin responses can be reduced by soaking hay in water. Proceedings of the 19th Equine Science Society Symposium Tucson (AZ); June, 2005. p. 293–8.
[29] Harris P, Bailey S, Elliot J, et al. Countermeasures for pasture-associated laminitis in ponies and horses. J Nutr 2006;136:2114S–21S.
[30] Longland A, Byrd B. Pasture nonstructural carbohydrates and equine laminitis. J Nutr 2006; 136:2099S–102S.
[31] Allen EA, Meyer W, Ralston SL, et al. Variation in soluble sugar content of pasture and turf grasses. Proceedings of the 19th Equine Science Society Symposium Tucson (AZ); June, 2005. p. 321–3.
[32] Splan R, Kronfeld D, Treiber K, et al. Genetic predisposition for laminitis in ponies. Proceedings of the 19th Equine Science Society Symposium (AZ); 2005. p. 219–20.
[33] Pagan JD, Geor RJ, Harris PA, et al. Effects of fat adaptation on glucose kinetics and substrate oxidation during low-intensity exercise. Equine Vet J Suppl 2002;(34):33–8.
[34] Orme CE, Harris RC, Marlin DJ, et al. Metabolic adaptation to fat-supplemented diet by the Thoroughbred horse. Br J Nutr 1997;78(3):443–58.
[35] Duren SE, Pagan JD, Harris PA, et al. Time of feeding and fat supplementation affect plasma concentrations of insulin and metabolites during exercise. Equine Vet J Suppl 1999;30:479–84.
[36] Freestone JF, Beadle R, Shoemaker K, et al. Improved insulin sensitivity in hyperinsulinaemic ponies through physical conditioning and controlled feed intake. Equine Vet J 1992; 24(3):187–90.
[37] Powell DM, Reedy SE, Sessions DR. Effect of short term exercise training on insulin sensitivity in obese and lean mares. Equine Vet J Suppl 2002;34:81–4.
[38] Black A, Ralston SL, Shapses SA, et al. Skeletal development in weanling horses in response to high dietary energy and exercise. J Anim Sci 1997;75(Suppl 1):170.
[39] Jeffcott LB, Field JR, McLean JG, et al. Glucose tolerance and insulin sensitivity in ponies and Standardbred horses. Equine Vet J 1986;18:97–101.

[40] Cubitt TA, Staniar WB, Kronfeld DS, et al. Insulin sensitivity of Thoroughbred foals increases with age and is affected by feed energy source. Proceedings of the 19th Equine Science Society Symposium Tucson (AZ); 2005. p. 137–8.
[41] Krusic L, Krusic-Kaplja A, Cestnik V, et al. Insulin response after oral glucose application in growing Lipizzaner foals. Proceedings of the 15th Equine Science Society Symposium Fort Woth (TX); 2005. p. 397–403.
[42] Ropp JK, Raub RH, Minton JE. The effect of dietary energy source on serum concentration of insulin-like growth factor-I growth hormone, insulin, glucose, and fat metabolites in weanling horses. J Anim Sci 2003;81(6):1581–9.
[43] Christensen RA, Malinowski K, Ralston SL, et al. Chronic effects of equine growth hormone (eGH) on postprandial changes in plasma glucose, nonesterified fatty acids and urea nitrogen in aged mares. J Anim Sci 1996;74(Suppl 1):226.
[44] Christensen RA, Malinowski K, Ralston SL, et al. Chronic effects of equine growth hormone (eGH) on plasma insulin, insulin-like growth factor-I and thyroid hormones in aged mares. J Anim Sci 1996;74(Suppl 1):226.
[45] Lindner A, Will Y, Chrispeels J. [Reference values for cortisol, T4 and T-uptake in different horse groups using the fluorescence polarization immunoassay (FPIA)] [in German]. Berl Munch Tierarztl Wochenschr 1990;103(12):411–6.
[46] Gibbs P, Cohen N. Early management of race-bred weanlings and yearlings on farms. J Equine Vet Sci 2001;21:279–83.
[47] Ralston SL, Duarte SR, Brady S. Growth rates of warmblood weanlings and yearlings. Proc 18th Equine Nutr Physiol Symp 2003;250.
[48] Ott EA. Influence of dietary fat and time of hay feeding on growth and development of yearling horses. Proceedings of 15th Equine Nutrition and Physiology Symposium 1997;150–2.
[49] Cymbaluk NF, Christison GI. Effects of diet and climate on growing horses. J Anim Sci 1989;67(1):48–59.
[50] Glade MJ, Reimers TJ. Effects of dietary energy supply on serum thyroxine, tri-iodothyronine and insulin concentrations in young horses. J Endocrinol 1985;104(1):93–8.
[51] Thompson KN, Jackson SG, Baker JP. The influence of high planes of nutrition on skeletal growth and development of weanling horses. J Anim Sci 1988;66(10):2459–67.
[52] Savage CJ, McCarthy RN, Jeffcott LB. Effects of dietary energy and protein on induction of dyschondroplasia in foals. Equine Vet J 1993;16:74–9.
[53] Hintz HF. Effect of energy and protein deprivation on body weight and height gains of young horses. Eq Prac 1992;14:7–8.
[54] Hintz HF. Influence of feeding on contracted tendons. Pferdeherilkunde 1996;12:343–4.
[55] Schryver HF, Meakim DW, Lowe JE, et al. Growth and calcium metabolism in horses fed varying levels of protein. Equine Vet J 1987;19:280–7.
[56] Cymbaluk NF, Christison GI. Effects of dietary energy and phosphorus content on blood chemistry and development of growing horses. J Anim Sci 1989;67(4):951–8.
[57] Murray MJ. The pathogenesis and prevalence of gastric ulceration in foals and horses. Vet Med 1991;86:815–9.
[58] Murray MJ, Eichorn ES. Effects of intermittent feed deprivation, intermittent feed deprivation with ranitidine administration and stall confinement with ad libitum access to hay on gastric ulceration in horses. Am J Vet Res 1996;57:1599–603.
[59] Nadeau JA, Andrews FM, Mathew AG, et al. Evaluation of diet as a cause of gastric ulcers in horses. Am J Vet Res 2000;61:784–90.
[60] Nadeau JA, Andrews FM, Patton CS, et al. Effects of hydrochloric, valeric and other volatile fatty acids on pathogenesis of ulcers in the nonglandular portion of the stomach of horses. Am J Vet Res 2003;64:413–7.
[61] Frank N, Andrews FM, Elliot SB, et al. Effects of dietary oils on the development of gastric ulcers in mares. Am J Vet Res 2003;66:2006–11.
[62] Dukti SA, Perkins S Murphy J, Barr B, et al. Prevalence of gastric squamous ulceration in horses with abdominal pain. Equine Vet J 2006;38(4):347–9.

[63] USDA. Part II: baseline reference of 1998 equine health and management. USDA: APHIS:VS, CEAH. Fort Collins (CO): National Animal Health Monitoring System; 1998. #N318.0400.
[64] Turner KK, Nielsen BD, O'Connor CI, et al. Bee pollen product supplementation to horses in training seems to improve feed intake: a pilot study. J Anim Physiol Ani Nutr (Berl) 2006; 90:414–20.
[65] O'Neill W, McKee S, Clarke AF. Immunological and haematinic consequences of feeding a standardized Echinacea (Echinacea angustifolia) extract to healthy horses. Equine Vet J 2002;34:222–7.
[66] O'Neill W, McKee S, Clarke AF. Flaxseed (Linum usitatissimum) supplementation associated with reduced skin test lesional area in horses with Culicoides hypersensitivity. Can J Vet Res 2002;66:272–7.
[67] Oomah BD, Mazza G, Kenaxcuk EO. Cyanogenic compounds in flaxseed. J Agric Food Chem 1992;40:1346–8.
[68] Munday R, Munday CM. Relative activities of organosulfur compounds derived from onions and garlic in increasing tissue activities of quinone reductase and glutathione transferase in rat tissues. Nutr Cancer 2001;40:205–10.
[69] Pearson W, Boermans HJ, Bettger WJ, et al. Association of maximum voluntary dietary intake of freeze-dried garlic with Heinz body anemia in horses. Am J Vet Res 2005;66:457–65.
[70] Liburt NR. Effects of ginger and cranberry extracts on markers of inflammation and performance following intense exercise in horses [masters thesis]. Rutgers, the State University of New Jersey, New Brunswick, NJ; 2005.
[71] Harman J. The toxicology of herbs in equine practice. Clin Tech Equine Pract 2002;1:74–80.
[72] Poppenga RH. Risks associated with the use of herbs and other dietary supplements. Vet Clin North Am Equine Pract 2001;17:455–77.
[73] Ralston SL. Digestive alterations in aged horses. J Equine Vet Sci 1989;9:203–5.
[74] Ralston SL, Breuer LH. Field evaluation of a feed formulated for geriatric horses. J Equine Vet Sci 1996;16:334–8.
[75] Ralston SL, Malinowski KM, Christensen R, et al. Digestion in the aged horse-re-visited. J Equine Vet Sci 2001;21(7):310–1.
[76] Henneke DR, Potter GD, Kreider JL, et al. Relationship between condition score, physical measurements and body fat percentage in mares. Equine Vet J 1983;15(4):371–2.
[77] Bertone AL, Ralston SL, Stashak TS. Fiber digestion and voluntary intake in horses after adaptation to extensive large-colon resection. Am J Vet Res 1989;50(9):1628–32.
[78] Bertone AL, van Soest PJ, Stashak TS. Digestion, fecal, and blood variables associated with extensive large colon resection in the horse. Am J Vet Res 1989;50(2):253–8.
[79] Ralston SL, Foster DL, Divers T, et al. Effect of dental correction on feed digestibility in horses. Equine Vet J 2001;33(4):390–3.
[80] Ralston SL, Nockels CF, Squires EL. Differences in diagnostic test results and hematologic data between aged and young horses. Am J Vet Res 1988;49:1387–92.
[81] McFarlane D, Sellon DC, Gaffney D, et al. Hematologic and serum biochemical variables and plasma corticotrophin concentrations in aged horses. Am J Vet Res 1998;59:1247–51.

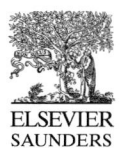

Common Procedures in Broodmare Practice: What Is the Evidence?

Steven P. Brinsko, DVM, MS, PhD

Department of Large Animal Clinical Sciences, College of Veterinary Medicine and Biomedical Sciences, Texas A&M University, College Station, TX 77843-4475, USA

Veterinary medicine is an art and a science. The art of veterinary medicine comprises those skills that are attained by study, practice, observation, and experience, including those arising from the exercise of the practitioner's intuitive faculties. The science of veterinary medicine encompasses the knowledge attained through observation and experimentation. Hopefully, this accumulated knowledge forms a base of evidence from which sound management practices can be developed.

Over the years, many of the procedures that have been adopted for use in the broodmare and stallion have been based on extrapolation from other species and the artful practices passed on from our predecessors and contemporaries. When scientific investigations fail to support those practices, however, or refute their validity, the science should not be ignored. This forum is too short to address procedures for broodmares and stallions; thus, this article examines a few clinically relevant questions pertaining to broodmare management. Described are several common practices in which the art and science of veterinary medicine may seem to be at odds.

Thyroid supplementation

Many clinical syndromes, including infertility, have been attributed to thyroid dysfunction. As a result, an unknown number of broodmares are supplemented with thyroxine (T_4) in an effort to improve fertility, regardless of whether or not they are showing clinical signs of hypothyroidism [1]. Anecdotal reports of the beneficial effects of T_4 supplementation in horses are largely unsubstantiated [2]. Whether or not hypothyroidism actually occurs in the horse is a controversial subject, but its prevalence is considered to be

---

E-mail address: sbrinsko@cvm.tamu.edu

rare, or at best uncommon, and documented cases of equine hypothyroidism are yet to be reported [2,3].

Even so, many broodmares are treated with T_4 because of a presumptive diagnosis of hypothyroidism. In broodmares, diagnosis of hypothyroidism is often based on the clinical signs of subfertility or failure to cycle normally in conjunction with low serum T_4 or triiodothyronine (T_3) levels, thereby prompting thyroid hormone supplementation. Measurement of the free fractions of thyroid hormones provides more useful information than measuring total amounts of circulating thyroid hormones; however, even these levels can be misleading when based on a single blood sample [1–3]. Serum T_3 and T_4 levels can vary widely in clinically normal animals. Furthermore, several factors, including time of day, diet, physiologic or pathologic condition, and certain drugs (phenylbutazone in particular), can influence the metabolism and measured level of thyroid hormones [1–3].

Part of the problem with interpreting results is that normal values vary among laboratories because of differences in assays, units of measurement, and the populations of horses used to establish normal reference ranges [2]. Compared with baseline measurements, thyroid-releasing hormone (TRH) or thyroid-stimulating hormone (TSH) stimulation tests are considered to be a superior method of testing thyroid function [2]. Unfortunately, the need for multiple blood sampling, along with the lack of availability of TRH and TSH and their prohibitive cost, preclude the routine use of these tests.

Some of the most compelling evidence against the need for thyroid supplementation to improve equine reproductive function comes from studies on thyroidectomized animals. Thyroidectomy of stallions affects libido, but semen characteristics and testicular histologic findings are normal [4]. Studies in mares resulted in similar findings, in that although behavioral characteristic were diminished by a thyroidectomy, they were not eliminated. In addition, thyroidectomized mares had similar estrous cycle lengths and luteinizing hormone (LH) and progestagen concentrations as control mares despite having undetectable levels of serum T_4 [5]. It should be noted that in these studies, sample sizes were small (n = 3 per group); therefore, the large amount of individual variation could have had an impact on the ability to demonstrate a statistically significant difference. In two seasons, three pregnancies in thyroidectomized mares resulted from one or two matings, including one from a thyroidectomized stallion. One of the thyroidectomized mares failed to become pregnant either year after being mated during two estrous cycles, however [5].

A cohort study involving 329 clinically normal Thoroughbred broodmares found no association between serum T_4 concentrations and pregnancy status in maiden, barren, or foaling mares 15 to 16 days after ovulation [6]. It should be noted, however, that 60 mares were receiving T_4 supplementation (44 of which became pregnant) and that T_4 measurements were based on a single blood sample. Subsequently, a prospective study involving 11 Thoroughbred and 68 Standardbred broodmares ranging in age from 2 to 22 years was performed [1]. A TRH response test was performed on all study mares before breeding while they were in diestrus. Baseline T_3 and T_4 levels varied widely among mares, but serum T_3 levels increased in all mares in response to TRH stimulation. Serum T_4 concentrations increased in all but 2 mares. By definition, this failure to respond to TRH stimulation would classify these 2 mares as having decreased thyroid function; however, one of these mares became pregnant, whereas the other did not. Overall, neither baseline nor stimulated serum T_3 and T_4 concentrations differed between mares that became pregnant and those that did not become pregnant. Authors of both of these studies questioned the practice of T_4 supplementation to broodmares in the absence of controlled studies demonstrating a relation between subfertility and reduced thyroid function.

When the relation between seasonal reproductive cyclicity and thyroid hormones was examined, it was found that mean T_4 concentrations were significantly higher in adult cyclic mares than in anestrous mares [7,8] but that T_3 concentrations were similar [8]. No significant differences have been detected for thyroid hormone concentrations between young (2- to 3-year-old) cyclic and anestrous mares. Mean T_3 and T_4 concentrations were higher in the first 60 to 90 days after parturition in mares resuming normal ovarian activity than in mares undergoing anestrus after foaling, and increases in T_3 and T_4 were associated with the first ovulation after foaling [8]. The authors concluded that the relation of seasonal reproductive activity and thyroid function does not indicate that the thyroid gland is involved in the control of seasonality. Additionally, they postulated that decreased T_3 and T_4 concentrations are a result of hypothalamic control, similar to that described for seasonal reproductive activity. From a physiologic perspective, this hypothesis is quite plausible, because thyroid hormone secretion is regulated by TSH from the anterior pituitary, which, in turn, is regulated by TRH from the hypothalamus.

Despite the lack of scientific evidence that thyroid hormone supplementation is necessary or beneficial, and because of anecdotal information claiming improvements in reproductive performance of older mares placed on thyroid hormone supplementation, the practice is likely to continue based on perceptions of efficacy as well as pressure from the popular demand to "do something" for subfertile mares. Nevertheless, any beneficial effects of thyroid supplementation for broodmares are probably the result of a generalized metabolic enhancement, particularly in aged euthyroid mares. Randomized controlled studies involving mares with low thyroid function documented by stimulation tests need to be performed to address the efficacy of thyroid hormone supplementation on reproductive performance.

Postbreeding antibiotic infusion

Transient mating-induced endometritis is a normal physiologic event. At the time of breeding, the mare's uterus is exposed to a wide variety of contaminants, including potentially pathogenic organisms [9]. As a result, whether mares are bred by natural service or by artificial insemination, an equally intense inflammatory response ensues. This occurs even when the cervix of genitally normal mares is breached at the time of breeding [10].

For many years, bacterial contamination of the uterus was believed to be the sole cause of postbreeding endometritis. It is now known that the inflammatory reaction is largely a result of the uterine response to spermatozoa, however, and seems to be a normal process by which sperm and other contaminants are eliminated from the uterus [11–14]. Physical uterine clearance seems to be an important part of the elimination process; mares that are susceptible to persistent mating-induced endometritis are unable to clear their uterus of contaminants effectively [15]. As a result of the continued antigenic stimulus in these mares, the inflammatory response is prolonged, leading to a hostile uterine environment, often with fluid accumulation. This, in turn, can impair survival of the embryo and can lead to premature luteolysis [16,17].

Despite evidence to the contrary, the mindset of a primary infectious cause of postbreeding endometritis endures. As a result, many mares are routinely infused with antibiotics after every mating. Many veterinarians and breeding managers justify this practice, because it is estimated that 10% to 15% of all broodmares may develop a pathologic form of persistent mating-induced endometritis [18]. Thus, based on the assumption that bacteria are a major contributing factor, it is also assumed that postbreeding antibiotic infusions can improve pregnancy rates. Nevertheless, is there scientific evidence that such a practice is necessary, or even effective, in broodmares?

The origin of the practice of postbreeding antibiotic infusion in mares probably arose, as many equine treatments have, through extrapolation from work in cattle. Early reports indicated that pregnancy rates in dairy cattle were improved, especially in repeat breeders, when cows received intrauterine infusions of antibiotics 24 to 48 hours after breeding [19,20]. Based on observations involving *Pseudomonas* sp in mares, and perhaps stimulated by the work in cattle, investigators suggested that postbreeding treatment probably prevented bacteria introduced at breeding from becoming established and preventing "conception" in mares of marginal breeding health [21]. Subsequently, many broodmare practitioners adopted this practice as a matter of routine.

Subsequent to the initial reports, however, it was recommended that controlled studies in dairy cattle be performed to validate the practice of postbreeding antibiotic infusions. A retrospective case-control study involving 3123 breedings in 32 Holstein herds found that breedings followed by antibiotic infusion were only 0.7 times as likely to result in pregnancy as breedings that were not followed by infusion [22].

Studies assessing the utility of postbreeding infusions have been attempted in broodmares. In one study, postbreeding antibiotic infusions improved pregnancy rates in mares having a condition described as "partial dilatation of the uterus" [23]. With postbreeding antibiotic infusions, 37 foals were obtained from 46 breedings of 30 affected mares. Of 25 affected mares that were never treated, 10 became pregnant and 15 remained barren. Twelve of the treated mares that were impregnated and eventually foaled subsequently remained barren when not treated.

These results as well as personal experience with two barren mares becoming pregnant after inadvertently receiving postbreeding antibiotic infusions prompted an investigation of the effect of postbreeding antibiotics on pregnancy rates over a 5-year period in Standardbred mares [24]. In that study, all mares that were not pregnant after being bred through two cycles (n = 186) were examined and infused with antibiotics 24 to 48 hours after being bred on the third cycle unless their cervix was closed at the time of examination. Mares were divided into four groups: normal mares (n = 45 treated, n = 36 nontreated), late foaling mares (n = 15 treated, n = 87 nontreated), barren mares with a positive culture (n = 39 treated, n = 23 nontreated), and barren mares with a negative culture (n = 23 treated, n = 18 nontreated). The proportion of live foals from all treated mares (59 [48%] of 122 mares) did not differ from the portion of live foals obtained from all nontreated mares (81 [49%] of 164 mares; $P = .96$). Antibiotic infusions tended to depress the foaling rate in normal mares (21 [46%] of 45 mares) compared with normal mares that were not treated (25 [69%] of 36 mares; $P = .07$), however. Foaling rates were similar ($P > .8$) within the late-foaling mare group, barren mare with positive culture group, and barren mare with negative culture group. What was most surprising was that postbreeding infusions did not improve foaling rates in the group of barren mares with positive cultures (21 [54%] of 39 treated mares versus 13 [57%] of 23 nontreated mares; $P = .95$), even though antibiotics were selected based on previous cultures and sensitivity patterns.

Once impaired uterine defense mechanisms were recognized as a major contributing factor in mares susceptible to persistent endometritis [25], several investigators directed their efforts to enhancing uterine defense mechanisms, including uterine clearance, in an effort to improve pregnancy rates. In two publications that shared data [26,27], investigators reported that postbreeding treatment (within 72 hours of mating) with antibiotics plus oxytocin yielded higher pregnancy rates ($P < .05$) on day 14 or 15 than those in mares that were not treated, treated with antibiotics alone, or treated with oxytocin alone; all three treatments resulted in higher pregnancy rates ($P < .01$) than in mares receiving no treatment. A critical examination of the evidence presented in the publications suggests that an error may have been made in the analyses, however, because the data presented in the text of the first publication do not coincide with the graphic presentation of the data in that report. In addition, reanalysis of the data presented in the second article does not agree with the published results. Specifically, χ^2 analysis of the data indicates that although higher pregnancy rates were obtained on days 13 to 15 in the mares receiving the combined postbreeding treatment of antibiotics plus oxytocin than in the mares receiving no treatment ($P < .05$), pregnancy rates were similar ($P > .1$) among the nontreated mares and the mares receiving antibiotics alone or oxytocin alone. Reanalysis of the data also indicates that pregnancy rates were similar ($P > .2$) among the mares receiving the three different postbreeding treatments.

Investigators examined the effects of adding autologous plasma to antibiotic infusions administered once at 12 to 36 hours after breeding [28]. Mares (141 maiden, 204 barren, and 560 lactating) were randomly assigned to one of three treatment groups: no treatment, antibiotic infusion, or antibiotic plus plasma infusion. Early per cycle pregnancy rate (14 to 16 days after breeding) and foaling rates were found to be higher ($P < .05$) in lactating mares treated with antibiotics and plasma than in lactating mares that were not treated or treated with antibiotics alone. Neither the use of antibiotics alone nor the use of antibiotics in combination with autologous plasma affected the early pregnancy rate or foaling rate in maiden mares. It was thus reported that in barren mares, treatment with antibiotics and plasma had a tendency ($P < .09$) to improve the pregnancy rate compared with nontreated mares and mares receiving antibiotics alone. Addition of autologous plasma to postbreeding antibiotic infusions is not widely practiced, however, possibly because the collection and processing of autologous plasma is too time-consuming and tedious to be practiced on a routine basis.

Because delayed uterine clearance is a significant problem in mares susceptible to persistent postbreeding endometritis [29,30], it would seem logical that aiding in the dilution and removal of uterine contaminants would be more beneficial than simply infusing antibiotics, especially because bacteria are only one of many potential antigenic stimuli present. Despite evidence that postbreeding lavage is a safe [31] and effective [32] method of removing mating-induced intrauterine fluid accumulations, it may not be routinely used on many breeding farms. This could be because practitioners believe that performing uterine lavage is too cumbersome and time-consuming. Yet, uterine lavage can be performed rapidly with a minimum of ancillary equipment [33]. Still, most practitioners find that it is far easier simply to infuse antibiotics with or without oxytocin as an adjunct therapy even though there is no hard evidence that it is beneficial, especially in maiden mares.

Progesterone supplementation in early pregnancy

It has become common practice for mares bred in the United States and several other countries to be administered progesterone or synthetic progestagens early in the postovulatory period. This is most often done in mares having a history of early embryonic loss or after embryo transfer. The rationale for this practice is to increase the chance of the mare maintaining pregnancy by supplementing allegedly low endogenous levels of progesterone.

There seems to be a wealth of anecdotal information about mares that have apparently not been able to get pregnant or have experienced early embryonic loss in the past and were subsequently able to become pregnant and maintain the pregnancy after receiving progesterone supplementation. As a result, several breeders and veterinarians have come to consider progesterone supplementation as standard practice for older subfertile mares and for use in embryo transfer programs. There seems to be little if any scientific evidence for the need for or the efficacy of this practice, however.

In normal mares, peripheral progesterone concentrations peak at 12 to 20 ng/mL around days 5 to 10 after ovulation but then decline to levels as low as 3 to 5 ng/mL by day 35 of pregnancy. At this time, support from the endometrial cups in the form of equine chorionic gonadotropin (eCG) boosts progesterone levels by inducing the formation of secondary corpora lutea after days 38 to 40 [34]. Mean serum progesterone concentrations of 4 ng/mL or greater are necessary to maintain pregnancy consistently in mares [35].

Clinicians monitoring progesterone levels after detection of pregnancy at days 14 to 16 in problem mares may be concerned by these low progesterone levels, and thus be prompted to institute progesterone supplementation. The primary question to be answered is whether or not waning progesterone level attributable to luteal insufficiency is a cause of early embryonic loss.

Several reports provide some presumptive evidence for luteal insufficiency being associated with early embryonic loss in mares [36–38]. In these reports, however, it is not possible to ascertain whether the reduced levels of progesterone arose from primary luteal insufficiency or as a result of defective embryos providing insufficient signaling for maternal recognition of pregnancy to occur. Others examining pregnancy loss at earlier time frames found that the major source of pregnancy wastage in the mare occurs before day 12; however, they were unable to find an association between pregnancy status and progesterone concentration [39]. In human beings, it has been shown that 60% of embryos lost in the first 12 weeks of gestation have gross chromosomal abnormalities [40], and chromosomal abnormalities account for at least 15% of embryonic deaths in the pig [41]. It is likely that similar chromosomal aberrations are responsible for early embryonic loss in mares [42].

It has been shown that the use of altrenogest (Regumate) can successfully salvage pregnancies in cases of experimentally induced luteal insufficiency [43]. Investigators have been able to maintain pregnancy in 5 of 5 mares administered a luteolytic dose of prostaglandin $F_{2\alpha}$ ($PGF_{2\alpha}$) on day 18 by starting altrenogest therapy on day 16; other progestagens were unable to maintain pregnancies in 20 similarly treated mares.

Other investigators have provided compelling evidence that luteal insufficiency is not a cause of early embryonic loss in mares, however [44]. Progesterone was measured at 2-day intervals in 179 mares beginning on days

16 to 18 of pregnancy. Seventeen of these mares lost their pregnancies between days 17 and 42. In only 1 of these mares was progesterone found to have fallen before the pregnancy loss, and in 14 of the mares, progesterone levels remained at normal levels until 4 to 10 days after they lost their pregnancy. The authors concluded that pregnancy loss in the mare between days 18 and 45 is rarely caused by insufficient progesterone. Indeed, based on work from several laboratories, the practice of progesterone supplementation for early pregnancy maintenance in the mare has been repeatedly questioned [34,42,45].

Supplemental progestagen therapy is routinely used in many embryo transfer programs, especially since transcervical transfer has been more widely employed. It is generally thought that nonsurgical embryo transfer may result in lower pregnancy rates with less experienced practitioners [46]. One of the factors commonly used to explain this is luteal insufficiency, which may occur as a result of $PGF_{2\alpha}$ release caused by manipulation of the cervix during transfer. Therefore, progesterone supplementation is routinely used, even by experienced practitioners, to improve posttransfer pregnancy rates by overcoming potentially lower progesterone levels in recipients. Although administration of progesterone up to 4 days after luteolysis can rescue pregnancies [47], the luteolytic pathway does not seem to be involved in pregnancy failure as a result of cervical manipulation. This is known because cervical dilatation to 4.5 cm on day 7 after ovulation did not result in $PGF_{2\alpha}$ release [48]. Although cervical dilatation resulted in lower progesterone levels than in control mares, concentrations did not drop to less than 4 ng/mL until day 14 after ovulation and insertion of the catheter into the cervix without dilatation did not result in significant changes in progesterone concentrations or cycle length [48]. Furthermore, cervical dilatation up to 4.5 cm on day 7 after ovulation had no adverse effects on pregnancy rates [49].

It has also been shown that progesterone levels do not differ between recipient mares that remain pregnant after transfer and those that are found to be nonpregnant, regardless of whether the transfer is performed transcervically [46] or surgically [50]. Higher or faster rising progesterone concentrations also do not increase the likelihood of the recipient becoming pregnant [46].

Although there is no clinical or experimental evidence indicating that progesterone deficiency is a significant cause of pregnancy loss in the mare, large numbers of mares are administered progestagens in the belief that hormonal supplementation can rescue an otherwise doomed conceptus [34]. Still, of all the possible causes of pregnancy failure, presumed hormonal deficiency is the only one in which therapy can logically be applied. This seems to have led to the premise of "better to do something than nothing." The veterinary literature still lacks well-designed controlled studies comparing pregnancy rates in recipient mares receiving similar quality embryos with and without progesterone supplementation.

Treatment of retained placenta

A retained placenta is considered to be the most common postpartum complication encountered in the broodmare [51,52]. The incidence of this condition after normal foaling in the general population of mares has been reported to range from 2% to 17% [53–56] but can be as high as 54% in draft breeds [57]. The incidence of a retained placenta increases with dystocia, especially when a fetotomy or caesarean section is performed [55,58,59].

A retained placenta has long been recognized as having the potential to affect the reproductive and general health of the mare adversely. Sequelae of a retained placenta reportedly vary from no clinical abnormalities to severe conditions, including toxic metritis, septicemia, laminitis, and death [60,61]. Discrepancy exists in the literature and among opinions of practitioners as to the normal time course in which the placenta is passed by the mare, however. As a result, there is also a lack of universal agreement as to when the placenta is considered to be pathologically retained.

The normal time for expulsion of the equine placenta after parturition has been reported as within 30 minutes [62], from 30 minutes to 3 hours [52,54], within 45 minutes [63], within the first hour [64], by 2 hours [65,66], by 3 hours [67], within 1.5 to 6 hours [68], and longer than 12 hours [61]. A "considerable number" of mares seem to expel the fetal membranes spontaneously between 8 and 24 hours postpartum [55].

When and how to intervene in cases of a retained placenta have had a long history of diverse opinion. Consequently, the time at which the placenta is considered to be pathologically retained and when treatment should be initiated varies widely. Until the recent publication of clinical trials [57,69,70], virtually all the available literature regarding a retained placenta in the mare has been based on personal experience, retrospective descriptions, and anecdotal evidence, with little to no experimental data to support the claims.

Varying opinions exist. One investigator suggests that if the placenta has not been passed by 1.5 hours, it is likely to be retained for 24 to 48 hours [51]. In the 1930s, stud grooms were instructed to seek assistance if the placenta had not passed in 10 hours [60]. In the 1970s and 1980s, another investigator considered 6 hours as the time after which the placenta should be considered retained [68], and this opinion was restated as recently as 2005 [67]. Even so, it seems that the majority opinion is that the placenta should be considered pathologically retained if it has not been expelled by 3 hours after parturition [52,53,63,71–73]. Nevertheless, a statement from a 1980 text on equine reproduction still rings true: "There are no criteria by which to define retention of the afterbirth as pathological" [74].

Neither does there seem to be a consensus on, or evidence for, a "best" method of treatment for placental retention or the time at which removal of the placental should be attempted. As early as the 1930s, attempting manual removal at 10 hours postpartum was recommended, with the caveat that if the placenta was firmly attached and fresh blood was found on the operator's hand, removal should be postponed for an additional 6 to 10 hours lest hemorrhage result [60]. Subsequently, several divergent opinions regarding the time at which (manual) removal of the placenta should be attempted were published [75], ranging from within 3 to 6 hours of parturition [55]; to longer than 8 hours [65]; to 10 hours, removing as much of the placenta as could be easily detached and then returning 3 to 4 days later when any remaining portions could usually be freed [74]; to a "customary" 12 hours [53]; to 12 to 20 hours after foaling [76]; and to 12 hours, with the caveat that manual removal should be delayed if the placenta was firmly attached [71].

Even so, at the same time that recommendations for the proper time for removal of the placental were being made, veterinarians noted that there were significant variations in a mare's response to having her placenta retained. In addition, they also noted that removal of the placenta itself could have adverse effects on the mare's uterus. For example, it was noted that many mares did not expel the placenta for up to 24 hours after a normal birth yet came to no harm and, furthermore, that there were several cases in which early intervention was harmful. One mare with a retained placenta died within 36 hours after foaling, whereas another mare retained part of the placenta for 6 days with no ill effect except for a chocolate-colored discharge. Even individuals with long experience in practice changed their opinions over time. For example, in 1949, Claiborne Farm's long-time resident veterinarian, Sager [71], stated that he ordinarily waited for 12 hours and then attempted manual removal; however, 2 decades later, he reversed this opinion and stated that he was opposed to manual removal of the membranes because it was better to wait for the membranes to slough than to damage the uterus, because this could be harmful or even dangerous. Still, he also stated that no harm would result if the placenta came away easily with gentle traction on the extruding portion [63].

The ideal method of removal of a retained placenta has not been determined. Although the use of oxytocin is currently favored by most practitioners as at least part of the treatment regimen for a retained placenta, until relatively recently, this has not always been so.

Manual removal was the probably the first method used to treat a retained placenta and is still widely practiced in some areas [69]. Over the years, several approaches have been used for manual removal of the placenta. These include applying traction to the free portion of the membranes, placing the hand between the allantochorion and the uterus to detach the membranes, twisting the membranes like a rope, massaging the uterus through the placental membrane (to avoid direct contact with the uterus) [71], and pushing a wooden ring cranially around the outside of the allantochorion while traction is applied to the membranes [77]. Although concerns about damage to the uterine endometrium from manual removal have been routinely expressed [51,58,78], in a randomized clinical trial, the reproductive performance of mares that underwent manual removal of the placenta more than 7 hours after parturition (n = 30) did not differ from that of mares that did not have their placentas manually removed (n = 24) [69]. It should be noted that all mares in the study received oxytocin treatment before manual removal of the placenta.

The use of oxytocin (Pituitrin or posterior-pituitary extract) was found to be beneficial in the treatment of a retained placenta more than 60 years ago [64,75]. The percentage of mares retaining the fetal membranes 8 hours or longer was lower on a farm where oxytocin was administered starting 2 hours postpartum compared with a farm where no oxytocin was used to treat retained fetal membranes [56].

Despite an apparent consensus on the utility of oxytocin for the treatment of a retained placenta, there remains a considerable discrepancy in dosage amount and interval. Despite frequent reports of mares experiencing significant discomfort [55,75,79], relatively high doses of oxytocin injected as a bolus were used for decades [51,55,61,63,66,75,80]. The label dose of oxytocin from most suppliers continues to remain at 60 to 100 IU for obstetric use in the mare.

Single large doses of oxytocin frequently seemed to result in spasmodic uterine contractions that were of little value [55]. As a result of these observations, recommendations were made to treat mares with a retained placenta by administering oxytocin intramuscularly at a dose of 20 IU at an interval of 1 to 2 hours [78] or preferably by adding oxytocin at a rate of 30 to 60 IU to saline at a rate of 1 to 2 L and administering this mixture by slow intravenous infusion over 30 to 60 minutes [55,58,68,79]. At the end of the infusion, the membranes were easily detached in 15 of 21 mares [55]. The infusion method of oxytocin treatment was deemed to be more physiologic than the large bolus method because it caused less discomfort to the mare [58,81] and, based on histologic examination, resulted in the release of more intact chorionic villi from the endometrial crypts [58]. The higher dose (60 IU) of oxytocin infused over the longer period (60 minutes) was considered to yield the best results [55].

Other investigators have reported that mares retaining their placenta longer than 3 hours postpartum had significantly lower serum calcium levels within 12 hours of foaling than mares that did not retain their placenta [70]. They also found that more mares expelled their entire placenta within 2 hours of treatment when 50 IU of oxytocin was dissolved in 450 mL of calcium-magnesium-borogluconate solution and infused over 15 minutes (34 of 53 mares) than when the infusion contained oxytocin dissolved in saline (26 of 59 mares). This type of objective evidence is certainly worth noting when clinicians are deciding on treatment strategies for a retained placenta.

Yet another technique for removal of the placenta involves distending the allantochorionic space with 9 to 12 L of warm (37°C) fluid by means of a stomach tube and pump [73]. After distention, the tube is removed and the membranes are held closed while the mare attempts to expel the fluid, with or without the aid of exogenous oxytocin. The workers who described this technique reported that mares would release the placenta in 15 to 30 minutes as a result of endogenous oxytocin release, as evidenced by milk streaming from the teats of treated mares. Removal using this technique resulted in complete expulsion of the membranes with the microvilli intact, as evidenced by histologic examination.

Lavaging or "douching" of the uterus was used at least as early as the 1930s as an adjunct therapy in the treatment of a retained placenta, especially when remnants of the fetal membranes were left after manual removal was attempted [60]. The rationale for uterine lavage is to remove bacteria and debris from the uterus of mares at risk of developing or having metritis, thereby reducing contamination and providing a less favorable environment for bacterial growth [52,82,83]. It has long been asserted that removal of uterine fluids and debris by siphoning is advantageous [54,60,61,63], although even as late as the mid-1980s, lavage of the uterus after removal of the placenta was considered by some to be a questionable practice [54].

The importance of exercise in helping the mare to expel accumulated fluid and enhance uterine involution was recognized in 1949 [71]. This simple and effective adjunct to medical therapy may be overlooked; however, there also seem to have been no studies conducted to evaluate the efficacy of this treatment.

A variety of media have been used for postpartum uterine lavage in the mare, including a soapy solution containing mercuric iodide [60], water [67,69], warm (45.9°C) water containing antiseptics [63], and saline with [55] and without [52,67,68,82] antibiotics added. Concerns have been raised about the use of antiseptics when flushing the uterus out of fear of damaging the endometrium and reducing phagocytosis [68,79], and this warning has been repeated by others in reviews of the treatment of a retained placenta. Although povidone-iodine concentrations of 2% or greater have been shown to induce a severe inflammatory response in the equine endometrium [84], concentrations of 0.2% or less are not detrimental to peripheral equine neutrophil function [85]. In addition, uterine lavage with a 0.05% povidone-iodine solution did not alter the relative frequency of neutrophils, lymphocytes, or glands in endometrial biopsy samples [86], nor did it reduce pregnancy rates when performed 4 hours after insemination [31]. Therefore, the blanket statement that antiseptics should not be used in postpartum uterine lavage must be viewed in light of the concentration and type of antiseptics used.

Potentially life-threatening sequelae can occur from placental retention as well as from the uterine damage that occurs in situations that contribute to a retained placenta, such as dystocia and the duration of and methods used to correct dystocia, and from uterine damage that may occur from attempted removal of the membranes [72,87]. Because of fear of such sequelae, the prophylactic use of antimicrobials, such as sulfanilamide, began to be used by some practitioners in cases of a retained placenta shortly after they became available for medical use [64]; however, it does not seem that this practice was widespread initially. By the late 1960s and early 1970s, intrauterine and systemic antimicrobial therapy seems to have been a common practice in the treatment of a retained placenta [51,55,61,63,82,88], and this practice has been widely continued [52,54,56,59,66–68,74,77,78,89]. Recently, however, there has been a movement away from the use of intrauterine antibiotics [90]. Although a variety of antimicrobials have been used over the years, choices should be based on sensitivity of the causative organisms and the efficacy of the drug in the target tissues, taking the mode of administration into consideration.

Antibiotic treatment is especially important in mares with or at risk of developing toxic metritis. In these cases, antibiotics with a gram-negative spectrum seem to be most appropriate [90]. The uterine environment is most favorable for the development of gram-negative bacterial infection in the early puerperal period; gram-positive organisms seem to contribute to infection later [68]. In six mares with a retained placenta [91] and 14 fatal cases of septic metritis [72], *Escherichia coli* was isolated from the uterus in every case. A combination of penicillin and gentamicin [92] or trimethoprim sulfa [66] seems to be the most common systemic antibiotic currently used when postpartum mares are at risk of endotoxemia and laminitis.

In conjunction with antimicrobial therapy, anti-inflammatory drugs, such as the cyclooxygenase inhibitors phenylbutazone and flunixin meglumine, are often administered for the prevention and treatment of endotoxemia and laminitis. Because significant damage to the hoof lamina can occur before any clinical signs of laminitis are apparent, measures to prevent laminitis are often implemented when mares are considered to be at risk [93]. Although antihistamines were once recommended by some [51], others subsequently found them to be of no benefit in the prevention or cure of laminitis [55]. Phenylbutazone was found to be useful in postpartum mares developing laminitis, however [68]. Many practitioners currently use flunixin meglumine at an antiendotoxic dose (0.25 mg/kg administered intravenously every 8 hours).

A relatively recent study raised concerns that the antiprostaglandin effects of flunixin meglumine may actually increase the risk of mares retaining their placenta [94]. Mares administered flunixin meglumine 8 hours and 1 hour before induction of parturition maintained their placentas longer than mares that did not receive flunixin meglumine. However, the longest interval from parturition to passage of the placenta in these mares was only 3.2 hours. Therefore, in mares with a retained placenta, use of flunixin meglumine for its antiendotoxic and anti-inflammatory effects would seem to outweigh concerns regarding prolonging placental retention.

In summary, although many veterinarians have been taught to regard every retained placenta in the mare as an emergency requiring treatment directed at prompt expulsion or prophylaxis against endotoxemia and laminitis, the validity of these assertions is questionable in mares that foal normally. There have been no controlled studies to determine the maximum time that a normal foaling mare can retain the placenta before being at risk of illness or adverse affects on reproductive performance; nevertheless, many practitioners institute aggressive therapy if the placenta has not passed within 3 to 4 hours of parturition. Conversely, there is ample anecdotal evidence of apparently normal foaling mares retaining the fetal membranes for periods of 24 hours [58,75] to 6 days with no ill effects other than a vulvar discharge [76]. This can be at least partially explained by the fact that, as Blanchard and colleagues [95] showed, the normal postparturient uterus is capable of restricting the absorption of lethal quantities of endotoxin. In all likelihood, the occurrence and severity of complications often associated with a retained placenta are related to the degree of endometrial damage experienced by the mare. Whether any normal foaling mare that retains the placenta for more than 3 hours requires treatment is still a matter of debate.

Summary

The procedures presented in this article are commonly performed in broodmare practice. Nevertheless, there is little scientific evidence to support their continued use. For some, in fact, there is evidence that the practice is neither necessary nor medically beneficial. Ideally, optimum strategies for managing the mare's reproductive system should be based on prospective studies and clinical trials rather than on retrospective reports and uncontrolled case series. Systematic reviews that detail the methodology used in the reviewed articles, as opposed to uncritical summaries of relevant information, are sorely needed. If circumstances involved in broodmare practice make randomized controlled trials unfeasible, alternative designs, such as prospective matched-pair trials, should be developed and used.

Currently, however, it seems that many practitioners base treatments more on anecdotal information from colleagues than on the scientific literature. In addition, the procedures are often of financial benefit to the practitioner, even if they are not directly beneficial to the mare. Thus, many of these practices are likely to continue despite the lack of evidence substantiating their necessity.

References

[1] Meredith TB, Dobrinski I. Thyroid function and pregnancy status in broodmares. J Am Vet Med Assoc 2004;224:892–4.
[2] Breuhaus B. Review of thyroid function and dysfunction in adult horses. Presented at the 50th Annual Convention of the American Association of Equine Practitioners. Denver (CO); 2004. p. 334–7.

[3] Messer NT. Thyroid dysfunction in horses. Presented at the 40th Annual Convention of the American Association of Equine Practitioners. Vancouver (BC); 1994. p. 153–4.
[4] Lowe JE, Baldwin BH, Foote RH, et al. Semen characteristics in thyroidectomized stallions. J Reprod Fertil Suppl 1975;23:81–6.
[5] Lowe JE, Foote RH, Baldwin BH, et al. Reproductive patterns in cyclic and pregnant thyroidectomized mares. J Reprod Fertil Suppl 1987;35:281–8.
[6] Gutierrez CV, Riddle WT, Bramlage LR. Serum thyroxine concentrations and pregnancy rates 15 to 16 days after ovulation in broodmares. J Am Vet Med Assoc 2002;220:64–6.
[7] Fitzgerald BP, Davison LA. Thyroxine concentrations are elevated in mares which continue to exhibit estrous cycles during the nonbreeding season. J Equine Vet Sci 1998;18:48–51.
[8] Huszenicza G, Nagy P, Juhász J, et al. Relationship between thyroid function and seasonal reproductive activity in mares. J Reprod Fertil Suppl 2000;56:163–72.
[9] Kenney RM, Bergman RV, Cooper WL, et al. Minimal contamination techniques for breeding mares. Technique and preliminary findings. Presented at the 21st Annual Convention of the American Association of Equine Practitioners. Boston; 1975. p. 327–6.
[10] Nikolakopuolos E, Watson ED. Does artificial insemination with chilled, extended semen reduce the antigenic challenge to the mare's uterus compared with natural service? Theriogenology 1997;47:583–90.
[11] Kotilainen T, Huhtinen M, Katila T. Sperm induced leukocytosis in the equine uterus. Theriogenology 1994;41:629–36.
[12] Troedsson MHT, Stieger BN, Ibrahim NM, et al. Mechanism of sperm-induced endometritis in the mare [abstract #307]. Biol Reprod 1995;52(Suppl 1):133.
[13] Troedsson MHT, Liu IKM, Crabo BG. Sperm transport and survival in the mare: a review. Theriogenology 1998;50:807–18.
[14] Troedsson MHT. Uterine clearance and resistance to persistent endometritis in the mare. Theriogenology 1999;52:461–71.
[15] Evans MJ, Hamer JM, Gason LM, et al. Factors affecting uterine clearance of inoculated materials in mares. J Reprod Fertil Suppl 1987;35:327–34.
[16] Peterson FB, McFeely RA, David JSE. Studies on the pathogenesis of endometritis in the mare. Presented at the 15th Annual Convention of the American Association of Equine Practitioners. Houston (TX); 1969. p. 279–87.
[17] Neely DP, Kindahl H, Stabenfeldt GH, et al. Prostaglandin release patterns in the mare: physiological, pathophysiological and therapeutic responses. J Reprod Fertil Suppl 1979;27:181–9.
[18] Troedsson MHT. Mating-induced endometritis. Presented at the 9th Annual Hagyard Bluegrass Equine Symposium. Lexington (KY); 2006. p. 43–7.
[19] Lindley DC. Intra-uterine antibiotic therapy postservice in infertile dairy cattle. J Am Vet Med Assoc 1954;124:187–9.
[20] Oxender WD, Seguin BE. Bovine intrauterine therapy. J Am Vet Med Assoc 1976;168:217–9.
[21] Hughes JP, Loy RG, Asbury AC, et al. The occurrence of *Pseudomonas* in the reproductive tract of mares and its effect on fertility. Cornell Vet 1966;54:593–610.
[22] Dohoo IR. A retrospective evaluation of postbreeding infusions in dairy cattle. Can J Comp Med 1894;48:6–9.
[23] Knudsen O. Partial dilatation of the uterus as a cause of sterility in the mare. Cornell Vet 1964;54:423–38.
[24] Wearly WK, Murdick PW, Hensel JD. A five year study of the use of post-breeding treatment in mares in a Standardbred stud. Presented at the 17th Annual Convention of the American Association of Equine Practitioners, Chicago; 1971. p. 89–96.
[25] Watson ED. Uterine defense mechanisms in mares resistant and susceptible to persistent endometritis: a review. Equine Vet J 1988;20:397–400.
[26] Pycock JF. Assessment of oxytocin and intrauterine antibiotics on intrauterine fluid and pregnancy rates in the mare. Presented at the 40th Annual Convention of the American Association of Equine Practitioners. Vancouver (Canada); 1994. p. 19–20.

[27] Pycock JF, Newcombe JR. Assessment of the effect of three treatments to remove intrauterine fluid on pregnancy rate in the mare. Vet Rec 1996;138:320–3.
[28] Pascoe DR. Effect of adding autologous plasma to an intrauterine antibiotic therapy after breeding on pregnancy rates in mares. Biol Reprod 1995;Mono 1:539–43.
[29] Troedsson MHT, Liu IKM. Uterine clearance of non-antigenic markers (Cr^{51}) in response to bacterial challenge in mares potentially susceptible to and resistant to chronic uterine infection. J Reprod Fertil Suppl 1991;44:283–8.
[30] Troedsson MHT, Liu IKM. Measurement of total volume and protein concentration of intrauterine secretion after intrauterine inoculation of bacteria in mares that were either resistant or susceptible to chronic infection. Am J Vet Res 1992;53:1641–4.
[31] Brinsko SP, Varner DD, Blanchard TL. The effect of uterine lavage on pregnancy rate in mares when performed four hours post insemination. Theriogenology 1991;35:1111–9.
[32] Knutti B, Pycock JF, Van Der Weijden GC, et al. The influence of early postbreeding uterine lavage on pregnancy rate in mares with intrauterine fluid accumulations after breeding. Equine Veterinary Education 2000;12:267–70.
[33] Brinsko SP. How to perform uterine lavage: indications and practical techniques. Presented at the 47th Annual Convention of the American Association of Equine Practitioners. San Diego (CA); 2001. p. 407–11.
[34] Allen WR. Luteal deficiency and embryo mortality in the mare. Reprod Domest Anim 2001; 36:121–31.
[35] Shideler RK, Squires EL, Voss JL, et al. Exogenous progestin therapy for maintenance of pregnancy in ovariectomized mares. Presented at the 27th Annual Convention of the American Association of Equine Practitioners. New Orleans (LA); 1981. p. 211–9.
[36] Ginther OJ. Embryonic loss in mares: incidence, time of occurrence, and hormonal involvement. Theriogenology 1985;23:77–89.
[37] Darenius K, Fredriksson G, Kindahl H. Allyl trenbolone and flunixin meglumine treatment of mares with repeated embryonic loss. Equine Vet J Suppl 1989;8:35–9.
[38] Bergfelt DR, Woods JA, Ginther OJ. Role of the embryonic vesicle and progesterone in embryonic loss in mares. J Reprod Fertil 1992;95:339–47.
[39] Forde D, Keenan L, Wade J, et al. Reproductive wastage in the mare and its relationship to progesterone in early pregnancy. J Reprod Fertil Suppl 1987;35:493–5.
[40] Boue' J, Boue' A, Lazar P. Retrospective and prospective epidemiological studies of 1500 karyotyped spontaneous human abortions. Teratology 1975;12:11–26.
[41] McFeely RA. Chromosomal abnormalities in early embryos of the pig. J Reprod Fertil 1967; 13:579–81.
[42] Allen WR. Is your progesterone therapy really necessary? Equine Vet J 1984;16:496–8.
[43] McKinnon AO, Lescun TB, Walker JH, et al. The inability of some synthetic progestagens to maintain pregnancy in the mare. Equine Vet J 2000;32:83–5.
[44] Irvine CHG, Sutton P, Turner JE, et al. Changes in plasma progesterone concentrations from days 17 to 42 of gestation in mares maintaining or losing pregnancy. Equine Vet J 1990;22:104–6.
[45] Allen WR. Progesterone and the pregnant mare: unanswered chestnuts. Equine Vet J 1993; 25:90–1.
[46] Stout TAE, Tremoleda JL, Knapp J, et al. Does compromised luteal function contribute to failure to establish pregnancy after non-surgical embryo transfer? In: Havemeyer Foundation Monograph Series 14, Proceedings of the 6th International Symposium on Equine Embryo Transfer. Rio De Janeiro (Brazil); 2004. p. 8–9.
[47] Kastelic JP, Adams GP, Ginther OJ. Role of progesterone in mobility, fixation, orientation, and survival of the equine embryonic vesicle. Theriogenology 1987;27:655–63.
[48] Handler J, Königshofer M, Kindahl H, et al. Secretion patterns of oxytocin and PGF2α-metabolite in response to cervical dilatation in cyclic mares. Theriogenology 2003;59:1381–91.
[49] Handler J, Gomes T, Waelchli RO, et al. Influence of cervical dilatation on pregnancy rates and embryonic development in inseminated mares. Theriogenology 2002;58:671–4.

[50] McCue PM, Vanderwall DK, Keith SL, et al. Equine embryo transfer: influence of endogenous progesterone concentration in recipients on pregnancy outcome [abstract]. Theriogenology 1999;51:267.
[51] Asbury AC. Management of the foaling mare. Presented at the 18th Annual Convention of the American Association of Equine Practitioners. San Francisco (CA); 1972. p. 487–90.
[52] Blanchard TL, Varner DD. Therapy for retained placenta in the mare. Vet Med 1993;88:55–9.
[53] Jennings WE. Some common problems in horse breeding. Cornell Vet 1941;31:197–216.
[54] Roberts SJ. Injuries and diseases of the puerperal period. In: Veterinary obstetrics and genital diseases (theriogenology). Woodstock (VT): Roberts SJ; 1986. p. 382–3.
[55] Vandeplassche M, Spincemaille J, Bouters R. Aetiology, pathogenesis and treatment of retained placenta in the mare. Equine Vet J 1971;3:144–7.
[56] Provencher R, Threllfall WR, Murdick PW, et al. Retained fetal membranes in the mare: a retrospective study. Can Vet J 1988;29:903–10.
[57] Sevinga M, Barkema HW, Stryhn H, et al. Retained placenta in Friesian mares: incidence, and potential risk factors with special emphasis on gestation length. Theriogenology 2004; 61:851–9.
[58] Vandeplassche M, Spincemaille J, Bouters R, et al. Some aspects of equine obstetrics. Equine Vet J 1972;4:105–9.
[59] Freeman DE, Hungerford LL, Schaeffer D, et al. Caesarean section and other methods for assisted delivery: comparison of effects on mare mortality and complications. Equine Vet J 1999;31:203–7.
[60] Heatley TG. A few notes on retention of the afterbirth in the mare. Vet Rec 1936;48:760–1.
[61] Alexander RW. Excessive retainment of the placenta in a mare. Vet Rec 1971;89:175–6.
[62] Williams WL. Veterinary obstetrics. Ithaca (NY): Williams; 1943.
[63] Sager FC. Management and medical treatment of uterine disease. J Am Vet Med Assoc 1968; 153:1567–9.
[64] Fincher MG. Retained placenta. J Am Vet Med Assoc 1941;99:395–404.
[65] Shipely WD, Bergen WC. Care of the foaling mare and foal. Vet Med Small Anim Clin 1969; 64:63–70.
[66] Card CE. Management of the pregnant mare. In: Samper JC, editor. Equine breeding management and artificial insemination. Philadelphia: WB Saunders; 2000. p. 247–66.
[67] England CW. Retained placenta. In: Fertility and obstetrics in the horse. 3rd edition. Oxford (UK): Blackwell; 2005. p. 173–7.
[68] Vandeplassche M, Bouters R, Spincemaille J, et al. Observations on involution and puerperal endometritis in mares. Irish Veterinary Journal 1983;37:126–32.
[69] Sevinga M, Barkema HW, Hesselink JW. Reproductive performance of Friesian mares after retained placenta and manual removal of the placenta. Theriogenology 2002;57:923–30.
[70] Sevinga M, Barkema HW, Hesselink JW. Serum calcium and magnesium concentrations and the use of a calcium-magnesium-borogluconate solution in the treatment of Friesian mares with retained placenta. Theriogenology 2002;57:941–7.
[71] Sager FC. Examination and care of the genital tract of the brood mare. J Am Vet Med Assoc 1949;115:450–5.
[72] Prickett ME. Septic metritis in postparturient mares. Mod Vet Pract 1970;51:42–5.
[73] Burns SJ, Judge NG, Martin JE, et al. Management of retained placenta in mares. Presented at the 23rd Annual Convention of the American Association of Equine Practitioners. Lexington (KY); 1977. p. 381–90.
[74] Rossdale PD, Ricketts SW. Birth. In: Equine stud farm medicine. 2nd edition. Philadelphia: Lea & Febiger; 1980. p. 220–76.
[75] Wright JG. Parturition in the mare. J Comp Pathol 1943;53:212–9.
[76] Kelly EV. Retained placenta in the mare. Vet Rec 1944;56:296.
[77] Threlfall WR, Provencher R, Carleton CL. Retained fetal membranes in the mare. Presented at the 33rd Annual Convention of the American Association of Equine Practitioners, Lexington (KY); 1987. p. 649–56.

[78] Vandeplassche M. Obstetrician's view of the physiology of equine parturition and dystocia. Equine Vet J 1980;12:45–9.
[79] Arthur GH. Wright's veterinary obstetrics. 3rd edition. London: Balliere, Tindal & Cox; 1964.
[80] White TE. Retained placenta. Mod Vet Pract 1980;61:87.
[81] Cox JE. Excessive retainment of the placenta in a mare. Vet Rec 1971;89:252–3.
[82] Blanchard TL, Varner DD, Scrutchfield WL, et al. Management of dystocia in mares: retained placenta, metritis, and laminitis. Compendium Continuing Education for Veterinarians 1990;12:563–71.
[83] Vowles GB. A case of caesarian section in the mare. Vet Rec 1975;96:155.
[84] Van Dyk E, Lange AL. Die skakelike gevolg van intra-uterine toediening van jodium by merries. J S Afr Vet Assoc 1986;57:205–10.
[85] Watson ED. Effect of povidone-iodine on in vitro locomotion of equine neutrophils. Equine Vet J 1987;193:226–8.
[86] Brinsko SP, Varner DD, Blanchard TL, et al. The effect of postbreeding uterine lavage on pregnancy rate in mares. Theriogenology 1990;33:465–75.
[87] Blanchard TL, Bierschwal CJ, Youngquist RS, et al. Sequelae to percutaneous fetotomy in the mare. J Am Vet Med Assoc 1983;182:1127.
[88] Mason TA. Retention of the placenta in the mare. Vet Rec 1971;89:546.
[89] Blanchard TL, Elmore RG, Varner DD, et al. Dystocia, toxic metritis and laminitis in mares. Presented at the 33rd Annual Convention of the American Association of Equine Practitioners, Lexington (KY); 1987. p. 641–8.
[90] Frazer GS. Recent advancements in equine obstetrics. Presented at the society for Theriogenology Annual Conference & SFT/ACT Symposium. Lexington (KY); 2004. p. 61–92.
[91] Blanchard TL, Orsini JA, Garcia MC, et al. Influence of dystocia on white blood cell and blood neutrophil counts in mares. Theriogenology 1986;25:347–52.
[92] Shuster R, Traub-Dargatz J, Baxter G. Survey of diplomates of the American College of Veterinary Internal Medicine and the American College of Veterinary Surgeons regarding clinical aspects and treatment of endotoxemia in horses. J Am Vet Med Assoc 1997;210:87–91.
[93] Pollitt C, Kyaw-Tanner M, French K, et al. Equine laminitis. Presented at the 49th Annual Convention of the American Association of Equine Practitioners. New Orleans (LA); 2003. p. 103–15.
[94] Vivrette SL, Kindahl H, Munro CJ, et al. Effects of flunixin meglumine on pituitary effluent oxytocin, arginine vasopressin, and 15-ketodihydroprostaglandin $F_{2\alpha}$ concentrations and clinical parturient events during oxytocin-induced parturition in mares. Biol Reprod 1995; Mono 1:69–75.
[95] Blanchard TL, Elmore RG, Kinden DA, et al. Effect of intrauterine infusion of *Escherichia coli* endotoxin in postpartum pony mares. Am J Vet Res 1985;46:2157–62.

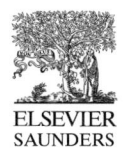

Evidence-Based Lameness Detection and Quantification

Kevin G. Keegan, DVM, MS

Department of Veterinary Medicine and Surgery, College of Veterinary Medicine, C163A Clydesdale Hall, 379 East Campus Drive, University of Missouri, Columbia, MO 65211, USA

Lameness is arguably the most important medical problem in horses. In one survey, limb lameness, hoof and foot problems, and "whole-body" lameness accounted for the first, fourth, and eighth most frequently reported health problems in horses [1]. Lameness has the highest annual incidence density of all medical problems in horses, with one half of all horse operations of 5 or more horses experiencing 1 or more cases of lameness per year [2]. Other sources estimate lameness incidence at 8.5 to 13.7 cases per 100 horses per year [3]. Assuming approximately 9.2 million horses in the United States [4] and an average of $432 spent on veterinary services per lameness incident [3], we can estimate that horse owners spend somewhere between $325 and $544 million per year on the diagnosis and treatment of lameness. The total annual financial loss to horse owners attributable to lameness, taking into consideration the cost of all loss of use and veterinary expenditures, is estimated to exceed $1 billion dollars per year [3].

Thus, to the horse owner and the horse trainer, lameness is the most important equine health issue they face [1]. Yet, less than 3% of horses die or are euthanized because of lameness. Furthermore, it is estimated that 70% of horses eventually recover from their lameness incidents [2]. This high rate of recovery should imply that the equine veterinarian is highly effective in the diagnosing and treating of equine lameness or that horses commonly get better without treatment or despite all the interventions performed on them. Evidence must be gathered with an eye toward clear and measurable diagnostic criteria, beginning with the ability to detect and quantify lameness definitively.

Although it may be the criterion of success that is most interesting and persuasive for a client, evaluating improvement or recovery from lameness

E-mail address: keegank@missouri.edu

0749-0739/07/$ - see front matter © 2007 Elsevier Inc. All rights reserved.
doi:10.1016/j.cveq.2007.04.008   *vetequine.theclinics.com*

using a benchmark of performance "success" is fraught with confounding factors, such as temperament, fortitude ("heart"), or conditioning as well as conditions that may be idiosyncratic to the individual animal, situation, or both. Some lame horses may even perform better than sound ones. Conversely, horses that have truly recovered from lameness may not perform well for other reasons, and it may thus be wrongly concluded that such performance "failure" is because the horse remains lame.

To objectify lameness measurement, some more defined scale of lameness quantification is necessary to mitigate these confounding factors. Quantifying lameness with defined scales is important for equine veterinarians to archive lameness severity for records accurately and to communicate with each other and with their equine clients effectively. Moreover, in many clinical reports and controlled studies, subjective evaluation of lameness has been used to assess improvement after treatment, with purported improvement then used to support continued use of that particular treatment. In the United Kingdom, lameness severity is quantified along an 11-point scale from 0, or no lameness, to 10, or maximum non–weight-bearing lameness [5]. A stricter and more criteria-based scale that has become the de facto standard in the United States is the American Association of Equine Practitioners (AAEP) guidelines for grading lameness, with 0 indicating normal or sound and 5 representing maximum lameness with minimal weight bearing [6]. Practitioners in the United States routinely split the scale, however, and quantify lameness in gradations of 0.5; thus, in essence, the UK and US scales are similar. Just how good is subjective evaluation of lameness in horses?

Subjective evaluation of lameness in horses: how good is it?

First, it is necessary to examine the AAEP guidelines more closely. Grade 0 is defined as soundness or no lameness perceptible under any circumstances (eg, weight carrying, circling, inclines, hard surface); grade 1 as difficult to observe or not consistently apparent regardless of circumstances; grade 2 as difficult to observe at a walk or when trotting in a straight line but consistently apparent under certain circumstances; grade 3 as consistently observable at a trot under all circumstances; grade 4 as obvious with marked nodding, hitching, or shortened stride; and grade 5 as lameness so severe as to cause the animal to have minimal or no weight bearing in motion or at rest or an inability to move. Interestingly, although the grades are separated by defined criteria, only the criterion for grade 5 (non–weight-bearing lameness) contains an unmistakable nonrelative observation. Grades 0 through 3, and to a lesser extent grade 4, depend on what the examiner is looking at and how skillful he or she is at evaluating what he or she is observing. Differences in evaluators' experiences and skills may blur the boundaries between levels, such that clinically similar lameness severities may be judged as being much different. These criteria also do not address differentiation of the side (left versus right) of lameness, which may be difficult to determine when lameness is mild.

Until recently, few have attempted to assess the validity of subjective evaluation of lameness severity in horses. A study conducted using videotapes (front, rear, and side views) of 6 horses with navicular bursal-induced inflammation before and after distal interphalangeal joint anesthesia reported a 100% intraobserver agreement among four different observers for grading the lameness (median score = 2.5, range: 2–3.5 on a 4-point scale). In this study, an interobserver agreement was not reported, however [7]. Another videotape study using lateral views of 24 horses trotting on a treadmill reported that intraobserver agreement among six experts for detecting forelimb lameness and picking the correct limb in horses with mild (not seen in every stride) to moderate (seen in every stride) lameness was good ($\kappa = 0.61$ or 61% greater than chance) and what would be expected in a blind test for a medical condition of moderate difficulty [8]. Intraobserver agreement for seven nonexperts (interns and residents in training) was not as good ($\kappa = 0.41$) but was still acceptable. Interobserver agreement for experts and nonexperts was poor, however ($\kappa = 0.23$ and $\kappa = 0.21$, respectively). These findings can be interpreted to suggest that experts become more reliable than nonexperts in assigning lameness severity but that they are not necessarily more correct.

Interestingly, in the latter study, different combinations of objective measures of movement of the head, limb, and foot correlated with the different examiners' subjective lameness evaluations, thus suggesting that evaluators look at different things when evaluating lameness in horses and that this could be one explanation for the poor interobserver agreement. Although the lack of sound for evaluation of the pitch and loudness of hoof impact, only providing lateral view movement for assessment, and the unfamiliar setting to some observers of evaluating horses trotting on the treadmill may have artificially lowered interobserver agreement, these limitations were likely offset by other factors, such as being able to view the videotape many times and evaluating many consecutive strides with the horse close to the examiner.

A few equine centers in the United Kingdom have directly endeavored to address the issues of repeatability (intraobserver agreement) and reproducibility (interobserver agreement) as measures of reliability of subjective evaluation of lameness in horses. In the absence of a universally accepted "gold standard" for detection and quantification of lameness, although this is a debatable point, reliability of subjective evaluation of lameness may be considered an estimate of validity. Comparing two different subjective grading scales, a numeric rating scale (NRS) ranging from 0 (no lameness) to 5 (extreme lameness) and a verbal rating scale (VRS) with explicit adjectives describing what to look for (eg, marked hitching, nodding, shortened stride), it was reported that 16 experienced veterinary examiners were only moderately repeatable or reliable (56%–60% total agreement) in assessing lameness severity regardless of the type of scale used [9–11]. A limitation of the study was that that no sound was presented on the examined videotapes and that 17 of 20 horses had hind limb lameness, which is thought by some to be more difficult to evaluate in general than forelimb lameness. Font and rear views and movement during lunging were evaluated, however, and each evaluator was specifically trained in the use of the observational scales used in the investigation.

Another study evaluated intra- and interindividual agreement using 19 moderately lame horses (scores given by all assessors ranged from 0–4 of a possible 10) [12]. One experienced veterinarian evaluated the horses by a full clinical examination and videotape evaluation (walk and trot in straight line and lunging on two different surfaces in both directions with audio included) on the first occasion and then by videotape on three subsequent occasions over a 9-month period; three veterinarians evaluated all videotapes of the horses on all dates; and one veterinarian evaluated the same videotapes on two separate occasions. Two different scores were given for the lameness at each time of evaluation; a numeric score ranging from 0 (no lameness) to 10 (non–weight-bearing lameness) and a "global score" representing change in lameness (worse, same, improved, or sound). Intraindividual agreement over time and in blind evaluations for the numeric grading and global scoring scales was good (κ range: 0.58–0.79); however, only the global scoring scale resulted in acceptable interindividual agreement ($\kappa = 0.60$).

The effect of not blinding evaluators to treatment on reliability of subjective evaluation of lameness was shown in an investigation in which 18 individuals (four experienced veterinarians, four nonexperienced veterinarians, and 10 veterinary students) subjectively evaluated videotapes of seven lame (grade 0.5–3 on the split AAEP guidelines scale) horses trotting toward and away from them [13]. In one experiment, the evaluators were completely blinded to treatment, unaware that the particular sequence being viewed might have been after a nerve block. In another separate experiment, the evaluators were not blinded and were shown sequences of the same horse, in succession, before and after the nerve block. The grade of lameness given to a horse at a particular time was influenced by whether or not the evaluator knew that a nerve block had been administered, illustrating a typical "hindsight bias." Expectation influenced evaluation. The same type of bias may be active when a veterinarian expects or an owner or trainer wants the lameness to be improved. Although calculation of κ (agreement greater than chance) was not done in this study, the authors concluded that consistency (intraobserver agreement) of assessments made by the individual observers was good. Interobserver agreement between experts was reasonable (± 1 grade) but was poor between nonexperts and students.

It should be pointed out that in none of these recent reports was there included in the architecture of the study an assessment of agreement on the selection of the side of lameness. In these studies, it was not reported whether or not there was indeed 100% agreement on selection of the correct side; whether it was assumed that agreement on the side of lameness was 100% when it was not; or whether the side of lameness was established beforehand, such that evaluators were not truly masked to the side of lameness. Selection of the correct side of lameness is more difficult for lameness of mild severity and, in general, for hind limb lameness compared with forelimb lameness.

Although none of these studies are perfect and each can be justifiably critiqued by picking one or two defects in the study architecture (eg, not using enough horses, not including individuals with all levels of lameness severity, evaluating a videotape, evaluating a videotape without sound, evaluating horses moving on a treadmill, not incorporating selection of side in the lameness scale), their consensus suggests that subjective lameness evaluation by one individual should not be the gold standard when lameness severity is the dependent variable of interest. When subjective scoring or grading methods of lameness evaluation are used, a less precise but more accurate method would be to take the mean value of more than one expert evaluator. To date, however, no study has been completed evaluating the intra- and interobserver agreement of more than one observer when completing a full overground lameness evaluation. Such a study is needed before subjective evaluation of experts can be reliably used as the gold standard for lameness evaluation in horses.

Objective evaluation of lameness in horses

Soundness and lameness in horses can be objectively quantified through biomechanics, which applies mechanical principles to the study of biologic entities—in this case, the horse in motion. Biomechanical analysis can be conducted from one of two different but related perspectives: kinematics and kinetics. Kinematics is concerned with the study of the description of motion. Kinetics, conversely, is concerned with the study of the action of forces. Kinematics describes motion, and kinetics explains motion. Kinematics evaluates motion characteristics spatially (eg, height, displacement) and temporally (eg, duration, rate) without direct reference to forces. Kinetic evaluation attempts to define and measure the forces causing a particular movement. Kinetic analysis of a moving body for lameness evaluation is easy to comprehend; increased lameness results in decreased weight bearing and a resultant decrease in ground reaction force acting on the limb. Kinetic analysis is not as intuitive or easy to visualize as kinematic analysis, however, because the human eye cannot see force. Forces acting on the body are translated, or "transduced," primarily into motion of that body. Nevertheless, both approaches, kinematics and kinetics, can be useful objective means to detect and quantify soundness and lameness in horses. For practical purposes of reviewing techniques suitable for clinical trials, in this article, the author discusses only the most common noninvasive techniques. Other techniques that require the horse to wear heavy equipment, to have long wires attached to its torso or limbs, or to be tethered to recording devices are not discussed.

Kinetic methods

The most available and common method of kinetic gait analysis in horses is the stationary force plate. In most natural conditions and induced lameness models, increasing severity of lameness in a limb correlates with decreasing peak vertical ground reaction force (pVGRF) acting on that limb. Other force plate measures that correlate well (negatively) with severity in lameness include vertical impulse (area under the vertical force curve), braking (negative horizontal) force and impulse, and propulsive (positive horizontal) force and impulse. Mean pVGRF on the forelimb of a sound horse trotting at approximately 3 m/s over eight strides was reported to be just less than 10 N/kg, with a 7% decrease for every 0.5 grade in subjective lameness scale [14]. This is comparable with data from other experimental studies. For example, in horses with navicular disease, an increase in mean pVGRF between 9% and 13% was measured in both forelimbs over six strides 6 hours after treatment with anti-inflammatory medication (phenylbutazone or flunixin meglumine) [15]. At a body weight–normalized baseline value of 9.79 N/kg, pVGRF had the highest sensitivity and specificity (both 81%) for detection of lameness of any measured force plate parameter [14]. This is partially because the coefficients of variation of time- and body weight–normalized pVGRF within and between horses are less than 10% [14] and because there is a high degree of symmetry in pVGRF between the right and left limbs at the walk and the trot [16].

For unilateral forelimb lameness, a decrease in mean pVGRF in the lame forelimb is accompanied by increases in mean pVGRF in the contralateral forelimb and both hind limbs at the walk [13] and in the contralateral forelimb and hind limb at the trot [16]. For unilateral hind limb lameness, a decrease in mean pVGRF in the lame hind limb is accompanied by increases in mean pVGRF in both forelimbs at the walk [13] but little change in the other limbs at the trot [17]. If the velocity of the trot can be stringently controlled and if enough valid strikes are collected, mean pVGRF asymmetry can even detect "subclinical" lameness, that is, lameness not seen by the naked eye [14].

Unfortunately, there is one caveat for the use of pVGRF as the sole objective measure or gold standard of lameness detection and quantification in horses. Some lameness conditions have caused not a decrease in mean pVGRF but a change in the shape of the VGRF signal. For example, it has been reported that mean forelimb pVGRF asymmetry in trotting horses with mild (less than grade 1 on a 5-point AAEP scale) induced superficial digital flexor tendinopathy or naturally occurring navicular disease did not differentiate soundness from lameness [18]. Instead, the shape of the VGRF curve changed with a decrease in VGRF in the cranial (superficial digital flexor tenopathy) or caudal (navicular disease) phase of stance. Information gathered from basic morphometric and biomechanics research leads to knowledge about when particular limb structures are active during the different phases of stance. Thus, the shape of the VGRF curve could potentially contain some meaningful information to assist in localization of lameness within the affected limb.

There are other disadvantages of using the stationary force plate as the gold standard in lameness clinical trials. Capturing enough valid (strike in center of plate) and pure (no other limbs striking at the same time) strikes of the limb of interest with the horse moving within a small range of accepted velocities is difficult and time-consuming. All attempted trials do not result in a valid strike. Also, ground reaction forces are sensitive to torso and limb speed as well as to extraneous movement of the head (head tossing) for forelimb measurement in quadrupeds. If valid strikes are even partially determined by evaluating the resultant force tracings, which is frequently done, there is no protection from data selection bias, and the evaluator must therefore still be blinded to treatment group. Finally, not all lameness conditions can be expected to exhibit the same amount of pain on every stride or to have pain on every stride. Accurate detection of these types of lameness is only possible with techniques that evaluate many strides over longer periods.

Two potential methods of measuring VGRF over multiple continuous strides include a telemeterized force-measuring horseshoe and the force-measuring equine treadmill. Although many attempts have been made [19–22], a force-measuring shoe with a design that supplies a combination of true transduction of force and a small enough footprint and weight of sensor and electronics, such that the normal limb movement is not altered, has not yet been accomplished. The only force-measuring equine treadmill in regular use is at the University of Zurich Laboratory for Biomechanics in Zurich, Switzerland [23]. It incorporates multiple piezoelectric load-sensitive sensors in the treadmill platform and a positioning system (rubber strings attached to and running from the horse's hooves to off-treadmill angular encoders) to determine the force application point. This device has generated important information on the relation between VGRF and lameness, especially compensatory lameness in nonaffected limbs (see section on compensatory lameness), but it is custom-made and expensive and requires considerable expertise to use.

Force can also be indirectly transduced or measured by strain gauges mounted on the hoof walls [24,25]. Such a system could potentially substitute for a force-measuring horseshoe to measure clinical lameness objectively in horses over multiple successive strides, but a system with a resilient and repeatable hoof mounting technique has not been evaluated for this purpose. Hoof wall–mounted systems would also likely be subject to large variation with different foot shapes, the presence or absence of shoes, state of trimming, shoe type, and overground surface conditions, such that the association between lameness and hoof wall deformations would have to be described for multiple different combinations of conditions. Accelerometers or other inertial-type sensors (gyroscopes) attached to the limb or hoof wall can measure impact phenomena, such as impact vibration frequency and amplitude, which may be associated with lameness, but such devices do not measure the midstance pVGRF, the kinetic parameter most closely associated with lameness [26–28]. Information from hoof-mounted sensors can be transmitted wirelessly over significant distances using a variety of wireless chipsets and protocols; however, a suitable combination of small footprint (size), long range of high data rate transmission, and suitable analysis algorithms and software, specifically for lameness evaluation, is not yet readily available.

Kinematic methods

The second method of objective detection and quantification of lameness in horses is kinematic gait analysis. Many laboratories around the world have concentrated more on kinematic as opposed to kinetic gait analysis because of the ease of data collection from multiple successive strides. Tracking the position of parts of the body using stationary cameras and passive markers attached to the horse suffers from limited resolution from large fields of view; thus, acquisition of meaningful data from large numbers of successive strides currently requires that the horse be filmed when moving on a treadmill. The equipment for kinematic gait analysis is expensive and time-consuming to operate, and horses must be trained to load onto and move consistently on the treadmill. Once they are trained to the treadmill, however, the speed of movement can be controlled, which helps to decrease variation of movement between examinations. This increases the likelihood of finding smaller differences between treatments.

Motion pattern has been shown to depend greatly on speed, and to detect small differences in kinematic parameters with mild lameness, it should be consistent. Individual horses also exhibit lameness better at trots of different speeds and levels of effort. These speeds may not be possible without riding the horse or using a high-speed equine treadmill, which also highlights one potential limitation of evaluating lameness with the horse viewed in hand. In one study, 12 of 18 horses had the most consistent kinematic asymmetry, indicative of lameness, at a moderate-speed trot, whereas in 6 of the 18, asymmetric motion pattern consistency was highest (and ability to quantify lameness) at a high-speed trot [29]. Although the horse moves slightly differently on the treadmill than over ground, these differences are not reflected in differences in the most likely parameters of interest for detecting and quantifying lameness in horses.

Many kinematic gait parameters have been shown to correlate with severity of lameness in horses. Asymmetry of displacement, usually expressed as a difference or a ratio of the duration or range of motion between the right and left sides rather than as the absolute amplitude of the parameter, is generally of more value for evaluation of lameness in the individual animal at a specific time. Changes in the absolute amplitude of kinematic parameters are still potentially useful for determination of change in lameness from baseline evaluation, for example, before and after diagnostic anesthetic block or before and after treatment in the same horse.

The list of kinematic parameters with significantly different kinematic indices between soundness and lameness is long and varied. Lameness in the forelimb causes an increase in the asymmetry of vertical head movement (acceleration and displacement) between left and right forelimb strides [30,31]. Lameness in the hind limb causes increases in the asymmetry of whole-pelvic vertical acceleration and displacement between left and right hind limb strides and in total displacement of the left and right tubera coxae relative to each other [30,32–34]. When the lame hind limb is bearing weight during stance, the whole pelvis moves down less compared with the sound hind limb. Extensor muscles contract to decrease the downward momentum of the back half of the body and, consequently, the force on the affected limb during stance. The lame limb also pushes the whole pelvis up less during and after the last half of stance. This causes the whole pelvis to move up less after stance. The pelvis seems to rotate toward the lame side because the lack of propulsion forces the lame hind limb to flex more during swing. Other changes with lameness include decreased maximum fetlock extension and distal interphalangeal joint flexion at midstance, decreased retraction (caudal movement of the distal limb) of the forelimb (for forelimb lameness), decreased protraction (cranial movement of the distal limb) of the hind limb (for hind limb lameness), decreased tarsal flexion during stance, and increased stance phase duration (for mild to moderate lameness) [33,35–39].

Many other kinematic parameters have been reported to correlate with lameness depending on the specific lameness model or condition being studied. This has relevance for future investigations for using kinematic gait analysis to help locate lameness within the affected limb. For example, in one kinematic study, investigators found a significant decrease in forelimb protraction in horses with induced lameness in the forelimb heel but a significant increase in forelimb protraction in horses with induced lameness in the toe region of the forelimb hoof [39]. In a model of induced hoof lameness, a significant increase in proximal limb joint flexion (carpus for forelimb and tarsus for hind limb) during swing was seen [35], but in other studies using carpal-induced lameness (injection of irritants into the carpal joints), decreased flexion of the carpus during swing was reported [36]. Further study to determine if unique combinations of kinematic parameter changes can be mapped to specific lameness conditions within the limb is needed. This knowledge could be useful to equine practitioners for establishing differential diagnoses and then ruling in or out the true cause of lameness with additional diagnostic tests.

What kinematic evidence can be used to help detect lameness?

Against this background of a seemingly unlimited number of potential kinematic clues for the detection and quantification of lameness, an important question would be, "What are some general features of changes in kinematics with lameness?" As previously described, lameness in a limb is manifested by an increase in asymmetry of movement of the body and limbs, asymmetry in amplitude between the right and left sides, or asymmetry in amplitude between the same phases in the right and left strides.

No horse moves its torso and limbs perfectly symmetrically on every stride. Natural "leggedness," or asymmetry in equine gait, has been reported [4]. Leggedness, or "laterality," was hypothesized to be inherited in trotting Standardbred colts because it was shown to develop early in life before training commenced [41]. Later, after training for racing, the asymmetry, or leggedness, was amplified. Asymmetry of stride length and synchrony of contralateral forelimb and hind limb footfall timing, and presumably almost every kinematic parameter, have also been shown to be greatest when the horse is trotting at speeds near to its normal transition to the canter or gallop [40].

With this evidence, it is clear, for purposes of using kinematics as a measure of lameness in a clinical trial, that an index or threshold of asymmetry exists and should be determined for the particular kinematic parameter being used. Kinematic parameters with high natural asymmetries or with high stride-by-stride variability would less likely be sensitive indicators of lameness. There are an almost limitless number of potential kinematic variables that can be used to detect and quantify lameness in horses. For such information to be clinically useful, however, this potential list needs to be pared down to a more manageable one. Human eyes can record, and human brains can remember, only so much.

Using simultaneous videotape recordings of the left and right sides of 13 clinically sound horses at a slow (3.2 m/s) overground trot, kinematic symmetry indices (KSIs) were measured over five strides ranging from 0.82 to 0.99 for forelimb and hind limb displacement and greater than 0.95 for all joint angle measurements, except the distal interphalangeal joints (perfect symmetry, KSI = 1) [42]. The KSI was calculated by an intercorrelation method that, in effect, compared the shapes of the displacement and joint angle versus time curves of the various body and limb parts between the left and right sides. In a later study by the same laboratory comparing body and limb KSIs between 13 clinically sound horses and 24 lame horses, it was found that KSIs for proximal limb displacements were the most sensitive for determination of weight-bearing soundness and lameness [43]. In contrast and based on data from only 3 horses, asymmetry in vertical movements of distal limb parts was most pronounced when the lameness was thought to be a "swinging" limb lameness (one case of stringhalt and two carpal injuries) [42]. Vertical displacement asymmetries for the lame horses were more prominent than for joint angle measurements.

Deference to proximal limb asymmetries being more useful to distinguish lameness from soundness is supported by other experimental studies as well. Variability in limb joint patterns in sound horses was found to increase distally along the limb, with the fetlock and distal interphalangeal joints being the most variable, making tracking of the fetlock joint motion for lameness evaluation more difficult [44]. One study using 6 horses with induced carpal lameness (injection of amphotericin B) trotting on a treadmill (4 m/s) and computer-assisted kinematic analysis of gait found that head movement asymmetry was significantly changed after treatment but that there was no significant change in stride length, swing, stance phase duration, forelimb abduction, or carpal and fetlock range of motion [45]. In another study evaluating frog pressure–induced forelimb lameness, maximum fetlock extension at midstance, along with vertical head movement asymmetry, were sensitive indicators of lameness, but other distal limb parameters (stride duration, stance duration, and carpal joint angle extension during stance) were insensitive [39]. Stride length was not significantly changed after induction of carpal lameness until the lameness was considered moderate at the trot [36]. In an investigation of 12 horses with mild right or left forelimb lameness trotting on a treadmill and neural network classification of kinematic gait data, all the necessary and best information for the detection and differentiation (right or left) of forelimb lameness was found in the vertical movement of the head and foot [46]. Information from the other limb markers was not as good and added little to the level of correct classification afforded by the vertical head and foot movement alone. All these studies support the notion that evaluating head and torso movement rather than limb movement is more accurate for detecting and quantifying lameness in horses.

The two most studied and supportable indicators of hind limb lameness are the temporal vertical movement asymmetry of the whole pelvis, as illustrated by an imaginary point on the dorsal midline between the tubera sacrale, and vertical displacement asymmetry between the left and right hemipelves, as illustrated by imaginary points on the bony protuberances of the right and left tubera coxae (Fig. 1). Temporal vertical movement asymmetry of the whole pelvis can be described as lower height of the whole pelvis during sound limb stance compared with lame limb stance and higher height of the whole pelvis after sound limb push off as compared with lame limb push off. Vertical displacement asymmetry between the left and right hemipelves can be described as a greater total vertical movement of the lame side tuber coxae compared with the sound side tuber coxae. This looks like rotation of the pelvis toward the lame side. As early as 1987, using

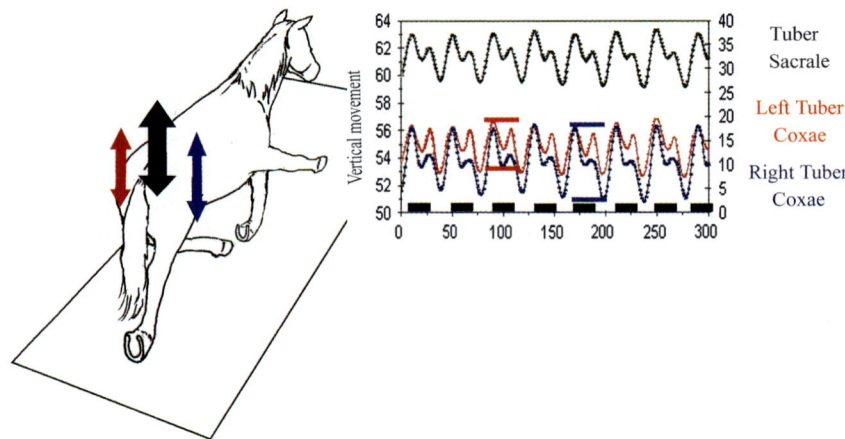

Fig. 1. Two methods of detecting hind limb lameness by observing pelvic movement. Black bars on the bottom of the graph indicate right hind limb stance. Method 1 is illustrated by the double black arrow and top black tracing in the graph, and method 2 is illustrated by red and blue arrows and correspondingly colored bottom tracings in the graph. In method 1, the whole pelvis, depicted as the position between the tubera sacrale, moves asymmetrically over time. In this right-sided hind limb lameness, the pelvis moves down less during the stance phase of the right hind limb and up less after the stance phase of the right hind limb. In method 2, one side of the pelvis, depicted as the position over the tuber coxae, displaces vertically more than the other side of the pelvis. In this right-sided lameness, note that the right tuber coxae (*blue arrow and tracing*) has greater vertical displacement than the left (*red arrow and trac*ing).

simple standard videotape equipment and attaching homemade markers to the right and left tubera coxae of 13 horses with naturally occurring hind limb lameness, increased total vertical movement of the tuber coxae during one complete stride on the side of hind limb lameness was demonstrated [32]. Conversely, a computer-assisted kinematic gait analysis of a sole pressure–induced model of hind limb lameness of horses walking and trotting on a treadmill found that vertical displacement and acceleration of the dorsal midline of the pelvis were the best indicators of hind limb lameness, with acceleration and displacement amplitude becoming less during stance of the lame limb [30]. Changes in vertical acceleration and displacement of markers on the tubera coxae were less sensitive to the induction of lameness. Another computer-assisted kinematic gait analysis, this one evaluating 15 strides of a model of distal tarsal arthritis induced by injection of *Escherichia coli* lipopolysaccharide endotoxin in 8 horses trotting on a treadmill, found significant differences in the ratio of right-to-left tubera coxae vertical excursion but no significant difference in minimum height of the dorsal midline of the sacrum between right and left stances [33]. With a different model of induced hind limb lameness (frog pressure), however, and when random pelvic movement was accounted for with a curve-fitting error-correction algorithm, this same laboratory found that dorsal pelvic height asymmetry between left and right strides was a sensitive measure for detection and quantification of hind limb lameness [34]. With this model and with studying more horses (n = 17) over a greater number of consecutive strides (80–90 strides), differences in the maximum height of the dorsum of the pelvis between right and left strides, which can be thought of as asymmetric propulsion of the hind limbs, was slightly more sensitive than differences in the minimum height of the dorsum of the pelvis between right and left strides, which can be thought of as asymmetric braking of the hind limbs. In other words, evaluation of how forcefully the horse pushed up the whole pelvis, and rear half of the torso, with each hind limb was more useful at detecting and quantifying hind limb lameness than how forcefully the horse landed on each hind limb.

These studies support using head and torso movement, more specifically vertical head and torso movement, rather than limb movement as the basis for developing kinematic gait analysis technique into an objective lameness evaluation tool. Based on biomechanical first principles, it is logical to assume that lameness causes less downward movement of the body during the first part of the stance phase (braking) of the lame limb stride (if the pain of lameness is occurring in the first half of stance), less upward movement of the body during the second part of the stance phase (propulsion) of the lame limb stride (if the pain of lameness is occurring in the second half of stance), or both. In fact, this assumption was tested directly in a study that measured virtual body center of mass movement in lame horses trotting on a treadmill [47]. With lameness of grade 2 severity, vertical body center of mass decreased by 34% during the stance phase of the lame limb and increased 9% during the stance phase of the sound limb. Changes in movement of the body center of mass in the other directions, right to left and back to front, with lameness were of much smaller absolute and relative magnitude.

Other methods of kinematic analysis

Kinematic gait analysis is an attractive method of objective lameness evaluation. With currently available systems, however, it is convenient to collect multiple successive strides only by capturing the movement when the horse is trotting on a treadmill (Fig. 2). This is difficult to accomplish, because horses must be transported to a clinic or laboratory with a treadmill and then trained to the treadmill. This requires extra time and money, and if a large number of subjects are needed for a clinical trial, the costs can become prohibitive. To circumvent this problem, a few body sensor–based equine lameness evaluation systems with wireless transmission of motion data have been described, which would allow overground collection of kinematic data from multiple successive strides.

One system that has been described is a 50-Hz two-accelerometer system called the Equimetrix, which is worn on the body of the horse attached to a girth strap or saddle [48]. The signals are transmitted to a data logger on the horse and then wirelessly to a computer for analysis. This system

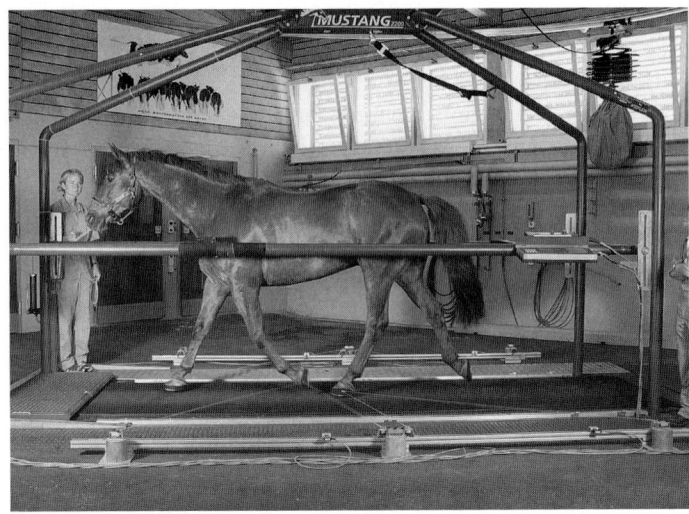

Fig. 2. Force-measuring treadmill, University of Zurich (Zurich, Switzerland).

measures dorsoventral and lateromedial accelerations of the torso. The acceleration signals during left and right weight bearing are processed by fast Fourier transform (fft) to calculate stride rate, and a peak detection algorithm selects strides. The shape of the acceleration signals is compared between left and right stances and from one stride to the next. Pain (lameness) during weight bearing in a limb reduces the correlation coefficient (shape similarity) of the acceleration signals between left and right strides (decreasing symmetry) and between successive strides (decreasing regularity).

Modified use of the Equimetrix, one with two accelerometers each on the pelvis and sternum, has been compared with the force-measuring treadmill at the University of Zurich and with subjective evaluation, using 32 horses trotting on the force-measuring treadmill [49]. Using approximately 25 strides for objective evaluation, correlation between all three evaluations (force-measuring treadmill, Equimetrix, and subjective evaluation) was only fair. For selection of group (sound, lame in the forelimb, or lame in the hind limb), significant correlation was found between measurement of pVGRF asymmetry and subjective evaluation ($r = 0.51$) and between the Equimetrix and subjective evaluation ($r = 0.47$) but not between measurement of pVGRF symmetry and the Equimetrix. For measurement of severity of lameness, correlations between the three types of lameness evaluation were nonsignificant. Correlation between raw pVGRF for the hind limbs and dorsoventral pelvic accelerations were higher and more significant than between raw pVGRF for the forelimbs and dorsoventral sternal accelerations.

The authors of this study, who have no commercial interest in the Equimetrix, explained the poor correlation between the Equimetrix and the force-measuring treadmill and between pVGRF of the forelimb and dorsoventral sternal accelerations on the complex phenomenon of body movement to compensate for lameness. Because the pelvis is linked to the hind limb in a direct bone-to-bone connection but the torso is linked to the forelimb by a soft tissue sling-like connection, lameness effect on sternal dorsoventral acceleration is reduced. Movement of the head on a long lever arm in the opposite direction of the torso with forelimb lameness also contributes to damping of forelimb lameness expression in torso movement. In support of this hypothesis, a study of six horses trotting on a treadmill with carpal lameness induced by injection of irritant found that head but not withers excursion decreased during the stance phase of the lame limb [45].

A different approach to an accelerometer-based system for detection of lameness has been described [50,51]. In this system, accelerometers are placed on the head (attached to the head halter) and dorsum of the pelvis (attached to a Velcro patch). Right and left stance phases are found by gyroscopes taped to the right fore limb and hind limb. Signals at a 200-Hz sampling frequency are wirelessly transmitted to a computer for analysis. Vertical acceleration signals are converted to displacement and processed in a curve-fitting error-correction approach to account for random movement and are then broken down into separate naturally expected and lameness-causing components. Symmetry of vertical head and pelvic movement is associated with angular velocity signals on the right fore limb and hind limb to determine right, left, or both limb involvement in lameness. Using eight horses with natural (before and after block) and induced (frog pressure) forelimb and hind limb lameness that, together, comprised 44 instances of evaluated trials with approximately 100 strides per trial, this system was compared with a camera and marker–based technique that has been previously tested for sensitivity in detecting mild lameness in the forelimb and hind limb. Correlations between the accelerometer-based and camera and marker–based systems was excellent ($r^2 = 0.94$ and $r^2 = 0.82$ for forelimb and hind limb lameness, respectively). Agreement between the two methods for detection of lameness was high ($\kappa = 0.76$ and $\kappa = 0.56$ for forelimb and hind limb lameness, respectively). The accelerometer-based system was considered by the authors to be more sensitive than the camera and marker–based system, because of the six total instances of disagreement between the two systems, five were instances of lameness that were detected by the accelerometer-based system but not by the camera and marker–based system and only one was an instance of lameness detected by the camera and marker–based system but not by the accelerometer-based system. Also, in the latter case, the horse was supposed to be sound (before lameness induction). Rotational movement toward the side of hind limb lameness was thought to contribute to greater sensitivity of the accelerometer-based system. A comparison of this accelerometer-based system with subjective evaluation of lameness by experts or with objective kinetic measures (force plate or force-measuring treadmill) and between overground and treadmill locomotion has not been reported.

Body sensor–based lameness evaluation systems with wireless transmission of data offer the best chance at realizing a relatively inexpensive, easy to use, and objective method of lameness detection and quantification in horses. Several laboratories and groups around the world are working on the development of body sensor–based objective lameness evaluation systems; however, as of the date of this publication, no results have been reported in peer-reviewed literature. At this time, there are at least three existing companies established that may soon be advertising or marketing wireless body sensor–based lameness evaluation systems for use in horses. More research and testing are sorely needed to determine, at least, sensitivity and specificity; more appropriately, positive and negative predictive values of these systems for lameness detection are also necessary. This requires testing on a normal cross section of the equine population so that the increased incidence of lameness in horses presented to a veterinary hospital does not inflate sensitivity and specificity. Further studies on relative agreement of these systems with subjective evaluation of experts and with kinetic (ground reaction force-measuring systems) technique should also be continued.

Compensatory lameness

Many times horses seem to have lameness in the front limbs and hind limbs at the same time. Two possible reasons are (1) true multiple limb lameness (ie, the horse indeed has pain in a front limb and a hind limb, possibly from two independent causes or possibly from pain in a limb occurring because of increased weight bearing secondary to decreased weight bearing on the primary or initially affected limb), and (2) false lameness in one limb, or the horse only has pain in one limb but shifts head and torso movement to compensate for decreased weight bearing on this affected limb, causing the appearance of lameness.

An unofficial equine veterinary law, the "law of sides," states that when horses have what seems to be an ipsilateral lameness, for example, left front and left hind, the primary true lameness is in the hind limb; furthermore, when horses have what seems to be a contralateral lameness, for example, the left forelimb and right hind limb, the primary true lameness is in the forelimb. Is there evidence to support this law? Evidence of the propensity and magnitude of compensatory lameness helps the equine veterinarian to detect the primarily affected limb correctly. The following is a summary of the objective evidence for the existence and propensity of compensatory lameness in the other "half" of the body.

Does a primary hind limb lameness cause an apparent (but false) ipsilateral forelimb lameness?

In one study, 13 horses with spontaneous hind limb lameness were videotaped [32]. All 13 showed lowering of the head lower than normal height when the lame hind limb was in the stance phase. Thus, all 13 horses, if using the "down on sound" methodology of evaluating forelimb lameness, had compensatory false ipsilateral forelimb lameness. Some but not all horses with sole pressure–induced hind limb lameness, evaluated by computer-assisted kinematic analysis of gait in horses trotting on a treadmill, showed that primary hind limb lameness had increased vertical head displacement amplitude and increased head acceleration when the lame hind limb was in the stance phase [30]. This implies that a readily apparent but false ipsilateral forelimb lameness occurs often in horses with primary hind limb lameness. In another computer-assisted kinematic study of horses trotting on a treadmill, 4 of 4 horses, regardless of the cause of lameness, had movements of the head that mimicked ipsilateral forelimb lameness [52]. A similar relation was demonstrated in horses with distal tarsal arthritis trotting over ground [42]. A false ipsilateral forelimb lameness was seen only after a hock flexion test, when the primary hind limb lameness was exacerbated.

Using the force-measuring treadmill and the sole pressure model of induced lameness in 8 horses, it was demonstrated that primary hind limb lameness caused the horse to shift vertical impulse (area under the VGRF curve) to the forelimbs and to the contralateral hind limb [17]. In the lame diagonal, the impulse shifted slightly (6.5%) to the forelimb when the lameness was of moderate severity (eg, the lameness was distinctly visible at the trot, wherein, however, the cadence of movement was not obviously disturbed). In the sound diagonal, the impulse shifted slightly (3.5%) to the hind limb when the lameness was of mild (visible on every stride at the trot) severity. The horse had decreased impulsion of the lame diagonal (-15%) even with lameness of subtle (not visible on every stride at the trot) severity, but compensated by increasing propulsion in the sound diagonal (5.7%) when lameness increased to mild severity. pVGRFs were only significantly different in the primarily affected hind limb. The authors of this study concluded that compensatory body movements prevented overload in the unaffected limbs. A later study using 17 horses with two different degrees of temporary induced (frog pressure) hind limb lameness and computer-assisted kinematic analysis of horses trotting on a treadmill found that primary hind limb lameness, even of moderate severity, induced a false ipsilateral compensatory forelimb lameness [53]. The false lameness was often of apparent greater severity than the primary hind limb lameness. In some horses, however, the false ipsilateral forelimb lameness was not seen.

Summary

Compilation of this current evidence indicates that equine practitioners should be aware of false compensatory forelimb lameness with primary hind limb lameness. This false compensatory lameness is always ipsilateral; thus, if a horse presents with an apparent simultaneous ipsilateral forelimb and hind limb lameness, even when the forelimb lameness seems of greater apparent intensity than the hind limb lameness, the hind limb lameness should be investigated first.

Does a primary forelimb lameness cause an apparent (but false) contralateral hind limb lameness?

The evidence for the other half of the law of sides is not as strong and somewhat conflicting. One investigation found that horses with primary induced forelimb lameness had decreased tubera sacrale displacement and acceleration when the lame forelimb and contralateral hind limb were in the stance phase. This implies a false but apparent contralateral hind limb lameness [30]. Another study had a similar conclusion but found that only 6 of 10 horses with primary forelimb lameness had compensatory movement of the pelvis that "looked like" contralateral hind limb lameness [52].

The opposite effect was seen with the force-measuring treadmill, however. Using this method of analysis, it was shown that primary forelimb lameness, even of mild severity, caused a decrease in pVGRF and impulse in the ipsilateral hind limb and an increase, when forelimb lameness was of moderate severity, in pVGRF and impulse in the contralateral hind limb [16]. These findings suggest the development of a false compensatory lameness in the ipsilateral hind limb, the opposite conclusion of the previous reports.

This apparent contradiction is explained in another study [53]. In that study, it was found that the side of apparent but false compensatory hind limb lameness depended on whether hind limb impact or propulsion was being evaluated. With forelimb lameness, at the trot, weight is shifted toward the diagonal hind limb. Thus, the pelvis moves down more during the lame diagonal stance phase. This looks like an ipsilateral hind limb lameness, because the pelvis moves down more during the contralateral hind limb stance compared with the ipsilateral hind limb stance. Vertical force and impulse of the hind limb in the sound diagonal is increased, however, presumably to keep the horse moving forward at the same overall speed. This looks like a contralateral hind limb lameness, because the hind limb in the sound diagonal, which is ipsilateral to the primary forelimb lameness, pushes up the pelvis less than the hind limb of the lame diagonal, which is contralateral to the primary forelimb lameness. Therefore, the false compensatory hind limb lameness is ipsilateral and contralateral, depending on whether one is evaluating how far the pelvis moves down or how far the pelvic moves up. Contrary to what is seen with a compensatory ipsilateral forelimb lameness, one that is easy to see with a primary hind limb lameness, the movements of a compensatory hind limb lameness with a primary forelimb lameness are small in amplitude and may be difficult to see with the unaided human eye.

Summary

Kinematic and kinetic gait analysis potentially offers veterinarians an objective method of determining equine limb lameness. Subjective analyses have been shown to be somewhat flawed, and there does not seem to be a high degree of intraobserver agreement when evaluating individual horses. In addition, recognition of the compensatory effects of primary lameness may be helpful for the practicing equine veterinarian. An apparent lameness in the forelimb and hind limb on the same side of the body should alert the veterinarian to the strong possibility of primary hind limb lameness and false compensatory forelimb lameness. Apparent lameness in the forelimb of one side of the body and in the hind limb of the other side can signify primary forelimb lameness or lameness in both limbs.

References

[1] Kaneene JB, Ross WA, Miller RA. The Michigan equine monitoring system. II. Frequencies and impact of selected health problems. Prev Vet Med 1997;29:277–92.
[2] USDA. Lameness and laminitis in U.S. horses. USDA:APHIS:VS, National Animal Health Monitoring System. Fort Collins (CO): 2000. #N318.0400.
[3] USDA. National economic cost of equine lameness, colic, and equine protozoal myeloencephalitis in the United States. USDA:APHIS:VS, National Health Monitoring System. Information sheet. Fort Collins (CO): October, 2001. #N348.1001.
[4] American Horse Council. The economic impact of the horse industry in the United States. Washington, DC: American Horse Council Publications; 2006.
[5] Wyn-Jones G. Equine lameness. Oxford (UK): Blackwell Scientific Publications; 1988. p. 5.
[6] AAEP, Guide for veterinary service and judging of equestrian events. 4th edition. Lexington (KY): American Association of Equine Practitioners; 1991. p. 19.
[7] Pleasant RS, Moll HD, Ley WB, et al. Intra-articular anesthesia of the distal interphalangeal joint alleviates lameness associated with the navicular bursa in horses. Vet Surg 1997;26: 137–40.
[8] Keegan KG, Wilson DA, Wilson DJ, et al. Evaluation of mild lameness in horses trotting on a treadmill: agreement by clinicians and interns or residents and correlation of their assessments with kinematic gait analysis. Am J Vet Res 1998;59:1370–7.
[9] Hewetson M, Christly RM, Hunt ID, et al. Investigations of the reliability of observational gait analysis for the assessment of lameness in horses. Vet Rec 2006;158:852–8.
[10] Fuller CJ, Bladon BM, Driver AJ, et al. The intra- and inter-assessor reliability of measurement of functional outcome by lameness scoring in horses. Vet J 2006;171:281–6.
[11] Arkell M, Archer RM, Guitian FJ, et al. Evidence of bias affecting the interpretation of the results of local anaesthetic nerve blocks when assessing lameness in horses. Vet Rec 2006;159: 346–9.
[12] Merkens HW, Schamhardt HC. Distribution of ground reaction forces of the concurrently loaded limbs in Dutch Warmblood horse at the normal walk. Equine Vet J 1988;20:209–13.
[13] Merkens HW, Schamhardt HC. Evaluation of equine locomotion during different degrees of experimentally induced lameness. II. Distribution of ground reaction force patterns of the concurrently loaded limbs. Equine Vet J Suppl 1988;Sep(6):107–12.
[14] Ishihara A, Bertone AL, Rajala-Schultz PJ. Association between subjective lameness grade and kinetic gait parameters in horses with experimentally induced forelimb lameness. Am J Vet Res 2005;66:1805–15.
[15] Erkert RS, MacAllister CG, Payton ME, et al. Use of force plate analysis to compare the analgesic effects of intravenous administration of phenylbutazone and flunixin meglumine in horses with navicular syndrome. Am J Vet Res 2005;66:284–8.
[16] Weishaupt MA, Wiestner T, Hogg HP, et al. Compensatory load distribution of horses with induced weight-bearing forelimb lameness trotting on a treadmill. Vet J 2006;171:135–46.

[17] Weishaupt MA, Wiestner T, Hogg HP, et al. Compensatory load redistribution of horse with induced weightbearing hindlimb lameness trotting on a treadmill. Equine Vet J 2004;36: 727–33.
[18] Willams GE, Silverman BW, Wilson AM, et al. Disease-specific changes in equine ground reaction force data documented by use of principal component analysis. Am J Vet Res 1999;60:549–55.
[19] Ratzlaff MH, Wilson PD, Hyde ML, et al. Relationship between locomotor forces, hoof position and joint motion during the support phase of the stride of galloping horses. Acta Anat (Basel) 1993;146:200–4.
[20] Roepstorff L, Drevemo S. Concept of a force-measuring horseshoe. Acta Anat (Basel) 1993; 146:114–9.
[21] Hjertén G, Drevemo S. Semi-quantitative analysis of hoof-strike in the horse. J Biomech 1994;27:997–1004.
[22] Kai M, Aoki O, Hiraga A, et al. Use of an instrument sandwiched between the hoof and shoe to measure vertical ground reaction forces and three-dimensional acceleration at the walk, trot, and canter in horses. Am J Vet Res 2000;61:979–85.
[23] Weishaupt M, Hogg HP, Wiestner T, et al. Instrumented treadmill for measuring vertical ground reaction forces in horses. Am J Vet Res 2002;63:520–7.
[24] Thomason JJ, McClinchey HL, Jofriet JC. Analysis of strain and stress in the equine hoof capsule using finite element methods: comparison with principal strains recorded in vivo. Equine Vet J 2002;34:719–25.
[25] Thomason JJ, Bignell WW, Batiste D, et al. Effects of hoof shape, body mass and velocity on surface strain in the wall of the unshod forefoot of Standardbreds trotting on a treadmill. Equine and Comparative Exercise Physiology 2004;1:87–97.
[26] Gustås P, Johnson C, Roepstorff L, et al. Relationships between fore- and hindlimb ground reaction force and hoof deceleration patterns in trotting horses. Equine Vet J 2004;36: 737–42.
[27] Parsons KJ, Wilson AM. The use of MP3 recorders to log data from equine hoof mounted accelerometers. Equine Vet J 2006;38:675–80.
[28] Keegan KG, Satterley JM, Skubic M, et al. Use of gyroscopic sensors for objective evaluation of trimming and shoeing to alter time between heel and toe lift-off at end of the stance phase in horses walking and trotting on a treadmill. Am J Vet Res 2005;66: 2046–54.
[29] Peham C, Licka T, Mayr A, et al. Speed dependency of motion pattern consistency. J Biomech 1998;31:769–72.
[30] Buchner HHF, Savelberg HHCM, Schamhardt HC, et al. Head and trunk movement adaptations in horses with experimentally induced fore- and hindlimb lameness. Equine Vet J 1996;28:71–6.
[31] Keegan KG, Pai PF, Wilson DA, et al. Signal decomposition method of evaluating head movement to measure induced forelimb lameness in horses trotting on a treadmill. Equine Vet J 2001;33:446–51.
[32] May SA, Wyn-Jones G. Identification of hindleg lameness. Equine Vet J 1987;19:185–8.
[33] Kramer J, Keegan KG, Wilson DA, et al. Kinematics of the hindlimb in trotting horses after induced lameness of the distal intertarsal and tarsometatarsal joints and intra-articular administration of anesthetic. Am J Vet Res 2000;61:1031–6.
[34] Kramer J, Keegan KG, Kelmer G, et al. Objective determination of pelvic movement during hind limb lameness by use of a signal decomposition method and pelvic height differences. Am J Vet Res 2004;65:741–7.
[35] Buchner HHF, Savelberg HHCM, Schamhardt HC, et al. Limb movement adaptations in horses with experimentally induced fore- and hindlimb lameness. Equine Vet J 1996;28: 63–70.
[36] Back W, Barneveld A, van Weeren PR, et al. Kinematic gait analysis in equine carpal lameness. Acta Anat 1993;146:86–9.

[37] Galisteo AM, Cano MR, Morales JL, et al. Kinematics in horses at the trot before and after induced forelimb supporting lameness. Equine Vet J Suppl 1997;23:97–101.
[38] Keegan KG, Wilson DJ, Wilson DA, et al. Effects of anesthesia of the palmar digital nerves on kinematic gait analysis in horses with and without navicular disease. Am J Vet Res 1997; 58:218–23.
[39] Keegan KG, Wilson DA, Smith BK, et al. Changes in kinematic variables seen with lameness induced by applying pressure to the frog and to the toe in adult horses trotting on a treadmill. Am J Vet Res 2000;61:612–9.
[40] Drevemo S, Fredricson I, Dalin G, et al. Equine locomotion: 2. The analysis of coordination between limbs of trotting Standardbreds. Equine Vet J 1980;12:66–70.
[41] Drevemo S, Fredricson I, Hjertén G, et al. Early development of gait asymmetries in trotting Standardbred colts. Equine Vet J 1987;19:189–91.
[42] Pourcelot P, Audigié F, Degueurce C, et al. Kinematic symmetry index: a method for quantifying the horse locomotion symmetry using kinematic data. Vet Res 1997;28:525–38.
[43] Audigié F, Pourcelot P, Degueurce C, et al. Kinematic analysis of the symmetry of limb movements in lame trotting horses. Equine Vet J Suppl 2001;33:128–34.
[44] Degueurce C, Pourcelot P, Audigié F, et al. Variability of the limb joint patterns of sound horses at trot. Equine Vet J Suppl 1997;23:89–92.
[45] Peloso JG, Stick JA, Soutas-Little RW, et al. Computer-assisted three-dimensional gait analysis of amphotericin-induced carpal lameness in horses. Am J Vet Res 1993;54:1535–43.
[46] Keegan KG, Arafat S, Skubic M, et al. Determination and differentiation (right vs left) of equine forelimb lameness using continuous wavelet transformation and neural network classification of kinematic data. Am J Vet Res 2003;64:1376–81.
[47] Buchner HHF, Obermuller S, Scheidl M. Body center of mass movement in the lame horse. Equine Vet J Suppl 2001;33:122–7.
[48] Barrey E, Desbrosse F. Lameness detection using an accelerometric device. Pferdeheilkunde 1996;12:617–22.
[49] Weishaupt MA, Wiestner T, Hogg HP, et al. Assessment of gait irregularities in the horse: eye vs gait analysis. Equine Vet J Suppl 2001;33:135–40.
[50] Keegan KG, Yonezawa Y, Pai PF, et al. Telemeterized accelerometer-based system for the detection of lameness in horses. Biomed Sci Instrum 2002;38:107–12.
[51] Keegan KG, Yonezawa Y, Pai PF, et al. Sensor based system of equine motion analysis for the detection and quantification of forelimb and hindlimb lameness in horses. Am J Vet Res 2004;65:665–70.
[52] Uhlir C, Licka T, Kubber P, et al. Compensatory movements of horses with a stance phase lameness. Equine Vet J Suppl 1997;23:102–5.
[53] Kelmer G, Keegan KG, Kramer J, et al. Computer-assisted kinematic evaluation of induced compensatory lameness in horses trotting on a treadmill. Am J Vet Res 2005;66:646–55.

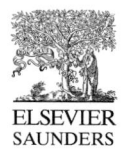

An Evidence-Based Assessment of the Biomechanical Effects of the Common Shoeing and Farriery Techniques

Ehud Eliashar, BSc, DVM, MRCVS

Department of Veterinary Clinical Sciences, The Royal Veterinary College, Hawkshead Lane, North Mymms, Hatfield, AL9 7TA, United Kingdom

Horses are commonly used as high-performance athletes. Originally, the main reason for applying shoes to horses was to protect the feet against excessive wear [1]. Over the years, numerous types of shoes and corrective farriery techniques have been developed in an attempt to influence performance or as a therapeutic aid to treat lameness. The ways in which horses are shod, however, are still similar to the techniques of centuries ago, no matter what the purpose of the shoes [2]. Most of these techniques rely largely on traditional empiric craftsmanship rather than on scientific evidence. This is mainly because relatively little research has been performed into the fundamental aspects of shoeing, resulting in a lack of basic scientific knowledge.

The past two decades have provided equine veterinarians with new information relating to limb biomechanics and the effects of various farriery methods, however, including so-called "corrective" ones. Obtaining much of this information became possible once computers, combined with force plates, pressure mats, and motion analysis systems, became available. This then allowed for finer analysis of the effects of various shoeing interventions in prospective biomechanical studies.

There is a fine line between maximal performance and overload injuries. When overload occurs, injury follows and the clinical sign observed is lameness. The horse's attempt to unload the painful limb creates the lameness that we observe. Because of the relatively simple anatomic arrangement of the distal limb, however, the horse has only a limited scope by which it can alter its gait. Furthermore, because the horse still has to support its weight, the ability to compensate and redistribute the load is limited [3].

E-mail address: eeliashar@rvc.ac.uk

Similarly, corrective shoeing and farriery techniques attempt to unload a specific site or to shorten the duration that a specific site is bearing weight. The effect of a particular shoe or farriery technique can be assessed during the propulsion phase or the stance phase of the stride. The latter phase is generally considered more important from a lameness point of view, because it is during this phase that the limb is subjected to external forces.

Of course, regaining soundness is not the only reason for which improved or different hoof or shoe conformations are used. Attempts to affect performance by altering hoof conformation have long been practiced. Classic examples are the historical practice of trimming the foot of racehorses, such that a lower heel and longer toe are achieved to promote a "longer" stride [4], or the attempt to hasten breakover by modifying the way the hooves are trimmed or shod [5–9].

The aim of this article is to review the progress made in the field of distal limb biomechanics. By understanding limb biomechanics, it is then possible to review the rationale behind a few of the more common techniques that veterinarians routinely use when treating their patients and to evaluate the evidence in support of them.

Basic biomechanical terminology

During stance, the limb is subjected to an external impact force by the ground. This external impact is called the ground reaction force (GRF), the magnitude of which depends on the horse's weight and speed of movement. The main effect of the GRF is to extend the distal interphalangeal (DIP) joint. For ease of mathematic calculations, the GRF is considered to act at a single point under the foot. This point is called the point of zero moment (PZM) or point of force (PoF) [10,11]. This point is not positioned directly under the center of rotation of the DIP joint, however. Rather, it is positioned horizontally, away from the center of rotation of the joint. This creates a lever, or what is referred to as a "moment arm." The action of the GRF and its moment arm creates a torque (ie, a force that produces or tends to produce rotation or torsion). This torque is the extending moment of the DIP joint (Fig. 1).

The extending moment of the DIP joint is balanced by an equal flexing moment generated by the deep digital flexor tendon (DDFT). Another moment arm is created by the tendon running over the navicular bone [12]. As a result of the deviation of the DDFT around the navicular bone during the stance phase of the stride, the tendon compresses the navicular bone with a force that is proportional not only to the DDFT force but to the angle of deviation of the DDFT around the bone [5,13,14]. By measuring the surface area of the flexor cortex of the navicular bone, the stress imposed on the bone by the DDFT throughout stance can be calculated [14,15].

Toward the end of stance, the PZM, the point at which the GRF is measured, moves toward the toe, because the heels are gradually unloading at

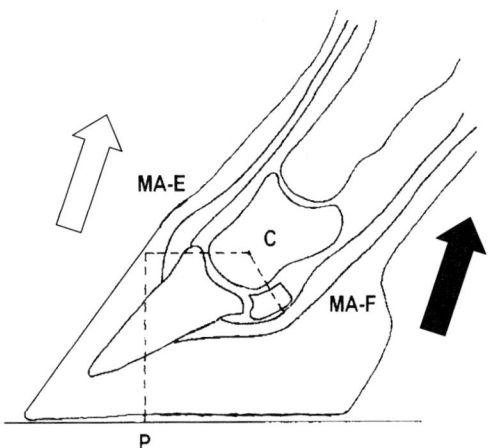

Fig. 1. Various moments acting to extend and flex the DIP joint are shown. C, center of rotation of the DIP joint; MA-E, extending moment arm of the DIP joint; MA-F, flexing moment arm of the DIP joint. The white arrow shows the extending moment of the DIP joint, and the black arrow shows the flexing moment of the DIP joint.

this time. When the PZM reaches the toe, the DIP joint moment arm cannot increase further because the moment arm can go no farther forward on the hoof. As a result, the extending moment falls off in line with the reducing GRF. At this stage, the flexing moment exceeds the extending moment, and the DIP joint flexes (ie, the heels leave the ground). This period at the terminal part of the stance phase is called breakover. During breakover, the time from heel-off to toe-off, the heel rotates around the toe [5,16].

The position of the PZM, GRF, and extending moment on the DIP joint can be determined using a combination of force plate and kinematic motion analysis [11]. Combining this with measurements taken from radiographs of the foot enables calculations on the force and stress exerted by the DDFT on the navicular bone during stance [5,13–15]. The addition of a pressure mat to the force plate and motion analysis system [17,18] allows for better definition of the forces applied to the entire solar surface during stance rather than at just a single point (eg, PZM).

Biomechanical studies vary in the way they are conducted and are affected by many variables. The horses studied can be sound or lame, standing or moving, on various surfaces or on treadmills, and at different speeds or gaits. In vitro studies using cadaver limbs can also be performed, although these studies may differ in the length of the limb depending on the level at which it was disarticulated from the body. The investigated change can be subtle, such as when the effects of normal hoof growth and wear are evaluated, or exaggerated, such as when using wedges or special shoes, with horses receiving an inconsistent amount of time, if any, to adjust to the change. The instrumentation used for the study as well as the way in which various points of interest on the limb are marked is also variable.

Regardless of the method of investigation chosen, the data collected can be used to calculate the resultant effects on many gait parameters, such as foot flight, stride length, foot landing, joint angles, stance duration, hoof roll, the external forces applied to the foot during stance, the forces exerted on various structures, and many more. The evaluation of such data must be made with an eye toward the variables involved with each individual study, however.

Effects of applying a shoe

The application of a standard steel shoe to a balanced foot has a minimal effect on the location of the PoF during stance. With a shoe, the PoF is located closer to the center of the foot in early stance and its excursion toward the lateral heel is smaller in magnitude [11].

The weight added to the distal limb by the shoe may have more significant effects on the horse's limb, however. The weight of a shoe increases inertia; that is, it decreases the ability of the limb to resist changes in its velocity. The weight of the shoe thus creates some changes to the gait, primarily to variables of the swing phase at high speed [19–21]. These changes in the swing phase are suggested to improve swing phase retraction (pulling up of the limb) as well as the animation of the trot [21]. In fact, many changes may occur in response to the weight of a shoe, including a slight increase in the loading of a limb, a slightly quicker rotation of the hoof segment, a less vertical hoof lifting [1], and an increase in the force exerted on the navicular bone by the DDFT by as much as 14% [13].

Shoeing also alters the concussion-dampening mechanism of the distal limb [22,23], resulting in an increase in the amount of impact on the hoof [1,24]. This increase in impact does not seem to extend to the upper limb, however, because it is largely attenuated at the interface between the hoof wall and distal phalanx. At the level of the metacarpophalangeal (MCP) joint, the difference between shod and unshod conditions is minimal [24].

Normally, when a horse's foot lands at the beginning of the stance phase, there is a certain amount of slide before the foot grips the ground. The duration and distance that a horse's foot slides after impact are not significantly affected by shoes made of different material [25]. Deceleration force (ie, the rate at which the force decreases at impact) can be affected with certain materials, however. This suggests that horses may have to alter their gait to compensate for the grip characteristics of the shoe so as to maintain a constant slip time and distance [25].

Shoeing also elevates the hoof from the ground surface by supporting the hoof wall. This results in less expansion of the palmar aspect of the hoof wall when compared with the unshod horse, although the heel still expands even without contact of the frog with the ground [26]. Shoeing also attenuates contraction of the wall at the heel during the late stages of the stance phase [26]. Without a shoe, hoof wall compression at the toe and quarter remains more constant and less in magnitude than with a shoe. Furthermore, at low weight-bearing loads, shoeing places increased pressure on the frog; that pressure decreases total hoof wall weight bearing and causes palmar movement of the distal phalanx [27]. However, the significance of the effects described previously on the hoof, the clinical relevance of the effects of certain shoes, and the relation of these effects to long-term future hoof health are not yet completely understood.

Hoof balance and biomechanics

It is important to distinguish between conformation and balance. Both are frequently mentioned in reference to the shape and size of the distal limb and the spatial relations between its different elements [28,29]. Conformation describes the general shape, size, and static relations of the distal limb [28]. Balance embraces the shape and function of the foot in relation to the ground as well as to skeletal structures of the limb, at rest and at exercise [30]. Each foot should have a conformation that maximizes its mechanical efficiency, and when such conformation is thought to have been achieved by trimming the foot, the foot is said to be balanced [29].

For years, veterinarians and farriers have been trying to define the "ideal" hoof balance that a "normal" sound horse should have. At present, it seems that the debate is far from reaching a unified conclusion. It is thus not surprising that several techniques have been described for assessing hoof balance. "Geometric" balance is defined as the attempt to make the hoof as symmetric as possible around its sagittal solar plane, which is positioned in a prescribed position in relation to the rest of the foot. "Dynamic" balance is defined as a conformation that allows the foot to contact the ground in a prescribed pattern [29]. Other techniques assess balance in relation to a reference point or a formula.

Although the debate over conformation and balance is beyond the scope of this article, it is important to explore how various alterations in hoof conformation affect foot biomechanics if veterinarians intend to make such alterations effectively for the benefit of the horse. The following sections describe the various responses to altered conformation. Because it is common for more than one structure or area to be affected by any particular change, the information is largely presented in terms of specific manipulations and their effect on isolated areas or structures.

Change in ground contact area

The common concept has defined the solar surface of the hoof wall as the primary weight-bearing surface of the foot, with the distal phalanx totally suspended and not participating in weight bearing. Characteristics of hoof conformation in feral horses have been used to question this concept [6]. Experimentally, unshod sound horses kept on pasture have a weight-bearing load distribution of a four- or three-point pattern [29]. In the four-point pattern, the major contact points are at the heel and lateral and medial to the toe, whereas in the three-point pattern, the latter two points are replaced by a single continuous contact area across the dorsal surface of the toe [29]. When these horses are stood on a deformable surface, the load distribution is principally solar; the bearing surface of the wall at the toe and heel has lower contact than the sole. An abrasive surface causes the solar pattern of load distribution to change rapidly, with loss of the three- or four-point pattern and increased contact of the peripheral wall, bars, and frog [29]. It thus seems that friction is responsible for balance in unshod feet, and that the balance is different depending on the amount of friction. Trimming results in a significant increase in contact surface area, which is characterized by an increased uniformity of wall contact, increase in the contact of the peripheral sole, and appearance of contact of the frog and bars; however, shoeing does not change this any further [29].

Egg-bar shoes are probably the most common farriery technique used to increase the ground contact area with shoes. The rationales for their application include an attempt to bring about a more correct weight distribution and to provide extra support to the heel [31,32]. This type of shoe is still used routinely by veterinarians and farriers as part of the treatment regimen for horses with navicular syndrome. Egg-bar shoes are suggested to have some effects on unloading the distal limb [33] and cause a negligible slight reduction in the maximal strain of the DDFT, but they also seem to increase the strain of the suspensory ligament (SL) [32]. Egg-bar shoes do not have any effect on the force exerted by the DDFT on the navicular bone in sound horses [13], but in some clinically affected horses, mainly those with a collapsed heel conformation, a significant reduction in the force and stress exerted on the navicular bone is observed [3]. The mechanism by which these shoes work is unclear but may result from distribution of the load over a greater area under the heel or reinforcement of the flexible palmar regions of the foot [3].

Contouring the lateral branch of a conventional shoe toward the center of the foot induces greater mean lateral roll of the hoof during the first half of breakover at the trot. This effect does not occur at the walk, however, and this small effect dissipates during the second half of breakover [34].

Changes in the sagittal plane

Changes in the dorsopalmar plane in the dorsal direction, such as in the broken forward/club-footed horse, or in the palmar direction, such as in the flat-footed/broken back/long toe–low heel horse, have received much attention from veterinarians and farriers. This is likely because of the widely suggested involvement of such abnormalities in the pathophysiology of many foot ailments, such as conditions involving the navicular apparatus [9,35].

Naturally, the processes of hoof growth and wear are balanced. This allows an unshod horse to maintain the shape and size of its feet, although the size and shape are directly influenced by the characteristics of the surface on which the horse lives as well as the friction between the surface and the sole [6,29]. In the domesticated shod horse, however, friction occurs between the expanding heel and the shoe and induces greater wear at the heel compared with that at the toe. Over time, this results in changes in hoof balance [18,36].

As the hoof grows in the shod horse, the dorsal hoof angle typically becomes shallower by a mean of 3.5° over a period of 8 weeks, the PZM moves in a palmar/plantar direction, and the hoof rolls in a more lateral direction (especially in the hind limbs) [18]. Furthermore, hoof growth results in extension of the DIP joint, whereas there is no significant change in the angle at the PIP joint [36]. However, the change in the location of the PZM is less than that predicted by direct measurements of the change in hoof morphometry [18]. This, in turn, suggests that a compensatory mechanism, which is not entirely understood, prevents the force and stress exerted by the DDFT on the navicular bone from increasing too much. A hypothesis has been suggested for such a compensatory mechanism, which involves an increase in the dorsal angle (smaller extension) of the MCP or metatarsophalangeal joint, a reduction in the angle of deviation of the DDFT around the joint, and a decrease in its tension [37]. In the hind limbs, another suggested compensatory mechanism to prevent the force on the navicular bone from increasing over time is the ability of the horse to change breakover direction laterally [37,38], moving the location of the PZM to a more lateral position at late stance and hence shortening the extending moment arm at the DIP joint [18].

Artificial manipulations

Although the studies mentioned previously have looked at the effect of naturally occurring changes of hoof conformation, similar changes, commonly more exaggerated, have also been investigated. These changes are most commonly made with the use of wedges or, alternatively, by using special shoes. Among other things, these manipulations attempt to induce change in toe length, change in the position or shape of the toe, change in heel or toe height, or change in ground contact area.

Change in heel or toe height

Heel height and shape have received a considerable amount of attention, mainly because of the evidence of the close association of imbalance involving low heels and navicular syndrome [9,35] that has been observed in more than 70% of clinically affected horses [35]. Over the years, investigations, both in vivo and in vitro, were made looking at the effect of change in heel height on various biomechanical parameters. Generally, it is accepted that increasing heel height induces flexion of the DIP and proximal interphalangeal (PIP) joints and extension of the MCP joint. Results from various studies regarding the change in flexion or extension of the PIP and MCP joints are conflicting, however, mainly because of the different experimental protocols. Furthermore, studies that relate these changes to the treatment of clinical conditions are still lacking, and, finally, some of the studies have been done in ponies, and thus, the validity of extrapolation of the findings to horses is unknown.

Effects on stance characteristics

An upright heel promotes a more pronounced heel-first landing [9], whereas a toe-first landing is seen with a long-toe–low-heel conformation [39]. With toe wedges, hoof impact is more dorsal on the lateral side, whereas it occurs more palmar with heel wedges [40]; however, the GRF is unchanged [13]. The PoF is displaced medially in early stance with a heel or toe wedge, but there is no apparent change in midstance [11], probably because the limb is exposed to the maximal GRF during that stage. Although stance duration is not affected by the application of a wedge [11,40,41], relative lengths of different periods of stance can be affected [40,41]. In late stance, movement of the PoF toward the toe occurs later with a heel wedge, resulting in delayed unloading of the heel [11,40,41] and shortening of breakover duration by approximately 1.5% of stance duration [40]. On a treadmill, however, the duration of breakover is unchanged [41], and the clinical relevance of any such change is unknown. Furthermore, on a treadmill, heel wedges promoted lateral rotation of the DIP joint [41]; however, it is unknown yet whether this occurs on the ground as well.

Effects on the distal interphalangeal joint

Various in vitro studies using cadaver limbs as well as in vivo studies in standing horses have demonstrated that raising the heels results in flexion of the DIP joint by approximately 1° for every 1° increase in height, whereas toe elevation induces a similar but opposite change [42,43]. When assessed in moving horses, heel wedges significantly increase and delay maximal flexion, and maximal extension of the DIP joint is significantly reduced [40,41]. Apart from the effect that such change has on surrounding soft tissues (mainly the DDFT), heel elevation increases the pressure within the DIP joint and alters the articular contact area. It has been hypothesized that this may lead to greater localized "wear and tear" on the joint surface, possibly predisposing the horse to an increased risk of arthritis [44]; however, no such predisposition has ever been demonstrated in clinical research.

Effects on the proximal interphalangeal joint

The PIP joint has a rather considerable range of movement (35°–56°) during the stride of horses running in a slow trot [1,45,46]. Traditionally, it has been perceived that at the point of contact with the ground, the PIP joint attains a nearly perfect tight-fitting position, remaining immobile throughout the stance phase, keeping the proximal and middle phalanges in a straight line [47]. As a result, the mathematic model for biomechanical analysis of the distal limb routinely assumes that the proximal and middle phalanges act as a single unit [12]. However, radiographic measurements have demonstrated a direct influence of a wedge, used to elevate the heel or the toe in standing horses, on the measured angles of the PIP joint [42,43]. Unfortunately, these radiographically measured changes are different from those measured using skin markers; this is attributable to a large movement of the skin markers in relation to the bones underneath, thus creating inaccurate measurements [42,48].

To overcome this discrepancy, surgically positioned markers were placed in the digital bones. This model of cadaver limbs loaded in a press demonstrated that raising the heels by 6° to 12° significantly increased the range of flexion of the PIP joint in high loads. Conversely, toe wedges induce extension of the joint and reduce the amplitude of flexion [48]. Similar experimental settings in vivo identified that heel wedges significantly increased maximal flexion and decreased maximal extension of the PIP joint [40,41].

Effects on the metacarpophalangeal joint

This joint received attention mainly because of the suggested relation of its angular position and the associated palmar or plantar soft tissues, mainly the SL and superficial digital flexor tendon (SDFT). The effects of toe and heel elevation on the function of this joint are still largely controversial, however, and there is clear disagreement between the results of studies using quasistatic radiographs and biomechanical data.

More than three decades ago, it was suggested that heel calks, which elevate the heels, reduce the strain in the SDFT and SL because of the reduced maximal extension of the MCP joint during stance [49]. Elevating the heel with a 5° heel wedge caused a significant reduction in maximal extension of the MCP joint at the trot but not at the walk [33]; however, no effect was seen at the trot with a 6° wedge in another study [13]. In vitro heel elevation of a single forelimb showed that as elevation increased, the extension of the MCP joint increased as well in a fairly linear fashion [50]. It must be noted that the changes demonstrated in the in vitro study were much greater than in the in vivo studies, probably because the limb was sectioned above the carpus, thus allowing for some loss in tension in the flexor tendons.

Markers placed surgically in the bones indicated that that a 1° increase in toe angle using a heel wedge induces MCP joint extension by 0.24° [42]. In a similar setup, using heel wedges, studying the three-dimensional movement of the MCP joint in walking horses during neutral loading, the extension of the MCP joint was 38.4° ± 8.7°, which was associated with lateral axial rotation of the proximal phalanx, and the extension of the MCP joint during stance was significantly increased [40,51]. Conversely, in horses trotting on a treadmill, heel wedges had no significant effect on flexion and extension of the MCP joint [41]. The authors of this treadmill study suggested that the effect of the wedge at the trot was totally absorbed by the interphalangeal joints. However, only three horses were used in the study and the assessment was made on a treadmill, which is known to induce some changes in the gait [52].

Effects on tendon strains

Reduction in strain of a tendon or ligament of the distal limb is commonly recommended for horses that have incurred various injuries. Over the years, many studies have looked at the correlations between change in balance or conformation and the forces to which tendons and ligaments are subjected. Most of these studies have concentrated on the MCP joint angle and SDFT or SL strain, or on the angle of the DIP joint and DDFT strain as well as the force exerted by the DDFT on the navicular bone.

An initial report suggested that heel calks reduce the strain of the SDFT and SL during stance [49]. Since that study, most studies, in vitro [53,54] and in vivo [32], have demonstrated no significant change or an opposite effect (increased strain). In one study, increasing the hoof angle from 40° to 70° made no change in SDFT or SL strain but decreased DDFT strain while standing or at the walk [53]. In another investigation, strain gauges were implanted into the flexor tendons and SL in the forelimb of five ponies and strain was recorded at the walk [32]. This study demonstrated that a toe wedge reduced strain in the SDFT and SL and significantly increased strain in the accessory ligament of the deep digital flexor tendon (ALDDFT), whereas a heel wedge decreased strain in the DDFT and ALDDFT, increased strain in the SL, but caused no change in SDFT strain [32]. The latter finding was in agreement with a study that found no change in SDFT strain at the walk with heel elevation of 10° [55]. In toto, the results of these studies suggest that in vivo change in tendon strain is different from that measured in vitro; thus, in vitro limb loading has only a limited value for assessing tendon function in vivo [56].

Increasing heel height by 6° with the use of a wedge decreases the force exerted on the navicular bone by the DDFT by 24% [13], mainly as a result of reduction in the extending moment arm of the DIP joint but also as a result in a flatter angle of deviation of the tendon around the navicular bone. A similar relation between the angle of the distal phalanx to the ground and the force and stress exerted by the DDFT on the navicular bone was identified in another study [14], showing that for every 1° increase in the angle of the distal phalanx, the calculated force and stress on the navicular bone were 6% lower. These changes were also attributable to a reduction in DIP moment arm and angle of deviation of the DDFT around the navicular bone. Furthermore, no correlation has been found between the ratio of heel and toe angles (define as heel collapse index) and the force and stress exerted on the navicular bone; however, these parameters were found to be well correlated to the height index (defined as the ratio of heel-to-toe height). It was therefore concluded that the latter might be a better clinical indicator of force on the navicular bone than simply looking at hoof angles.

With heel wedges, forces on the MCP joint both increase and decrease. The contribution of the DDFT to the total moment of force at the MCP joint reduces by 21%, whereas the combined contribution of the SDFT and SL increases by 5% [13]. Because the SL force is directly related to the angle of the MCP joint, and this angle did not change significantly, the increase in the combined load with wedges can be attributed fully to the SDFT. The increase in flexion of the PIP joint after application of a wedge may contribute partially to relaxation of the DDFT and may affect the tension in SDFT [40].

Finally, although most authors agree that heel wedges reduce strain in the DDFT and, subsequently, the force and stress exerted on the navicular bone, it is important to emphasize that heel wedges do not unload the heels [11]. Hence, it is recommended that their use in horses with collapsed heels has to be time limited or the condition may worsen.

Change in toe position or length

Alterations of toe position or length can be made by trimming of the hoof or by application of shoes with a different toe profile. Using high-speed cinematography, the notion that trimming feet with a more acute angle, thus creating a longer toe and increasing stride length has been refuted [39,57]. Although toe length or angle does not affect the duration of the stance phase in the barefooted horse, breakover duration is significantly prolonged with a longer toe [13]. However, in comparison to conventional plain steel shoes, breakover is not significantly different when rocker-toe, rolled toe, or square toe shoes are used [16]. Similar findings were demonstrated with the use of a motion analysis system and force plate, demonstrating that there are no differences between rocker-toed and standard flat shoes with respect to the duration or ease of breakover or the proximity of breakover to the center of the toe [58]. Rocker-toed shoes do not influence the stride characteristics of sound Dutch Warmblood horses, and there seems to be no objective ground for the use of rocker-toed shoes in sound horses [58].

Another study compared the effects of different toe profiles using toe-clip shoes, quarter-clip shoes pulled to the white line, and natural balance shoes [5]. The further back the toe position, the shorter was the moment arm of the GRF on the DIP joint. Similar to the previous studies, the duration of breakover was not significantly different between the three types of shoes, and neither was the force exerted on the navicular bone [5]. Combining a pressure mat with the analysis system, it has been demonstrated that stance time and breakover duration as well as cumulative extending moment of the DIP joint are similar with conventional or rolled-toe shoes [59]. Peak DIP joint moment is 14% smaller with the rolled-toe shoe, however, and hoof movement seems to be smoother and more gradual, suggesting a better possibility of the horse for correct coordination [59]. Although this may imply that using a shoe of this type is ideal for every horse, there is no clinical evidence to support such a notion.

Changes in the frontal plane

The most common clinical presentation of horses with mediolateral imbalance (ie, uneven height of the hoof wall from the ground when viewed from the dorsal aspect) is "sheared heels" [60], which is thought to develop because of uneven forces acting on the bulbs of the heel during stance. In sound horses, a 6-mm wedge placed to alter the mediolateral balance moves the PZM toward the elevated side of the foot [11]. This indicates that the elevated side sustains a higher load, thus supporting the notion that in horses with such abnormal mediolateral imbalance, the change in load distribution may be the reason for structural breakdown between the bulbs of the heel [11]. Imbalance in this plane affects structures that are more proximal as well. A 12° lateral wedge induces a combination of axial rotation of the proximal phalanx and widening of the opposite side of the MCP joint [51]. It has been suggested that even though the amplitude of these changes is small, their biomechanical effects should be considered to improve the understanding of MCP joint injuries and the rationale of exercise and corrective farriery in lame horses.

Another commonly applied farriery technique attempting to change force distribution in the frontal plane is the application of lateral extension shoes to horses with osteoarthritis of the small tarsal joints (bone spavin). The aim in this technique is to assist these horses to unload the dorsomedial aspect of the small tarsal joints by redistributing their weight to a more caudolateral aspect of the foot [61]. However, the efficacy of these extensions as a treatment was found to be questionable. Twenty-millimeter wide lateral extensions applied to horses clinically affected with osteoarthritis of the small tarsal joints were found to have only a little consistent effect on the position of the PZM during stance as well as on the degree of lameness [62].

Foot biomechanics of lame horses

The limb of the lame horse is lifted off the ground in a more flexed orientation, with the foot higher, and limb placing and loading occur more slowly [3]. Stance phase duration increases with experimentally induced lameness in some studies [63–65], but other studies fail to demonstrate this correlation or they identify the opposite [66–68]. Peak limb loading may be somewhat less on the affected limb of a lame horse [3], and this is compensated for primarily by the contralateral limb and, to a lesser extent, by the concurrently loaded limbs [69] during the stance and swing phases of the lame limb [70], without overloading of the other limbs [71]. The most reliable change in foot dynamics during lameness is a decreased extension of the MCP joint during stance; other changes are less specific to the origin of pain [72]. Results of different studies seem to be inconsistent, however, possibly because of the differences in the lameness models evaluated. Inducing lameness by pressure to various parts of the sole may not produce similar biomechanical effects as those of a clinically affected horse [72].

Horses with navicular disease have abnormal limb-loading force patterns compared with sound horses [15,73]. The peak DDFT force and the peak stress exerted by the DDFT on the navicular bone are similar between normal horses and those with navicular syndrome [15]. In early stance, however, the force and stress in the diseased horses are approximately double the values of that in normal horses. The increased force and stress are assumed to result from higher forces in the deep digital flexor muscle as the horses attempt to unload their heels [15]. This mechanism is thought to result in the classic toe-first gait seen in some horses with navicular disease and is suggested to cause a vicious cycle promoting further damage [15].

In laminitic ponies, with 6° to 13° rotation of distal phalanx, the GRF is 13% lower, mostly because of their reduced speed of movement [74]. The PZM is located palmar to the center of rotation of the DIP joint during the first 40% of stance, and DDFT force reaches its peak later in stance compared with that in normal sound ponies. Although the peak DDFT force is, on average, 40% smaller in late stance because of the action of its accessory ligament, it is similar to that in normal ponies [74]. This supports the strategy of stall confinement during the active stage of laminitis to minimize the risk of further separation of the bone from the damaged laminae.

Conformation, shoeing, and injuries

Only a limited number of studies describing the relation between conformation, farriery techniques, and injuries have been published, and the data are conflicting at times. Changes in conformation, particularly a long toe, low heel, and sloping pastern, have been reported to be important in the occurrence of carpal fractures [75]. Another study found that as the heels become more underrun compared with the angle of the hoof at the toe, the odds of carpal effusion increase but there is no association with carpal fractures [76]. An increased difference in toe and heel angles may be a risk factor for failure of the suspensory apparatus, and the difference [77] or ratio [76] between these two angles seems to be more important than is toe or heel angle alone [77]. Conversely, it has also been claimed that hoof angle has no effect on musculoskeletal disease [76]. An increased risk of tendonitis of the SDFT was found to be related to a more upright (less extended) conformation of the MCP joint in a large group of National Hunt racehorses [78].

In racehorses, toe grabs have been suggested to be a potential risk factor for fatal musculoskeletal injuries, failure of the suspensory apparatus, and condylar fractures, with the magnitudes of these associations increasing with increased height of the toe grabs [79]. These findings are also disputed, however, because another study found that although the odds of injury in racehorses running with toe grabs are 1.5 times the odds of those without, the difference is insignificant [80]. Regardless, it has been suggested that the resultant increased height of the toe decreases the functional angle of the shod foot, delays breakover, and thus increases the lever arm on the PIP and MCP joints, thereby increasing the strain in the SL and predisposing horses to injury [79].

Despite the identified relation between the angle of the distal phalanx and the force and stress exerted by the DDFT on the navicular bone [14], no significant differences were found in the angle of the distal phalanx in horses of mixed breeds, with and without deep digital flexor tendonitis in the digit [81]. In Thoroughbred horses with DDFT lesions, there was a trend toward more acute distal phalanx angles when these horses were compared with clinically sound Thoroughbred horses.

Summary

Incorporation of more advanced analysis systems in recent years has provided veterinarians with abundant new information related to the various effects of common shoeing and farriery techniques on foot and lower limb biomechanics. It is quite obvious however, that some aspects are still controversial or unclear. Among these controversies are the effects of change in heel height on the angles of the PIP and MCP joints and on the strains of the flexor tendons and SL. Comparisons of unshod and shod horses are rare, but the use of analysis systems, such as the pressure mat, may help to clarify debate about the purported benefits of shoeing horses versus leaving them barefoot. Fine analysis of the distal limb seems to be limited by the complex anatomy. Indeed, it seems that a full understanding of the function of smaller structures, such as the distal sesamoidean or collateral ligaments, may only be achieved with the use of computer simulation.

Finally, it should be noted that from an evidence-based perspective, most studies that have been performed evaluating the biomechanical effects of the common shoeing and farriery techniques have been performed using sound horses, and many others have been in vitro studies. Thus, although the information obtained from such studies is interesting, its direct clinical relevance is speculative and the strength of evidence is not as strong as is desirable. There is a significant deficit in veterinary knowledge regarding the effects of shoeing and farriery techniques on clinically affected lame horses or horses with identified clinical conditions. Hopefully, future studies are planned to bridge this gap comparing clinically lame horses with sound ones as controls or in prospective designs assessing the long-term effects of any particular technique.

References

[1] Roepstorff L, Johnston C, Drevemo S. The effect of shoeing on kinetics and kinematics during the stance phase. Equine Vet J Suppl 1999;30:279–85.
[2] Van Heel MC, Moleman M, Barneveld A, et al. Changes in location of centre of pressure and hoof-unrollment pattern in relation to an 8-week shoeing interval in the horse. Equine Vet J 2005;37:536–40.
[3] Wilson AM, McGuigan MP, Pardoe C. The biomechanical effects of wedged, eggbar and extension shoes in sound and lame horses. Proceedings of the American Association of Equine Practitioners 2001;47:339–43.
[4] Finnochio EJ. Pitfalls in shoeing for gait. The Horse Digest 1984;24–6.
[5] Eliashar E, McGuigan MP, Rogers KA, et al. A comparison of three horseshoeing styles on the kinetics of breakover in sound horses. Equine Vet J 2002;34:184–90.
[6] Ovnicek G, Erfle JB. Wild horse hoof patterns offer a formula for preventing and treating lameness. Proceedings of the American Association of Equine Practitioners 1995;41:258–60.
[7] Stashak TS. Navicular syndrome (navicular disease). In: White NA, Moore JN, editors. Current techniques in equine surgery and lameness. 2nd edition. Philadelphia: W.B Saunders Co; 1998. p. 537–43.
[8] Turner TA. Shoeing principles for the management of navicular disease in horses. J Am Vet Med Assoc 1986;189:298–301.
[9] Wright IM, Douglas J. Biomechanical considerations in the treatment of navicular disease. Vet Rec 1993;133:109–14.
[10] Nigg BM, Herzog W. Biomechanics of the musculoskeletal system. Chichester, England: John Riley and Sons; 1994.
[11] Wilson AM, Seelig TJ, Shield RA, et al. The effect of foot imbalance on point of force application in the horse. Equine Vet J 1998;30:540–5.
[12] Bartel DL, Schryver HF, Lowe JE, et al. Locomotion in the horse: a procedure for computing the internal forces in the digit. Am J Vet Res 1978;39:1721–7.
[13] Willemen MA, Savelberg HH, Barneveld A. The effect of orthopaedic shoeing on the force exerted by the deep digital flexor tendon on the navicular bone in horses. Equine Vet J 1999; 31:25–30.
[14] Eliashar E, McGuigan MP, Wilson AM. Relationship of foot conformation and force applied to the navicular bone of sound horses at the trot. Equine Vet J 2004;36:431–5.
[15] Wilson AM, McGuigan MP, Fouracre L, et al. The force and contact stress on the navicular bone during trot locomotion in sound horses and horses with navicular disease. Equine Vet J 2001;33:159–65.
[16] Clayton HM, Sigafoos R, Curle RD. Effect of three shoe types on the duration of breakover in sound trotting horses. Journal of Equine Veterinary Science 1991;11:129–32.
[17] Rogers CW, Back W. Wedge and eggbar shoes change the pressure distribution under the hoof of the forelimb in the square standing horse. Journal of Equine Veterinary Science 2003;23:306–9.
[18] van Heel MC, Barneveld A, van Weeren PR, et al. Dynamic pressure measurements for the detailed study of hoof balance: the effect of trimming. Equine Vet J 2004;36:778–82.
[19] Willemen MA, Savelberg HHCM, Bruin G, et al. The effect of toe weights on linear and temporal stride characteristics of Standardbred trotters. Vet Q 1994;16(Suppl 2):S97–100.
[20] Singelton WH, Clayton HM, Lanovaz JL, et al. Effects of shoeing on forelimb phase kinetics of trotting horses. Vet Comp Orthop Traumatol 2003;16:16–20.
[21] Willemen MA, Savelberg HHCM, Barneveld A. The improvement of the gait quality of sound trotting horses by normal shoeing and its effect on the load of the lower limb. Livest Prod Sci 1998;52:145–53.

[22] Benoit P, Barrey E, Regnault JC, et al. Comparison of the damping effect of different shoeing by the measurement of hoof acceleration. Acta Anat 1993;146:109–13.
[23] Dyhre-Poulsen P, Smedegaard HH, Roed J, et al. Equine hoof function investigated by pressure transducers inside the hoof and accelerometers mounted on the first phalanx. Equine Vet J 1994;26:326–66.
[24] Willemen MA, Jacobs MW, Schamhardt HC. In vitro transmission and attenuation of impact vibrations in the distal forelimb. Equine Vet J Suppl 1999;30:245–8.
[25] Pardoe CH, McGuigan MP, Rogers KM, et al. The effect of shoe material on the kinetics and kinematics of foot slip at impact on concrete. Equine Vet J Suppl 2001;33:70–3.
[26] Roepstorff L, Johnston C, Drevemo S. In vivo and in vitro heel expansion in relation to shoeing and frog pressure. Equine Vet J Suppl 2001;54–7.
[27] Olivier A, Wannenburg J, Gottschalk RD, et al. The effect of frog pressure and downward vertical load on hoof wall weight-bearing and third phalanx displacement in the horse—an in vitro study. J S Afr Vet Assoc 2001;72:217–27.
[28] Parks A. Form and function of the equine digit. Veterinary Clinics of North America Equine Practice 2003;19:285–308.
[29] Hood DM, Taylor D, Wagner IP. Effects of ground surface deformability, trimming, and shoeing on quasistatic hoof loading patterns in horses. Am J Vet Res 2001;62:895–900.
[30] Parks AH. Foot balance, conformation, and lameness. In: Ross MW, Dyson SJ, editors. Diagnosis and management of lameness in the horse. Philadelphia: Saunders; 2003. p. 250–61.
[31] Østblom LC, Lund C, Melsen F. Navicular bone disease: results of treatment using egg-bar shoeing technique. Equine Vet J 1984;16:203–6.
[32] Riemersma DJ, van den Bogert AJ, Jansen MO, et al. Influence of shoeing on ground reaction forces and tendon strains in the forelimbs of ponies. Equine Vet J 1996;28:126–32.
[33] Scheffer CJ, Back W. Effects of 'navicular' shoeing on equine distal forelimb kinematics on different track surface. Vet Q 2001;23:191–5.
[34] Keegan KG, Satterley JM, Skubic M, et al. Use of gyroscopic sensors for objective evaluation of trimming and shoeing to alter time between heel and toe lift-off at end of the stance phase in horses walking and trotting on a treadmill. Am J Vet Res 2005;66:2046–54.
[35] Wright IM. A study of 118 cases of navicular disease: clinical features. Equine Vet J 1993;25:488–92.
[36] Moleman M, van Heel MC, van Weeren PR, et al. Hoof growth between two shoeing sessions leads to a substantial increase of the moment about the distal, but not the proximal, interphalangeal joint. Equine Vet J 2006;38:170–4.
[37] van Heel MC, van Weeren PR, Back W. Compensation for changes in hoof conformation between shoeing sessions through the adaptation of angular kinematics of the distal segments of the limbs of horses. Am J Vet Res 2006;67:1199–203.
[38] Back W, Schamhardt HC, Hartman W, et al. Kinematic differences between the distal portions of the forelimbs and hind limbs of horses at the trot. Am J Vet Res 1995;56:1522–8.
[39] Clayton HM. The effect of an acute hoof wall angulation on the stride kinematics of trotting horses. Equine Vet J Suppl 1990;9:86–90.
[40] Chateau H, Degueurce C, Denoix JM. Effects of 6 degree elevation of the heels on 3D kinematics of the distal portion of the forelimb in the walking horse. Equine Vet J 2004;36:649–54.
[41] Chateau H, Degueurce C, Denoix JM. Three-dimensional kinematics of the distal forelimb in horses trotting on a treadmill and effects of elevation of heel and toe. Equine Vet J 2006;38:164–9.
[42] Crevier-Denoix N, Roosen C, Dardillat C, et al. Effects of heel and toe elevation upon the digital joint angles in the standing horse. Equine Vet J Suppl 2001;33:74–8.
[43] Bushe T, Turner TA, Poulos PW, et al. The effect of hoof angle on coffin, pastern and fetlock joint angles. Proceedings of the American Association of Equine Practitioners 1987;33:729–38.

[44] Viitanen M, Bird J, Smith R, et al. Biochemical characterisation of navicular hyaline cartilage, navicular fibrocartilage and the deep digital flexor tendon in horses with navicular disease. Res Vet Sci 2003;75:113–20.
[45] Clayton HM, Hodson E, Lanovaz JL. The forelimb in walking horses: 2. Net joint moments and joint powers. Equine Vet J 2000;32:295–300.
[46] Drevemo S, Johnston C, Roepstorff L, et al. Nerve block and intra-articular anaesthesia of the forelimb in the sound horse. Equine Vet J Suppl 1999;30:266–9.
[47] Rooney JR. The foreleg. In: Rooney JR, Robert E, editors. The mechanics of the horse. Melbourne (FL): Krieger Publishing Co; 1980. p. 39–64.
[48] Degueurce C, Chateau H, Jerbi H, et al. Three-dimensional kinematics of the proximal interphalangeal joint: effects of raising the heels or the toe. Equine Vet J Suppl 2001;33:79–83.
[49] Nilsson G, Fredrickson I, Drevemo S. Some procedures and tools in the diagnostics of distal equine lameness. Acta Vet Scand Suppl 1973;44:63–79.
[50] Rooney J. The angulation of the forefoot and pastern of the horse. Journal of Equine Veterinary Science 1984;4:138–43.
[51] Chateau H, Degueurce C, Jerbi H, et al. Normal three-dimensional behaviour of the metacarpophalangeal joint and the effect of uneven foot bearing. Equine Vet J Suppl 2001;33:84–8.
[52] Buchner HH, Savelberg HH, Schamhardt HC, et al. Kinematics of treadmill versus overground locomotion in horses. Vet Q 1994;16(Suppl 2):S87–90.
[53] Lochner FK, Milne DW, Mills EJ, et al. In vivo and in vitro measurement of tendon strain in the horse. Am J Vet Res 1980;41(12):1929–37.
[54] Thompson KN, Cheung TK, Silverman BS. The effect of toe angle on tendon, ligament and hoof wall strains in vitro. H Eq Vet Sci 1993;13(11):651–4.
[55] Stephens PR, Nunamaker DM, Butterweck DM. Application of a Hall-effect transducer for measurement of tendon strains in horses. Am J Vet Res 1989;50:1089–95.
[56] Riemersma DJ, van den Bogert AJ, Jansen MO, et al. Tendon strain in the forelimbs as a function of gait and ground characteristics and in vitro limb loading in ponies. Equine Vet J 1996;28:133–8.
[57] Clayton HM. Comparison of the stride of trotting horses trimmed with a normal and a broken-back hoof axis. Proceedings of the American Association of Equine Practitioners 1987;33:289–98.
[58] Willemen MA, Savelberg HH, Jacobs MW, et al. Biomechanical effects of rocker-toed shoes in sound horses. Vet Q 1996;18(Suppl 2):S75–8.
[59] van Heel MC, van Weeren PR, Back W. Shoeing sound warmblood horses with a rolled toe optimises hoof-unrollment and lowers peak loading during breakover. Equine Vet J 2006;38:258–62.
[60] O'Grady SE, Poupard DA. Proper physiologic horseshoeing. Vet Clin North Am Equine Pract 2003;19:333–51.
[61] Boswell JC, McGuigan PM, Schramme M, et al. The position of the point of zero moment relative to the foot in normal horses and horses suffering from osteoarthritis of the small tarsal joints (bone spavin). Presented at the 4th International Workshop Anim Locomot. Vienna, Austria, May 2000.
[62] Newman S, Rogers KM, Mcguigan PM, et al. The effect of corrective shoeing on the position of the point of zero moment relative to the foot in horses with osteoarthritis of the small tarsal joints (bone spavin). Proceedings of the British Equine Veterinary Association Cong 2000;198.
[63] Keegan KG, Wilson DJ, Wilson DA, et al. Effects of anesthesia of the palmar digital nerves on kinematic gait analysis in horses with and without navicular disease. Am J Vet Res 1997;58:218–23.
[64] Galisteo AM, Cano MR, Morales JL, et al. Kinematics in horses at the trot before and after an induced forelimb supporting lameness. Equine Vet J Suppl 1997;23:97–101.

[65] Huskamp B, Tietje S, Nowak M, et al. Fubungs- und bewegungsmuster gesunder und strahlbeinkranker pferde-gemessen mit dem Equine-Gait-Analysis-System (EGA-system). Pferdeheilkunde 1990;6:231–6 [in German].
[66] Peloso JG, Stick JA, Soutas-Little RW, et al. Computer-assisted three-dimensional gait analysis of amphotericin-induced carpal lameness in horses. Am J Vet Res 1993;54:1535–43.
[67] Clayton CM. Cinematographic analysis of the gait of lame horses. III: fractures of the third carpal bone. J Equine Vet Sci 1987;7:130–5.
[68] Clayton CM. Cinematographic analysis of the gait of lame horses. IV: degenerative joint disease of the distal intertarsal joint. J Equine Vet Sci 1987;7:274–8.
[69] Merkens HW, Schamhardt HC. Evaluation of equine locomotion during different degrees of experimentally induced lameness. II: distribution of ground reaction force patterns of the concurrently loaded limbs. Equine Vet J Suppl 1988;6:107–12.
[70] Merkens HW, Schamhardt HC. Evaluation of equine locomotion during different degrees of experimentally induced lameness. I: lameness model and quantification of ground reaction force patterns of the limbs. Equine Vet J Suppl 1988;6:99–106.
[71] Weishaupt MA. Compensatory load redistribution in forelimb and hind limb lameness. Proceedings of the American Association of Equine Practitioners 2005;51:141–8.
[72] Keegan KG, Wilson DA, Smith BK, et al. Changes in kinematic variables observed during pressure-induced forelimb lameness in adult horses trotting on a treadmill. Am J Vet Res 2000;61:612–9.
[73] Williams GE. Locomotor characteristics of horses with navicular disease. Am J Vet Res 2001;62:206–10.
[74] McGuigan MP, Walsh TC, Pardoe CH, et al. Deep digital flexor tendon force and digital mechanics in normal ponies and ponies with rotation of the distal phalanx as a sequel to laminitis. Equine Vet J 2005;37:161–5.
[75] Barr AR. Carpal conformation in relation to carpal chip fracture. Vet Rec 1994;134:646–50.
[76] Anderson TM, McIlwraith CW, Douay P. The role of conformation in musculoskeletal problems in the racing Thoroughbred. Equine Vet J 2004;36:571–5.
[77] Kane AJ, Stover SM, Gardner IA, et al. Hoof size, shape, and balance as possible risk factors for catastrophic musculoskeletal injury of Thoroughbred racehorses. Am J Vet Res 1998;59: 1545–52.
[78] Weller R, Pfau T, Verheyen K, et al. The effect of conformation on orthopaedic health and performance in a cohort of National Hunt racehorses: preliminary results. Equine Vet J 2006;38:622–7.
[79] Kane AJ, Stover SM, Gardner IA, et al. Horseshoe characteristics as possible risk factors for fatal musculoskeletal injury of Thoroughbred racehorses. Am J Vet Res 1996;57:1147–52.
[80] Hernandez JA, Scollay MC, Hawkins DL, et al. Evaluation of horseshoe characteristics and high-speed exercise history as possible risk factors for catastrophic musculoskeletal injury in Thoroughbred racehorses. Am J Vet Res 2005;66:1314–20.
[81] Smith SS, Dyson SJ, Murray RC, et al. Is there an association between distal phalanx angles and deep digital flexor tendon lesions? Proceedings: American Association of Equine Practitioners 2004;50:1454.

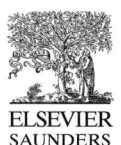

An Evidence-Based Approach to Selected Joint Therapies in Horses

Dean W. Richardson, DVM[a],*, Ricardo Loinaz, VMD[b]

[a]*University of Pennsylvania, School of Veterinary Medicine, New Bolton Center, 382 West Street Road, Kennett Square, PA 19348–1692, USA*
[b]*Urb. Tintillo Gardens, Suite 8 G-14, Guaynabo, PR 00966, USA*

Arthritis is common in human beings and horses; thus, it is hardly surprising that the treatments available so widely by prescription and over the counter in people have found their way into the equine market. The saturation of the equine industry with an enormous array of antiarthritis medications is readily witnessed by anyone who opens any magazine geared toward horse owners. There is constant pressure on veterinarians to treat performance-limiting joint problems successfully, preferably with something inexpensive, effective, and risk-free.

There is an enormous volume of published material about most of the agents used to treat or prevent arthritis. Unfortunately, most of the claims made by nearly all purveyors of arthritis medications in such media are largely unsubstantiated. In addition, the quality of the available information is highly inconsistent, making evidence-based recommendations difficult. This review concentrates on injectable polysulfated glycosaminoglycan (PSGAG), injectable hyaluronan (HA), and the common oral "nutraceutic" agents.

The use of nutraceutic agents in the treatment or management of osteoarthritis (OA) in the horse has become increasingly common. From a treatment standpoint, they are easy to administer and perceived as benign [1]. Their use is, however, controversial, because there is considerable variability in reports of their efficacy, and based on the literature examined in this review, there is a general consensus in the veterinary and human medical communities that high-quality studies providing true evidence of efficacy and elucidating the mechanisms of action of these substances are lacking [2–11]. Although there is an abundance of anecdotal evidence [12–14] from

* Corresponding author.
  E-mail address: dwr@vet.upenn.edu (D.W. Richardson).

practitioners who have found glucosamine (GS), chondroitin sulfate (CS), PSGAG, and HA products to be beneficial for patients with OA, considerable skepticism remains about these products [7,8,15,16]. The apparent basis of this skepticism is a combination of the clinical failure of these products to produce significant beneficial effects and the poor quality of available clinical trials. The latter are commonly limited by critical flaws in design, such as inadequate sample sizes, lack of randomization and blinding, and multiple potential sources of bias [6,7,17–19]. In addition, nutraceutic agents are recognized as supplements by the US Food and Drug Administration (FDA), and as such, they are not subjected to the same strict regulations as drugs are, which affects the purity of these substances and the ability of their efficacy to be consistently evaluated [1,20,21].

Oral nutraceutic agents: glucosamine and chondroitin sulfate

The paradox of oral nutraceutic (a "new" word made from combining the words nutrition and pharmaceutic) agents is that although they are remarkably successful commercially and there is no shortage in the quantity of reports evaluating efficacy, there is no consensus on their efficacy and, more remarkably, no real understanding of a possible mechanism for their proposed efficacy. The scientific information on the subject is plagued in particular with in vitro work showing effects of these agents at doses that cannot be proven to be attainable in vivo. In general, in vitro studies do not provide high-quality evidence of effectiveness; effects seen in the laboratory often cannot be extended to the living animal. A systematic review of 17 randomized controlled trials (RCTs) conducted on human patients reported that GS may be effective and safe in delaying the progression of OA and in ameliorating the symptoms of OA of the knee [19]. Although the authors provided detailed discussion of the selection criteria for studies included and how the data were pooled and interpreted, only 2 of the 17 RCTs were used in their statistical analysis and both had been conducted with GS sulfate salt only, which likely limits the ability to extrapolate the results of these studies to other GS products. A review from the *Cochrane Database of Systematic Reviews* [22] looked at 20 RCTs conducted for at least 2 to 3 months in human patients with knee and hip OA and reported inconsistent results regarding the efficacy of GS. Investigators found that, collectively, the studies showed modest benefits for GS over placebo in improving pain (28%) and function (21%) on Lequesne index scores but that there was marked heterogeneity in these results and that some of the outcome measures in the Western Ontario and McMaster Universities osteoarthritis (WOMAC) index did not reach statistical significance. This review also showed that those studies looking at a specific GS preparation (Rotta Pharmaceuticals, Monza Milan, Italy), and sponsored by the manufacturer of the product, reported better results with GS than those studies that did not use the same GS preparation and were independently funded. The same authors repeated the meta-analysis 4 years later and concluded that newer information was trending toward showing less positive effects [6].

A meta-analysis of 15 double-blind, placebo-controlled RCTs lasting at least 4 weeks reported that although moderate to large beneficial effects were seen with GS and CS over placebo, methodologic issues and publication bias had likely led to an overestimation of these effects and that the results from these studies were so heterogeneous that the meta-analysis itself was limited in quality [10]. Another meta-analysis examined 7 RCTs on CS treatment for OA and found that CS showed superior effects compared with placebo [11]. According to the authors, the results of the 7 studies were consistent throughout the different populations analyzed and major methodologic deficiencies or flaws were not detected in these publications. The authors recognize that in all the studies included in their analysis, however, CS was given concurrently to other analgesics, thus increasing the likelihood of a confounding effect influencing the validity of the results. A more recent meta-analysis specifically examining trials with CS concluded that there was no evidence of any efficacy in trials that were properly performed [23].

A comprehensive review on nutraceutic therapies for degenerative joint disease (DJD) concluded that there are too many conflicting reports and an overall lack of knowledge regarding the efficacy, safety, and mechanisms of action of nutraceutic agents [24]. Other investigators also supported the idea that there is a need for high-quality studies in horses to establish the efficacy of GS but claimed that there is enough clinical evidence to support the use of GS [25]. The general tone of multiple reviews confirms a lack of good evidence for efficacy of nutraceutic agents, but most authors suggest that there are no compelling reasons to discourage the use of GS and CS because they have been shown to be safe [6,7,10,19,26].

The quality of evidence provided by many reviews is questionable because of a lack of discussion of how studies were analyzed and selected and how the information gathered from different studies included in these reviews was pooled and interpreted.

Clinical trials, specifically long-term RCTs, on GS and CS are lacking in the veterinary literature. A 2-week, double-blind, placebo-controlled study of 8 horses with tarsal DJD given an oral supplement for "joint health" reported a more symmetric gait pattern in the supplement-treated group compared with the placebo group [27]. A lack of randomization, small sample size, short study period, and commercial sponsorship limit the quality of evidence derived from this study, however. Another clinical trial looked at the effects of a GS/CS product (Cosequin, Nutramax Laboratories, Inc., Edgewood, Maryland) on 25 horses diagnosed with DJD [28]. Horses weighing less than 545 kg were given GS/CS at a dose of 9 g and horses weighing more than 545 kg were given the treatment at a dose of 12 g, with both groups receiving treatment orally twice daily for 6 weeks. Investigators evaluated lameness, flexion, and stride length and found statistically significant improvements ($P < .0001$) in all three outcome measures in the first 2 weeks of the trial and further improvements, at slower rates, in lameness but not in flexion scores or stride length in the following 4 weeks of the study period. This study lacked a placebo group, there was no randomization or blinding of the examiners, and commercial sponsorship may have added an additional source of bias; therefore, the quality of evidence derived from these results is limited. A randomized, double-blind, placebo-controlled clinical trial looked at the effects of Cosequin in 14 horses with navicular syndrome [29]. Investigators reported significant ($P<.05$) improvements in lameness scores and clinical condition but no significant improvements ($P>.05$) in radiographic scores after 8 weeks of treatment. No obvious flaws in design were detected in this study other than small sample size and potential bias caused by sponsorship from the manufacturer of the tested product. Another RCT was conducted on 30 horses subjected to the complete Freund's adjuvant (CFA) model of carpitis and treated every 4 days for 4 weeks with 500-mg (mL) intramuscular injections of PSGAG, acetyl-D-glucosamine, or chondroitin monosulfate [30]. Investigators evaluated lameness scores, carpal flexion, stride length, and carpal circumference and found an overall statistically significant ($P<.0001$) treatment effect, with the PSGAG group having significantly increased improvements compared with the GS and CS groups. No significant differences were found between the GS and CS groups. The quality of these results is questionable, however, because PSGAG was used as a positive control and no negative control group was established. The authors claim that PSGAG has been established as an effective treatment, but it is not clear if comparing GS and CS with PSGAG limits the quality of this study. The short study period (4 weeks) is likely an additional limitation.

In the human literature, randomized, double-blind, placebo-controlled clinical trials also reported conflicting results. In a study of 98 patients with knee OA, investigators found no statistically significant differences between GS and placebo treatments in reducing pain, as assessed with a visual analogue scale (VAS), at 30 days at rest ($P = .66$) or walking ($P = .69$) [31]. No differences were found at 60 days, and no differences were found in the mean change from baseline VAS scores for the two treatments. A 6-month, double-blind, placebo-controlled RCT evaluated patients with OA who had been using a GS product for at least 2 months and had experienced significant improvements [32]. The patients were randomly allocated to a GS group or a placebo (discontinuation) group. Investigators looked at the incidence, duration, severity of disease flare-ups, and use of "rescue" analgesics. No statistically significant differences in any of the outcome measures were seen between those patients continued on GS and those receiving the placebo. In contrast, two long-term, double-blind, placebo-controlled, randomized clinical trials found that GS was significantly more effective than placebo at treating the symptoms of OA and that placebo-treated patients experienced significant joint space loss, whereas GS-treated patients did not [9,33]. These four studies [9,31–33] were similar in design, patient population and sample size, dosages of GS tested, and outcome measures evaluated. The two studies reporting no beneficial effects with GS treatment were independently funded studies, however, whereas the two studies reporting beneficial effects were sponsored by the manufacturers of the GS product used, potentially leading to publication bias. It is not clear how the heterogeneity in these results influences the quality of evidence that can be derived from these studies; furthermore, these studies are substantially different from those found in the equine literature, thus making extrapolation of reported results difficult.

Although reports of clinical efficacy have been variable, it has been almost universally concluded that GS and CS are as safe as placebo treatments; there have been few reports of adverse reactions. A study done on six healthy mares that were administered five times the minimum recommended dose for Cosequin for 35 days found no abnormal clinical changes attributable to the product [34]. Investigators found statistically significant ($P<.05$) increases in hemoglobin, hematocrit, and white blood cell counts, but these findings were not considered clinically significant. Although the authors suggested that the results indicated that Cosequin was safe even at higher than normal doses, real evidence found in this study is limited primarily because of a lack of a control group, a small sample size, and commercial sponsorship by the manufacturer of Cosequin as well as because statistically significant findings were described as clinically insignificant without a detailed discussion.

Several experimental studies in horses or equine tissues have attempted to elucidate the possible mechanisms of action of GS and CS. One study looked at the inhibitory effects of GS on interleukin (IL)-1–conditioned equine articular cartilage [35]. Investigators used recombinant equine IL-1 (reIL-1) because this has been shown to be present in high levels in diseased joints and to be responsible for inducing changes associated with OA, such as increased production of prostaglandin (PG) E_2, nitric oxide (NO), and matrix metalloproteinases (MMPs). Investigators cultured equine cartilage explants with reIL-1 and GS hydrogen chloride (HCl) at 0.25, 2.5, and 25 mg/mL and found that the highest dose had a statistically significant ($P<.001$) inhibitory effect on all enzymes associated with cartilage degradation measured in this experiment. The statistical significance described by the authors does not necessarily imply clinical significance, however, because a concentration of GS at 25 mg/mL is unlikely to be achieved in vivo. This problem of relating in vitro doses to achievable in vivo concentrations exists in many studies, and this seriously diminishes the quality of evidence.

Another study analyzed glycosaminoglycan (GAG) synthesis and total GAG content in equine cartilage explants (normal and cultured with human IL-1) that were treated with GS alone, CS alone, or a combination of GS/CS at 0, 12.5, 25, 125 or 250 μg/mL [36]. Investigators found that the highest dose of the GS/CS combination showed a statistically significant ($P<.0001$) reduction in total GAG release into the media in IL-1–conditioned cartilage.

This finding is potentially clinically significant because other investigators have reported that GAG levels were found to be higher in arthritic joints, which was indicative of cartilage degradation [37]. The authors indicated that a concentration of GS/CS of 250 μg/mL could be achieved in vivo, however, if 100% bioavailability was assumed or if multiple treatments with GS led to accumulation in the extracellular fluid. Oral bioavailability of GS and CS in horses is uncertain and not likely to approach 100%. Another study reported that GS, at a concentration of 10 μg/mL, reduced reIL-β–induced stimulation of MMP-13, aggrecanase 1, and junctional terminal kinase (JNK), which are enzymes that have been implicated in the pathogenesis of OA [38]. Investigators found that CS, however, did not show these inhibitory effects. This study is perhaps more valuable in terms of the evidence it provides to support the chondroprotective action of GS, because the concentrations used (2.5–10 μg/mL) approximate the in vivo concentrations feasible in horses after oral administration of GS. Another study found similar results and reported that GS at concentrations as low as 0.5 and 1.0 mg/mL inhibited PGE_2 and NO, respectively, and that CS at concentrations of 0.25 or 0.5 mg/mL did not inhibit these mediators of cartilage degradation [39]. Investigators found that the combination of GS at a dose of 1.0 mg/mL and CS at a dose of 0.5 mg/mL showed the most significant inhibition, suggesting a complimentary action between GS and CS. Two of the cited equine studies were sponsored by the manufacturers of the tested product, a potential source of bias [5,36]. All four studies used concentrations of GS and CS that are not certain to be achievable in vivo. Although this issue is acknowledged by the authors, it still limits the clinical significance of the reported results.

Principal questions regarding the use of oral nutraceutic agents in horses are whether or not they are absorbed and, if they are, what their "true" bioavailability is [40,41]. One study looked the oral bioavailability of low-molecular-weight CS and GS HCl in horses after oral and intravenous administration [41]. Bioavailability was determined by measuring total disaccharides in plasma. Because the purity of CS and GS products has been shown to be variable, the authors used products that, according to previous studies, were effective and met the label claims. Investigators performed two studies: study 1 (n = 10) looked at CS absorption, whereas study 2 (n = 2) looked at GS absorption. Study 1 horses received one of four different treatments, which consisted of intravenous CS (8 kDa), oral CS (8 kDa), intravenous CS (16.9 kDa), and oral CS (16.9 kDa), all with concurrent administration with GS, whereas study 2 horses received intravenous GS or oral GS. Results for study 1 showed that CS at doses of 8 and 16 kDa was absorbed but that the lower molecular weight had a higher numeric bioavailability (32% versus 22%), which was not regarded by the authors as statistically significant. Results for study 2 showed that after intravenous administration, GS concentration declined rapidly (half-life [$t_{1/2}$] = 0.83 hour) and that after oral administration, the bioavailability of GS was measured to be 2.5%, which the authors attributed to an extensive first-pass effect in the gastrointestinal tract or liver before systemic absorption. The authors concluded that the results of the study showed that CS and GS are both absorbed in horses, with CS having a higher rate of absorption and bioavailability than GS and possibly a mode of absorption that depends on molecular weight.

Unfortunately, the evidence for oral bioavailability derived from these results is limited, because in study 2, investigators used a dose of GS 5 to 10 times higher than the dose commonly given to horses, thus limiting the clinical significance of the results. In addition, the authors indicated that the 8-kDa preparations used were experimental preparations and not available commercially; because the highest bioavailability was achieved with this molecular weight (although the authors described this finding as statistically insignificant), it is not clear how this affects the clinical significance of the results. Another study evaluating synovial fluid levels and serum pharmacokinetics in horses after treatment with oral GS at clinically relevant doses in eight adult mares found that such doses resulted in serum and synovial fluid concentrations at least 500 times lower than those reported to have metabolic-modifying effects on chondrocytes in vitro [42].

A final consideration regarding oral nutraceutic agents evaluated in this review was the question regarding the purity of commonly used GS and CS products. Several authors have suggested that even if oral nutraceutic agents are indeed effective, it is difficult to evaluate and establish true evidence for this efficacy if the GS and CS contents of these products differ from what is claimed on their labels. A study done on 11 oral joint supplements containing GS, CS, or both analyzed the total sulfated GAG, keratin sulfate (KS), and HA contents of these products [21]. Results indicated that GS contents in 5 products containing GS only, according to their labels, ranged from 63.6% to 112.2% of label claims and that CS contents in 5 products containing CS only, according to their labels, ranged from 22.5% to 155.7% of label claims. According to the authors, the laboratory that performed the analysis was blinded as a way of preventing bias; however, no discussion of potential factors influencing the results is found in the article. A second study looked at the actual GS content by measuring glucosamine free base (GFB) of 23 equine oral joint supplements and found a range for GS content of 0% to 221.2% of label claims [20]. Investigators reported that 9 of the 23 products contained less GS than claimed by the manufacturers and that 4 of these products contained less than 30% of the expected GS content. Evidence regarding the use of oral nutraceutic agents is limited not only by conflicting reports of efficacy, modes of action, and bioavailability but by a lack of regulation of purity of these products.

The most recent meta-analysis that thoroughly evaluated all the available trials evaluating CS concluded that there was no indication of any efficacy in terms of pain relief for OA of the human knee and hip [23]. This analysis was particularly interesting, given that the "negative" conclusion is more firmly stated than previous analyses using similar techniques. The probable explanation for this is that the size and quality of studies have improved over time and that more rigidly structured trials without publication bias have trended markedly toward showing no effect. This historical trend in human beings may augur a similar evaluation of these drugs in horses as the quality of evidence improves.

Polysulfated glycosaminoglycan

PSGAG has been used as a licensed drug to treat various joint diseases in horses in North America for more than 20 years [43]. Before its licensing as Adequan (Luitpold Animal Health, Shirley, New York), it was widely imported from Europe, where it was sold for many years as Arteparon. Because the drug has been around and in use for so long, there have been numerous claims concerning its action and efficacy. It has been reported to induce articular cartilage matrix synthesis and to decrease matrix degradation [44]. Although PSGAG has been shown to have chondroprotective properties, anti-inflammatory activities, anabolic effects, and catabolic effects on articular cartilage, the exact mechanisms for these actions remain unclear and results reported in vitro have been largely undemonstrated in vivo [43–47].

Adverse reactions have also been reported with intra-articular administration of PSGAG. There is clinical and experiment evidence that PSGAG diminishes the joint's capacity to resist infection [44,48]. Furthermore, because of its heparin-like activity, PSGAG administration has been associated with complications in animals with a history of hypersensitivity, shock, and bleeding tendencies [44].

High-quality RCTs evaluating PSGAG are scarce in the equine literature [4,5,43–45,47], but because the drug has been available for a long time and has been heavily marketed, there are several studies that have attempted to prove its efficacy. A randomized, double-blind, placebo-controlled clinical trial compared the effects of PSGAG and sodium hyaluronate (SH) with a placebo treatment in horses with naturally occurring traumatic arthritis [46]. Investigators reported statistically significant improvements in lameness scores after 3 weeks of treatment in the PSGAG and SH groups when compared with the placebo group and found no significant differences between PSGAG and SH treatments. Although the study had a possibly adequate sample size (n = 77), the treatment groups were comparable and treated equally throughout the study period, and a placebo group was used, the duration of the study is recognized as short (a potential limitation) by the authors, and it is unclear if testing PSGAG and SH in the same study affected the validity of the authors' claims. Another randomized, double-blind, controlled clinical trial was done on 8 horses that had partial-thickness and full-thickness cartilage defects created surgically on one middle carpal joint and chemically induced cartilage defects created on the contralateral middle carpal joint [49]. Horses were randomly allocated to an intramuscular PSGAG (500 mg) or an intramuscular saline (2 mL) control group, with both groups receiving treatment every 4 days for a total of seven injections. Investigators looked at lameness scores, limb circumference, radiographic findings, and microscopic evaluation and did not find any significant differences between the PSGAG group and the control group, with the exception of slightly greater matrix staining intensity for GAG (safranin-O staining) in the joints of horses with chemically induced defects in the PSGAG-treated group. Investigators concluded that PSGAG did not show significant effects on healing articular cartilage lesions and showed only minor chondroprotective effects from chemically induced lesions. Although randomization was used, discussion of blinding for all parts of the postsurgical evaluation is lacking and the authors admit that the dose of PSGAG used may have been insufficient and the duration of the treatment period too short to allow for the beneficial effects of PSGAG reported in other studies to be demonstrated.

Another randomized, double-blind study looked at the effects of exercise and PSGAG treatment on the development of OA in ponies with osteochondral defects [50]. Eighteen ponies were randomized to two groups of 9 (one group of ponies was exercised and the other was not) in which 6 ponies were treated with 5 weekly intra-articular injections of PSGAG (250 mg) in one middle carpal joint and saline in the contralateral joint and 3 ponies received saline in both joints. Investigators looked at various parameters, including joint pain, radiographic signs, diagnostic ultrasound, synovial fluid analysis, and cytology. They found that exercised nonmedicated ponies were the most lame, whereas nonexercised nonmedicated ponies were the least lame; medication caused a significant decrease in lameness at 9 weeks in the exercised medicated ponies. Investigators also reported that PSGAG-treated ponies had less type II collagen relative to type I than nonmedicated ponies, indicating fibrous tissue deposition. The authors concluded that PSGAG mitigated the symptoms of OA in exercised ponies, particularly if given during the rehabilitation period and not immediately after surgery, because of its effects on the quality of the cartilage repair tissue. A similar study looked at the effects of exercise and PSGAG on radionuclide uptake on blood pool and delayed images as a measure of metabolic activity (bone remodeling) and progression of OA in ponies with osteochondral defects [51]. The authors of this study reported that exercise without PSGAG promoted increased bone remodeling, seen as an undesirable effect consistent with development of OA, and that intra-articular PSGAG seemed to counteract this effect and provided a protective effect against the development of OA. Although these two studies were described as RCTs and do not exhibit obvious flaws in their design, they were both sponsored by the manufacturer of PSGAG (Adequan). Furthermore, both studies evaluated several different factors (age, exercise, and medication effects), and although the authors claimed to have adjusted their statistical analysis to account for the possible interactions between these factors, the possibility of a confounding effect is likely increased.

Another study looked at the effects of PSGAG and SH compared with a saline (control) group on the biochemical composition of the repair tissue in ponies with full-thickness, arthroscopically induced osteochondral defects [52]. Investigators found no significant differences between treated and control groups with regard to total collagen content, uronic acid content, and the relative proportions of type I and type II collagen in the repair tissue. Any putative chondroprotective effects of PSGAG were not demonstrated in this study, because secondary "kissing" lesions were found in all joints examined. This study, however, lacked a description of a randomization and blinding process and a discussion of possible limitations to the study, including individual variation among the horses examined that might have influenced the results.

Some of the putative beneficial effects of PSGAG have been ascribed to its ability to inhibit enzymes of cartilage destruction, promote synthesis of endogenous HA, and inhibit mediators of inflammation in the horse [43–45,47,48]. One study looked at the effects of PSGAG on chondrocyte replication and on the synthesis and degradation of the matrix of articular cartilage and attempted to see if there was any evidence that arthritic equine articular cartilage was more sensitive to the effects of PSGAG than normal cartilage [53]. When cartilage explants were cultured with different concentrations of PSGAG, investigators found that low-molecular-weight PSGAG exhibited a dose-dependent stimulation of collagen synthesis in normal and arthritic articular cartilage, with the latter having a statistically significant ($P<.01$) greater response. At high doses of PSGAG (50 mg/mL), GAG degradation was significantly inhibited and extracellular matrix formation was stimulated, whereas at lower doses of PSGAG (12.5 mg/mL), chondrocyte replication was stimulated. The authors claim that the highest concentrations of PSGAG used in their study (25 and 50 mg/mL) approximate the concentrations of PSGAG found in the synovial fluid after intra-articular injection of 250 mg, a commonly used treatment dose. This is an important finding, because the authors are not only providing statistically significant but clinically significant results. If PSGAG were able to inhibit, at concentrations that are achievable in vivo, the degradation of articular cartilage, which is the defining process of OA, this would be evidence that PSGAG should be considered an effective treatment for OA [54–56]. The validity of this study and the quality of real evidence it provides, however, are potentially limited by commercial sponsorship from the manufacturers of the PSGAG product (Adequan) tested.

Unfortunately, these promising results have not been repeatable. A similar study [57] found a statistically significant ($P \leq .04$) decrease in proteoglycan synthesis in cartilage explants cultured with concentrations of PSGAG similar to those in the previously described study [53]. In addition, these investigators found that PSGAG had no influence on cartilage matrix degradation. The cartilage explant cultures used in this experiment came from four different horses, and four separate experiments were done with individual explants, forming an experimental block, which likely makes this study less subject to bias attributable to interindividual variation than the previous study described, but the small sample size (n = 4) is problematic for this kind of study. Another study was done with equine synoviocytes, whereby investigators looked at the effects of PSGAG and HA on PGE_2 production [58]. Synoviocytes from four horses with no macroscopic signs of joint disease were stimulated with lipopolysaccharide (LPS), which produced statistically significant ($P<.001$ for cells in the HA experiment and $P<.006$ for cells in the PSGAG experiment) increases in PGE_2 production in untreated cells. Cells were cultured with three different preparations of HA or different concentrations of PSGAG. Investigators found that PSGAG concentrations of 200, 2000, 10,000, and 20,000 µg/mL caused decreases in LPS-induced PGE_2 production but that only the two highest concentrations produced statistically significant ($P = .003$) decreases. According to the authors, these concentrations are achievable in vivo by intra-articular administration but not by intramuscular injection. This presents a clinically significant finding, because PGE_2 is an important mediator in inflammation and hyperalgesia [48,58]. It is not clear if the validity of these results is weakened by the use of a positive-control treatment (indomethacin, a nonsteroidal anti-inflammatory drug [NSAID]), however, because a true control population (not stimulated by LPS) and an LPS-stimulated and untreated population were maintained.

Another study looked at the ability of PSGAG to modulate the transcription of IL-1β, a mediator of OA, and to increase the steady-state mRNA levels, and thus synthesis, of major structural matrix molecules, such as type II procollagen and aggrecan core protein [59]. Investigators found that IL-1β significantly decreased steady-state mRNA of matrix molecules and increased that of MMPs, enzymes responsible for cartilage degradation [45–47,59]; PSGAG (Adequan) was apparently able to counteract these effects on cartilage in a dose-dependent way. Two similar studies looked at the inhibitory effects of PSGAG on stromelysin [60] and MMP-2,9 [40] enzymes, which are important mediators in the pathogenesis of OA. Investigators in the first study looked at the inhibitory activities of different substances used in the treatment of OA, including PSGAG, HA, and different NSAIDS, and found that only PSGAG, at a concentration (20 mg/mL) likely attainable in vivo in the fetlock joint, showed a statistically significant ($P<.001$) inhibitory effect. The second study used similar concentrations of PSGAG and found that at concentrations greater than 10 mg/mL, PSGAG had a statistically significant ($P<.05$) inhibitory effect on MMPs. The authors of this study, however, were reluctant to classify this finding as clinically significant, because it is unclear that PSGAG could remain in the joint space at high concentrations for a prolonged period.

Another obvious confounding issue with PSGAG is that virtually all the in vitro studies done with the drug have used concentrations that would only be achievable with intra-articular administration. The potential for adequate distribution of the drug to the affected joint(s) when it is given intramuscularly remains highly questionable. Some studies have shown that there may be some concentration of the intramuscularly injected drug in joint tissues [61,62]; however, the relevance of this minor concentrating effect is doubtful, because in vitro studies have not shown significant effects at such low doses.

Hyaluronan

HA has been suggested to impart viscosity to synovial fluid, lubricate unloaded joints, exert a direct anti-inflammatory effect [63], restore the rheologic properties of synovial fluid, and be a safe treatment for OA [63–65]. A review of the evolution of viscosupplementation, the use of an elastoviscous HA solution to replace synovial fluid components, reported that HA had been suggested to provide an analgesic effect to horses with traumatic arthritis, which was later confirmed by force plate gait analysis [64]. Another review on the use of intra-articular injection of HA found that most clinical studies showed that 60% to 75% of human patients given repeated injections of HA experienced significant clinical benefits that were longer lasting than those derived from corticosteroid injections and that, overall, HA was a well-tolerated treatment [66]. Similarly, an analysis of clinical studies done using a cross-linked high-molecular-weight HA product (Synvisc, Genzyme Corporation, Cambridge, Massachusetts) reported that HA, when injected as many as 6 to 10 times during the study period (3–4 weeks), was found to be significantly superior to placebo in improving the symptoms of OA. These reviews, however, do not include a discussion of the qualifications of the studies that were included, or excluded, and do not discuss the potential biases and limitations that may be included in these publications [64,66,67]. Indeed, a recent meta-analysis of 22 clinical trials found that intra-articular HA had a small effect compared with placebo and that publication bias and flaws in experimental design may have led to an overestimation of the benefits derived from HA treatment [3].

Clinical trials on HA have been done in horses since the 1970s. Some of the early studies done with intra-articular HA reported significant improvements in lameness, weight-bearing scores, and quality of the synovial fluid and reported no significant adverse reactions [68–71]. The evidence provided by these results is limited, however, because of a lack of description of randomization and blinding [69,70], absence of a control group [69,70], and use of a positive control group (corticosteroid) [68] or a historical control group (horses that had failed to respond to previous treatments) [71]. Another study looked at the effects of exogenous HA on joint function in horses with surgically induced chip fractures [53]. After induction of OA, investigators randomly allocated 25 horses to HA treatment groups using a single intra-articular injection of HA at a dose of 0 (saline, placebo group), 5, 10, 20, or 40 mg and then returned the horses to their daily exercise regimen, restricting all concurrent medications. Based on lameness examination and force plate testing, investigators found significant improvements in the 20-mg and 40-mg treated horses, because none of the horses in these two groups were lame after 2 weeks and soundness persisted for at least 4 weeks after treatment. Investigators used the mean peak vertical force (F_{max}) obtained from force plate testing as a reflection of weight bearing and joint function and found no statistically significant differences in the F_{max} of 20-mg and 40-mg HA-treated horses between the prearthritic values (before surgical induction) and posttreatment values at any point during the 4-week study period, suggesting that HA restored normal joint function. This in vitro finding may serve as clinically significant evidence because it supports the favorable results that have been noted by other investigators using HA.

Another study looked at the changes in the synovia in horses with normal joints and with surgically induced cartilage defects after treatment with SH or placebo (saline) and found no significant differences in endogenous hyaluronic acid concentration, protein concentration, or intrinsic viscosity between the two treatment groups [72]. Moreover, investigators found the elimination $t_{1/2}$ of HA to be approximately 96 hours in normal joints, which investigators concluded is likely too short for exogenous HA to replenish the synovial hyaluronic acid for any length of time. The quality of evidence of this study, however, is limited by a lack of discussion of the selection criteria for the 12 horses used, a likely inadequate sample size (n = 12), and a short-duration study period. The authors also suggest that further work is needed to determine if the effects of exogenous HA are not based on stimulating endogenous HA synthesis but rather on stimulating a higher quality and higher molecular weight HA (other studies have suggested that HA has a mode of action that depends on molecular weight).

One experimental study looked at the effects of exogenous HA on the synthesis and molecular size of endogenous HA in normal and osteoarthritic joints and found that exogenous HA influenced neither the rate of synthesis nor the hydrodynamic size of newly synthesized HA in either of the cell cultures (normal and arthritic) [73]. The authors recognized that their study may have been limited by not using a high-molecular-weight exogenous HA, which may have been needed to exert a stimulatory effect on endogenous HA. There seems to be no clear indication that the molecular weight of HA used for therapeutic purposes has clinical relevance, however [74].

A more recent randomized, blind, prospective study of racing Quarter Horses treated with intravenous HA found that HA-treated horses raced for longer before requiring intra-articular treatments and had a greater number of starts than placebo-treated horses [75]. This study was limited by the confounding effects of concurrent medications allowed by investigators, however. The authors recognized that the HA-treated horses were also receiving more PSGAG treatments than the placebo-treated horses, which the authors attributed to differences in trainer preferences. Another recently published prospective, randomized, double-blind, placebo-controlled clinical trial evaluated the efficacy of intra-articular HA for OA of the knee in human patients and found that HA was superior to placebo in ameliorating the signs of OA but found no differences in these effects between treatments lasting 3 weeks and treatments lasting 6 weeks [76]. The authors of this study provided detailed discussions of the selection criteria of the experimental subjects and of the statistical analysis and data interpretation, and methods of OA evaluation regarded in human medicine as standardized and objective (WOMAC index) were used, but the authors recognize that the study is limited by the absence of a control group.

Summary

The evidence-based medicine guidelines and rating systems used to evaluate the literature suggest that many important components must be considered in a study or publication to offer true evidence for the topic of interest [17,18,54,55]. Controlled trials should be randomized and blind, study groups should be comparable and treated equally throughout the study period, and results should be valid and, most importantly, clinically relevant. Statistical analyses conducted in clinical trials and experimental studies must be appropriate and discussed in terms of statistical and clinical significance. Selection bias and publication bias, sometimes associated with commercial sponsorship, must also be avoided or accounted for in clinical trials, and a detailed discussion of inclusion and exclusion criteria for the experimental subjects must be included. Systematic reviews and meta-analyses should also include a discussion of selection criteria for the studies that are used and a discussion of how all the data were pooled and interpreted. Any potential limitations in the individual studies reviewed and analyzed as well as heterogeneity in the collective results must also be reported.

Publications that met, to some extent, some of these criteria for evidence-based medicine were mostly found in the human literature. Most clinical trials found in the equine literature were short in duration, and inconsistencies in randomization and blinding were found. Long-term, randomized, double-blind, placebo-controlled clinical trials on nutraceutic agents, PSGAG, and HA were not found in the equine literature. Although some of the clinical trials found did not have obvious or major flaws in their design, all these studies were sponsored, in part, by the manufacturers of the different products that were tested. This was a common finding across all publication types reviewed for horses, and the influence this had on the results reported is unclear, but most publications reporting commercial sponsorship also reported beneficial effects for the products tested. A similar finding in 20 RCTs of human patients with OA was discussed in the *Cochrane Database of Systematic Reviews* [6].

Systematic reviews and meta-analyses were also lacking in the veterinary literature, and although some clinical and critical reviews were found, it is not clear that these types of publications provide adequate evidence because they do not discuss how the literature was selected and evaluated in the process of reviewing the current state of knowledge on nutraceutic agents, PSGAG, and HA. Although these reviews reference clinical trials and experimental studies done on the subject and briefly describe the potential qualifications and limitations of these studies, they do not provide additional significant information that may answer questions regarding the efficacy, safety, and clinical uses of the products discussed. Systematic reviews and meta-analyses found in the human literature were more consistent in following the criteria for evidence-based medicine discussed previously, but heterogeneity in results and potentially limiting factors, such as concurrent medications and confounding effects, may influence the quality of evidence derived from these publications. There is an enormous volume of literature on these agents that encompasses a spectrum of evidential quality. Conflicting results, flaws in experimental design, commercial sponsorship, and a lack of detailed descriptions regarding the experimental process make it unlikely that many of the publications found could be considered outstanding examples of evidence-based medicine. Accordingly, recommendations for the use of the products considered in this review are not made from a strong base of evidence, and considerably more research is necessary before a truly evidence-based prescription can be made.

References

[1] Trumble T. The use of nutraceuticals for osteoarthritis in horses. Vet Clin North Am Equine Pract 2005;21(3):575–97.
[2] Deal CL, Moskowitz RW. Nutraceuticals as therapeutic agents in osteoarthritis. The role of glucosamine, chondroitin sulfate, and collagen hydrolysate. Rheum Dis Clin North Am 1999;25(2):379–95.
[3] Lo G, et al. Intra-articular hyaluronic acid in treatment of knee osteoarthritis: a meta-analysis. J Am Med Assoc 2003;290(23):3115–21.
[4] McIlwraith C. Licensed medications, "generic" medications, compounding, and nutraceuticals: what has been scientifically validated, where do we encounter scientific mistruth, and where are we legally? Proceedings of the 50th Annu Conv Am Assoc Equine Pract 2004:50:p. 1–16.
[5] Neil KM, Caron JP, Orth MW. The role of glucosamine and chondroitin sulfate in treatment for and prevention of osteoarthritis in animals. J Am Vet Med Assoc 2005;226(7):1079–88.
[6] Towheed TE. Glucosamine therapy for treating osteoarthritis. Cochrane Database Syst Rev 2005;2:CD002946.
[7] McAlindon TE. Nutraceuticals: do they work and when should we use them? Best Pract Res Clin Rheumatol 2006;20(1):99–115.
[8] Chard J, Dieppe P. Glucosamine for osteoarthritis: magic, hype, or confusion? It's probably safe—but there's no good evidence that it works. Br Med J 2001;322(7300):1439–40.
[9] Reginster JY, et al. Long-term effects of glucosamine sulphate on osteoarthritis progression: a randomised, placebo-controlled clinical trial. Lancet 2001;357(9252):251–6.
[10] McAlindon TE, et al. Glucosamine and chondroitin for treatment of osteoarthritis: a systematic quality assessment and meta-analysis. JAMA 2000;283(11):1469–75.

[11] Leeb BF, et al. A metaanalysis of chondroitin sulfate in the treatment of osteoarthritis. J Rheumatol 2000;27(1):205–11.
[12] Hungerford DS, Jones LC. Glucosamine and chondroitin sulfate are effective in the management of osteoarthritis. J Arthroplasty 2003;18(3 Suppl 1):5–9.
[13] McIlwraith C. Should I recommend the use of oral glycosaminoglycans? Compend Contin Educ Pract Vet 1999;21(5):450–7.
[14] Sonnino D. Glucosamine for osteoarthritis: patients' welfare should be primary concern. Br Med J 2001;323:1003.
[15] Ramey DW. Skeptical of treatment with glucosamine and chondroitin sulfate [letter to editor]. J Am Vet Med Assoc 2005;226(11):1798–9.
[16] Verbruggen G. Chondroprotective drugs in degenerative joint diseases. Rheumatology 2006; 45(2):129–38.
[17] Rosenthal R. Evidence-based medicine concepts. Vet Clin North Am Small Anim Pract 2004;34:1–6.
[18] Glasziou P. Levels of evidence and grades of recommendation. Oxford Centre for Evidence Based Medicine. Available at: http://www.cebm.net/levels_of_evidence.asp; 2007.
[19] Poolsup N, et al. Glucosamine long-term treatment and the progression of knee osteoarthritis: systematic review of randomized controlled trials. Ann Pharmacother 2005;39(6):1080–7.
[20] Oke S, et al. Evaluation of glucosamine levels in commercial equine oral supplements for joints. Equine Vet J 2006;38(1):93–5.
[21] Ramey DW, et al. An analysis of glucosamine and chondroitin sulfate content in oral joint supplement products. J Equine Vet Sci 2002;22(3):125–7.
[22] Towheed TE. Glucosamine therapy for treating osteoarthritis. Cochrane Database Syst Rev 2001;1:CD002946.
[23] Reichenbach S, et al. Meta-analysis: chondroitin for osteoarthritis of the knee or hip. Ann Intern Med 2007;146:580–90.
[24] Goggs R, et al. Nutraceutical therapies for degenerative joint diseases: a critical review. Crit Rev Food Sci Nutr 2005;45(3):145–64.
[25] Hanson RR. Oral glycosaminoglycans in treatment of degenerative joint disease in horses. Equine Practice 1996;18(10):18–22.
[26] McAlindon TE, Biggee BA. Nutritional factors and osteoarthritis: recent developments. Curr Opin Rheumatol 2005;17(5):647–52.
[27] Clayton HM, Almeida PE, Prades M. Double-blind study of the effects of an oral supplement intended to support joint health in horses with tarsal degenerative joint disease. Proceedings of the 48th Annu Conv Am Assoc Equine Pract;2002:48. p. 314–17.
[28] Hanson R, Smalley L, Huff G. Oral treatment with a glucosamine-chondroitin sulfate compound for degenerative joint disease in horses: 25 cases. Equine Practice 1997;19(9):16–22.
[29] Hanson RR, Brawner W, Blaik M. Oral treatment with a nutraceutical (Cosequin®) for ameliorating signs of navicular syndrome in horses. Vet Ther 2001;2(2):148–59.
[30] White GW, et al. Efficacy of intramuscular chondroitin sulfate and compounded acetyl-D-glucosamine in a positive controlled study of equine carpitis. In proceedings of the 50th annual convention of the American association of equine practitioners, Denver (CO), 4–8 December, 2004. 2004, American association of equine practitioners (AAEP): Lexington. p. 264–9.
[31] Rindone JP, et al. Randomized, controlled trial of glucosamine for treating osteoarthritis of the knee. West J Med 2000;172(2):91–4.
[32] Cibere J, et al. Randomized, double-blind, placebo-controlled glucosamine discontinuation trial in knee osteoarthritis. Arthritis Rheum 2004;51(5):738–45.
[33] Pavelka K, et al. Glucosamine sulfate use and delay of progression of knee osteoarthritis: a 3-year, randomized, placebo-controlled, double-blind study. Arch Intern Med 2002;162(18): 2113–23.
[34] Kirker-Head C, Kirker-Head R. Safety of an oral chondroprotective agent in horses. Vet Ther 2001;2(4):345–53.

[35] Fenton JI, et al. Effect of glucosamine on interleukin-1-conditioned articular cartilage. Equine Vet J 2002;(Suppl 34):219–23.
[36] Dechant JE, et al. Effects of glucosamine hydrochloride and chondroitin sulphate, alone and in combination, on normal and interleukin-1 conditioned equine articular cartilage explant metabolism. Equine Vet J 2005;37(3):227–31.
[37] Alwan W, et al. Glycosaminoglycans in horses with osteoarthritis. Equine Vet J 1991;23(1): 44–7.
[38] Neil KM, et al. Effects of glucosamine and chondroitin sulfate on mediators of osteoarthritis in cultured equine chondrocytes stimulated by use of recombinant equine interleukin-1 beta. Am J Vet Res 2005;66(11):1861–9.
[39] Orth MW, Peters TL, Hawkins JN. Inhibition of articular cartilage degradation by glucosamine-HCl and chondroitin sulphate. Equine Vet J 2002;(Suppl 34):224–9.
[40] Clegg PD, Jones MD, Carte SD. The effect of drugs commonly used in the treatment of equine articular disorders on the activity of equine matrix metalloproteinase-2 and 9. J Vet Pharmacol Ther 1998;21(5):406–13.
[41] Du J, White N, Eddington N. The bioavailability and pharmacokinetics of glucosamine hydrochloride and chondroitin sulfate after oral and intravenous single dose administration in the horse. Biopharm Drug Dispos 2004;25:109–16.
[42] Laverty S, et al. Synovial fluid levels and serum pharmacokinetics in a large animal model following treatment with oral glucosamine at clinically relevant doses. Arthritis Rheum 2005;52(1):181–91.
[43] Trotter G. Sulfated glycosaminoglycans in equine joint diseases. Compend Cont Educ Pract Vet 1997;19(11):1292–5.
[44] Todhunter RJ, Lust G. Polysulfated glycosaminoglycan in the treatment of osteoarthritis. J Am Vet Med Assoc 1994;204(8):1245–51.
[45] Caron J. Intra-articular injections for joint disease in horses. Vet Clin North Am Equine Pract 2005;21(3):559–73.
[46] Gaustad G, LS. Comparison of polysulphated glycosaminoglycan and sodium hyaluronate with placebo in treatment of traumatic arthritis in horses. Equine Vet J 1995;27(5):356–362.
[47] Goodrich LR, Nixon AJ. Medical treatment of osteoarthritis in the horse—a review. Vet J 2006;171(1):51–69.
[48] McIlwraith CW, Frisbie DD, Kawcak CE. Current treatments for traumatic synovitis, capsulitis, and osteoarthritis. Proceedings at the 47th Annu Conv Am Assoc Equine Pract; 2001:47. p. 194–206.
[49] Trotter GW, et al. Effects of intramuscular polysulfated glycosaminoglycan on chemical and physical defects in equine articular cartilage. Can J Vet Res 1989;53(2):224–30.
[50] Todhunter RJ, et al. Effects of exercise and polysulfated glycosaminoglycan on repair of articular cartilage defects in the equine carpus. J Orthop Res 1993;11(6):782–95.
[51] Todhunter RJ, et al. Use of scintimetry to assess effects of exercise and polysulfated glycosaminoglycan on equine carpal joints with osteochondral defects. Am J Vet Res 1993;54(7): 997–1006.
[52] Barr ARS, et al. Influence of intra-articular sodium hyaluronate and polysulphated glycosaminoglycan on the biochemical composition of equine articular surface repair tissue. Equine Vet J 1994;26(1):40–2.
[53] Glade MJ. Polysulfated glycosaminoglycan accelerates net synthesis of collagen and glycosaminoglycans by arthritic equine cartilage tissues and chondrocytes. Am J Vet Res 1990; 51(5):779–85.
[54] Guyatt G, Sackett D, Cook D. How to use an article about therapy or prevention. A—are the results of the study valid? J Am Med Assoc 1993;270(21):2598–601.
[55] Guyatt G, Sackett D, Cook D. How to use an article about a therapy or prevention. B—what are the results and will they help me in caring for my patients. J Am Med Assoc 1994;271(1): 59–63.

[56] Jaeschke R, Guyatt G, Sackett D. How to use an article about a diagnostic test. A—are the results of the study valid? J Am Med Assoc 1994;271(5):389–91.
[57] Caron JP, Toppin DS, Block JA. Effect of polysulfated glycosaminoglycan on osteoarthritic equine articular cartilage in explant culture. Am J Vet Res 1993;54(7):1116–21.
[58] Frean SP, Lees P. Effects of polysulfated glycosaminoglycan and hyaluronan on prostaglandin E2 production by cultured equine synoviocytes. Am J Vet Res 2000;61(5):499–505.
[59] Mertens WD, MacLeod JN, Fubini SL. Polysulphated glycosaminoglycans modulate transcription of interleukin-1 beta treated chondrocytes in monolayer culture. Vet Comp Ortho Trauma 2003;16(2):93–8.
[60] May SA, Hooke RE, Lees P. The effect of drugs used in the treatment of osteoarthrosis on stromelysin (proteoglycanase) of equine synovial cell origin. Equine Vet J 1988;(Suppl 6):28–32.
[61] Andrews JL, Sutherland J, Ghosh P. Distribution and binding of glycosaminoglycan polysulfate to intervertebral disc, knee joint articular cartilage and meniscus. Arzneimittel-Forschung 1985;35(1):144–8.
[62] Muller W, et al. [In vivo study of the distribution, affinity for cartilage and metabolism of glycosaminoglycan polysulphate (GAGPS, Arteparon)]. Zeitschrift fur Rheumatologie 1983;42(6):355–61.
[63] Fortier L. Systemic therapies for joint disease in horses. Vet Clin North Am Equine Pract 2005;21(3):547–57.
[64] Balazs EA. Viscosupplementation for treatment of osteoarthritis: from initial discovery to current status and results. Surg Technol Int 2004;12:278–89.
[65] Kuroki K, Cook JL, Kreeger JM. Mechanisms of action and potential uses of hyaluronan in dogs with osteoarthritis. J Am Vet Med Assoc 2002;221(7):944–50.
[66] Peyron JG. Intraarticular hyaluronan injections in the treatment of osteoarthritis: state-of-the-art review. J Rheumatol Suppl 1993;39:10–5.
[67] Adams ME. An analysis of clinical studies of the use of crosslinked hyaluronan, hylan, in the treatment of osteoarthritis. J Rheumatol Suppl 1993;39:16–8.
[68] Asheim A, Lindblad G. Intra-articular treatment of arthritis in race-horses with sodium hyaluronate. Acta Vet Scand 1976;17(4):379–94.
[69] Auer J, et al. Effect of hyaluronic acid in naturally occurring and experimentally induced osteoarthritis. Am J Vet Res 1980;41(4):568–74.
[70] Rose R. The intra-articular use of sodium hyaluronate for the treatment of osteo-arthrosis in the horse. N Z Vet J 1979;27(1–2):5–8.
[71] Rydell N, Butler J, Balazs E. Hyaluronic acid in synovial fluid. VI. Effect of intra-articular injection of hyaluronic acid on the clinical symptoms of arthritis in track horses. Acta Vet Scan 1970;1970(11):2.
[72] Hilbert B, Rowley G, Antonas K. Changes in the synovia after the intra-articular injection of sodium hyaluronate into normal horse joints and after arthrotomy and experimental cartilage damage. Aust Vet J 1985;62(6):182–4.
[73] Lynch TM, et al. Influence of exogenous hyaluronan on synthesis of hyaluronan and collagenase by equine synoviocytes. Am J Vet Res 1998;59(7):888–92.
[74] Vitanzo P, Sennett B. Hyaluronans: is clinical effectiveness dependent on molecular weight? Am J Orthop 2006;35(9):421–8.
[75] McIlwraith CW, Goodman NL, Frisbie DD. Prospective study on the prophylactic value of intravenous hyaluronan in 2-year-old racing quarter horses. Proceedings of the 44th Annu Conv Am Assoc Equine Pract; 1998:44. p. 269–71.
[76] Petrella RJ, Petrella M. A prospective, randomized, double-blind, placebo controlled study to evaluate the efficacy of intraarticular hyaluronic acid for osteoarthritis of the knee. J Rheumatol 2006;33(5):951–6.

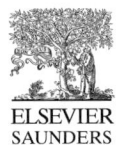

VETERINARY
CLINICS
Equine Practice

Evidence-Based Musculoskeletal Surgery in Horses

Stephanie S. Caston, DVM, LA,
Eric L. Reinertson, DVM, MS*

Department of Veterinary Clinical Sciences, College of Veterinary Medicine, Iowa State University, 1600 SE 16th Street, Ames, IA 50011, USA

Musculoskeletal disorders comprise a large portion of the conditions treated by equine veterinarians. Surgical intervention is the treatment of choice in many cases. The body of literature describing and exploring surgical correction of musculoskeletal disorders in horses is steadily growing but still lacking.

Despite this lack, use of an evidence-based approach for surgical management of these conditions should be the goal of equine surgeons. This is undertaken with the realization that most of what we have available are weaker sources of evidence [1–3]. Many publications in veterinary surgery can be categorized as class IV studies according to guidelines published for application of evidence-based methods [2,3]. These guidelines have been adapted to categorize and evaluate the quality of evidence produced from veterinary orthopedic research (Table 1) [3]. Although making decisions based on the relatively weak research is not necessarily wrong and, in some cases, is the only option, it is far from ideal.

In addition to the difficulties arising from making sound clinical decisions in the face of a lack of good evidence, making clinical decisions using evidence-based veterinary medicine (EBVM) can be complicated when one considers the other factors and variables involved in what constitutes an acceptable result after surgery. For example, such variables as the intended function after surgery, soundness to compete versus pasture sound, economic considerations, owner's acceptance of lameness, cosmesis, and client compliance regarding aftercare all influence the perception of what may be a successful outcome and, accordingly, a veterinarian's decision making-process

---

* Corresponding author.
  E-mail address: ereinert@iastate.edu (E.L. Reinertson).

Table 1
Evidence classes: guidelines for study categorization and the quality of evidence produced from veterinary orthopedic research

Evidence class	Study design	Examples/comments
I	Evidence derived from multiple, randomized, blind, placebo-controlled trials in the target species	Systematic reviews (ie, meta-analyses). Advantages of meta-analyses are objective appraisal, large number of subjects, improving estimates of association, assimilating large quantities of information, developing findings on a common scale, and improving the quality of primary research
II	Evidence derived from high-quality clinical trials using historical controls	Randomized controlled clinical studies on animals that developed the disease naturally and is performed in a laboratory setting. Historical controls are thought to be less reliable than randomized controls
III	Evidence derived from uncontrolled case series	Nonrandomized prospective case comparison studies. Examples include prospective comparison studies that are not truly randomized with limited subjective influence to prospective case series that include subjective clinical impressions to objective gait analysis
IV	Evidence derived from expert opinion or extrapolated from research or physiologic studies	Retrospective case comparison studies. This category possesses the most prominent source of information available today regarding cranial cruciate injuries and surgical repair. Studies on research subjects (non-client owned) are also included in this class

From Aragon CL, Budsberg SC. Applications of evidence-based medicine: cranial cruciate ligament injury repair in the dog. Vet Surg 2005;34:95; with permission.

before surgery. Even those attempting to embrace EBVM may have trouble practicing it according to formal guidelines outlined in some texts and articles [4]. Even though data may be meager or of lower quality, however, the surgeon can still make use of the philosophy of targeted questions and critical evaluation of information [5]. Being aware of the deficiencies in our body of research can only aid in improving it. In light of this, the goal of this article is to discuss some of the aspects of selected equine musculoskeletal operations and to review the information currently available to meet the needs of practitioners attempting to practice EBVM. It is beyond the necessary length and scope of this article to perform a systematic review of each section, but a critical review of available data should undoubtedly raise questions. Hopefully, these questions can be answered by future research and systematic reviews, and such information, when it is obtained, should provide a strong database of higher quality evidence for the equine practitioner.

Long bone fractures

Fractures of long bones in horses involve an incredible number of variables. The horse's signalment, configuration of the fracture, economic considerations, expected postoperative use, and availability of treatment (surgical expertise and equipment) are but a few of those variables that must be considered when planning long bone fracture repair. In addition, surgical repair of fractures in horses often works at the threshold of fixation devices' ability to stabilize the bone [6]. As implant development continues, some surgical techniques have been changing faster than many case numbers can accumulate. Because all these factors make repair choices limited, prospective studies may be difficult to design and carry out.

Publications describing surgical long bone fracture repair in horses tend to be case studies, case series, or in vitro or retrospective studies. Although we might desire evidence that includes randomized controlled trials, implant failure of any kind may necessitate humane euthanasia. As a result, many aspects of long bone repair in horses have been studied in vitro using cadaveric bone or bone substitutes. The available data in this instance consist of mostly class IV evidence, including retrospective case comparisons, case reports, and expert opinions. There is some available class III evidence (uncontrolled case series), but they are few in number.

For example, if we consider radius fractures, many examples are described in the literature as case reports and case series. Only two major retrospectives seem to have been published: one that discusses 47 cases [7] and one that discusses 15 cases [8]. One of the reasons for the paucity of information may lie in the difficulty faced in the treatment of radius fractures in horses, especially in adult horses. For instance, in the series of 15 cases, only 2 of the horses survived. In the series of 47 cases, 19 of the horses were humanely destroyed on presentation with no treatment attempted.

Traditionally, much of the available literature has described treating radius fractures with internal fixation using two dynamic compression plates and screws. More recently, some equine surgeons have begun using a dynamic condylar screw implant with a dynamic compression plate to repair distal radial fractures [9–11]. There is also one case report in the literature of successful fixation using this plate in an adult horse [9], and its use has been suggested to provide the most stable method of repair [10–12]. A recent in vitro study comparing the two methods of fixation failed to show a difference between the two implant systems in construct stiffness or failure loads, however [13]. Although such in vitro studies do not completely reflect clinical cases, they do at least highlight the possibility that expert opinion and case reports may be misleading.

Although some evidence, such as the preceding, may be lower on the evidence pyramid, it is all that is available, and is therefore valuable to veterinary practitioners in their decision-making process. It should also be valuable to equine surgeons treating a long bone fracture, in addition to the opinion and experience of the surgeon. Although there are certainly enormous difficulties in conducting controlled, double-blind, randomized studies of such conditions, alternative designs, such as prospective matched-pair trials, are feasible. In addition, continued implant development and research should help to provide practitioners with better evidence to support the use of different surgical techniques in the future.

Chip fractures

Osteochondral fragmentation, or chip fractures, occurs with frequency in Thoroughbred, Quarter Horse, and Standardbred racing horses as well as in performance horses of other disciplines. Chip fractures are commonly found in the carpus and fetlock and are thought to be generated by repeated trauma and hyperextension of the joints during high-speed training and racing [14]. Most studies addressing surgical treatment of this condition are of class III and IV quality. Based on these studies and reports, arthroscopic surgery to remove the fragments is considered the treatment of choice [15].

The results of surgery to remove carpal chip fractures are reported in several studies that explore horses' performance after removal [16–18]. Most evaluate return to racing, number of times placed in a race, earnings, and other variables before and after surgery. In most articles, there is no comparison population, and the reports are retrospective case series. Comparison between the same horse's performance before and after surgery may not accurately assess treatment outcome because of the influence of age, concurrent injuries, and other factors that affect performance. Many of those variables might be expected to have a negative impact on performance; yet, some of the horses improved their race level after surgery [16]. Still, it is dangerous to assume that the difference between a group's outcome before and after an intervention is solely attributable to the intervention. Changes may indicate the natural course of the disease. In this case, lacking other data, such as outcomes from untreated horses, we can use other publications that may provide evidence suggesting that the natural course of osteochondral fragmentation would be degenerative joint disease [19,20].

When evaluated, it seems that the database we have now supports the use of arthroscopic surgery to treat most chip fractures. Even so, the evidence is still mostly class IV. Prospective studies could give the veterinary surgeon stronger evidence that arthroscopic removal of fragments is indeed the best care for these patients as well as what other factors affect future performance. Other specific questions that might be posed, and answered, by continued research and an evidence-based approach to chip fractures include the following:

- How does fragment size and position affect the prognosis for return to racing?
- How does breed or race type affect the decision-making process when evaluating chip fractures?
- Does a certain degree of concurrent pathologic change in a joint negate possible benefits for removing a fragment?

Osteochondrosis

Osteochondrosis (OC) is a disease complex that occurs in young growing horses in which endochondral ossification is abnormal or disturbed. This results in irregular thickness of the cartilage, areas of weakness, and sometimes the development of loose or partially loose fragments or subchondral bone cysts [21]. Lesions occur in certain sites with predictability; many times, they are bilateral. Horses typically present with joint effusion, although there is none in some cases. The degree and grade of lameness can vary or be absent altogether.

Arthroscopic surgery to remove OC fragments, loose or devitalized cartilage, and debridement of the subchondral bone is deemed by most equine surgeons to be the treatment of choice [21]. Recently, reattachment of cartilage flaps has also been described [22]. Various surgical methods to treat subchondral bone cysts have been described in the literature, and it remains in question which treatment is likely to be optimal for horses with this condition.

The body of evidence supporting treatment of OC fragments by means of arthroscopic removal is fairly large yet relatively weak. There are many retrospective and a few prospective studies published that describe removal of OC fragments by means of arthroscopy [23–26]. The studies describe findings and follow-up in a retrospective manner, compare an operated population with a matched population, or compare pre- and postoperative performance. We still lack prospective studies in which the operated population is compared with a control group. A few articles compare an operated population with one treated by conservative methods (usually joint injection, rest, or nonsteroidal anti-inflammatory drugs [NSAIDs]). In a 1998 retrospective, the authors note that clinical signs of lameness, effusion, or both resolved in approximately 50% of surgically treated cases (21 cases that had follow-up), whereas such signs resolved in only 30% of conservatively treated cases (16 cases that had follow-up). Nevertheless, five (83%) of six horses treated with surgery and four (80%) of five conservatively treated horses that were presented with the complaint of lameness were still lame at the time of follow-up [24]. These two different aspects of the results are not explored; the poor value of these data is only compounded by low numbers and the comparison of OC in different joints and locations within the same study.

The research on subchondral bone cysts, as mentioned previously, is more varied than removal of the abnormal tissue by means of arthroscopy. Studies have been published describing arthroscopic debridement of the cyst [27], compacted cancellous bone grafting [28], and osteochondral grafting [29]. Arthroscopic intralesional corticosteroid injection is mentioned in textbooks and proceedings articles, and a recent retrospective was presented in which 55% of cases had a successful outcome [30]. It is difficult to compare the success of this or the other methods with that of another treatment, because successful outcome criteria can be different depending on the study design and breed or discipline of the study population. Having a control population to measure success with would be ideal. There is also a study that used a controlled experiment model in which defects were created in the medial femoral condyle [28]. Although this study was not performed on animals with naturally occurring disease, good experimental models are sorely needed in veterinary surgical studies. Filling the cystic cavity after debridement with such substances as tricalcium phosphate granules, biodegradable cements, and hydrogel/growth factor composites has also been described [31]. Other studies include retrospectives or case series in which follow-up is recorded but no comparison populations are evaluated along with the treated group.

In summary, for subchondral cystic lesions, it is unclear how effective our attempts at treatment are. In fact, there seems to be no agreement on the origin of the lesions [21,31]. Although a narrative literature review has also been published that compared cystic bone lesions in human beings and horses [32], unfortunately, no clear criteria for article inclusion were set and no statistical analysis of the data was performed. Many of the references reviewed in the article were of poor evidentiary value, including lectures, retrospectives, case studies, proceedings, and even a letter to the editor. This article is not a true systematic review or meta-analysis and is of little more value to EBVM practitioners than the mostly class IV materials that it reviews.

Questions regarding surgical care for horses with OC that could be answered by an evidence-based approach to the problem might include the following:

How often do lesions resolve or cease to be a clinical problem in a control group versus a treatment group or in X treatment group versus Y treatment group?

Using a defined measurable outcome, is surgical removal or debridement of OC lesions always the best way to treat these horses?

What detrimental effects might surgical intervention have?

Arthrodesis

Surgical arthrodesis of joints is sometimes chosen by veterinarians as a treatment for horses with joints affected by sepsis, degenerative joint disease, and injuries like fractures or luxation [33]. Horses with these conditions are often quite lame. Eliminating movement of the affected joint can make them comfortable and, in some cases, enable them to return to work. The joints that are amenable to fusion and, at the same time, maintain a good to excellent prognosis for athletic performance are widely accepted to be the proximal interphalangeal joints and the tarsometatarsal and distal intertarsal joints. Arthrodesis techniques have also been described for many other joints, yet the preponderance of evidence is made up by retrospective case series, case reports, and experimental studies on small numbers of normal horses.

Techniques for proximal interphalangeal joint arthrodesis have been well described and include the use of crossed [34] or parallel lag [34–38] screws traversing the joint, cartilage debridement and immobilization without internal fixation [38,39], lag screws in combination with plate fixation [40,41], or double-plate fixation [42]. Unsurprisingly, all the studies are retrospective case series except for one [34]. Nevertheless, the retrospective studies make it clear that the proximal interphalangeal joint can be surgically fused by several methods and that, in most cases, this procedure results in a more comfortable patient. Chemical arthrodesis, or the use of an intra-articularly administered chemical to produce cartilage destruction and subsequent ankylosis, has also been described in the pastern and small tarsal joints [43,44]. Recently, use of a plate and two lag screws has been recommended as the treatment of choice for arthrodesis of the pastern, even though the evidence comparing this technique with other techniques is lacking [33].

For the small tarsal joints, the most recent investigation studied the use of ethyl alcohol to facilitate ankylosis. This method was predated by intra-articular drilling, injection of monoiodoacetate, internal fixation, and laser surgery [44–49]. In addition, two experimental studies have recently been published comparing arthrodesis techniques in normal horses [50,51], evaluating the drilling technique compared with laser treatment, and drilling, laser surgery, and intra-articular monoiodoacetate in randomly assigned treatment groups. Both of these articles, although prospective and randomized studies, were performed in a small number of normal horses. They do compare surgical techniques in matched groups, however, and have definitive and quantitative measurement of outcome, including postmortem examinations.

Practitioners seeking evidence regarding surgical arthrodesis of any joint still largely depend on class IV evidence, although good evidence comparing techniques for pastern arthrodesis and distal tarsal joint arthrodesis may be on the horizon because of the relative frequency with which they are performed.

Angular limb deformities

Foals are commonly born with limb deformities, including angular deformities. These deformities are described using the joint in which deviation begins and as varus (medial deviation of the distal limb) or valgus (lateral deviation). Carpal valgus, fetlock varus, and tarsal valgus are the most common deformities found clinically [52]. Several methods have been used to correct angular limb deformities surgically, but in recent years, a more conservative approach has been advocated, because most foals have deformities that correct with time [53].

Growth retardation by transphyseal bridging and hemicircumferential periosteal transection and elevation (HCPTE) are the surgical methods used most commonly to treat angular deformities. Textbooks and other publications recommend HCPTE as the best surgical method for treatment of angular limb deformities in foals [52–54]. The study that introduced HCPTE for use in foals was an experimental model using six pony foals. The study was not blind, and there was no significant difference in growth at the distal radial physis after the procedure in principal limbs compared with controls [54]. Differences in angulation of the limbs were found to be significantly different; the greatest difference during the study in average angulation between control and principal limbs was 3.2°. It was concluded that an angulation was created in the principal limbs beyond that of the control limbs. Nevertheless, much of the literature concerning this procedure claims that a limb cannot be overcorrected with this procedure. In addition, most of the measured angulations throughout the study were within what would be considered normal ranges [55]. Furthermore, all the foals were 60 days of age or less, and most were 45 days of age or less. This is an age range when it would be expected that there would normally be change in angulation of limbs as the foal matures [53,54].

Thus, this and other evidence for HCPTE (mostly retrospective studies or case series) falls mostly into the category of class IV evidence. It is hard to use evidence-based medicine and recommend HCPTE based on principles of evidence-based medicine. Indeed, in answer to the question of what surgical procedure is most effective in correcting angular limb deformities in foals, and whether surgical intervention is necessary, we must currently answer, "We don't know."

The effectiveness of HCPTE for angular limb deformities is especially suspect in light of a few recently published studies. One is a randomized, controlled, blind study performed on normal foals in which angular limb deformities of 15° were created with transphyseal bridging [56]. One limb in each foal underwent HCPTE, and the other limb served as a control using a sham surgical procedure. All limbs straightened over the course of observation, and the mean angulation was not significantly different between treated or control legs at any point in the study [56]. In another study, there was no difference between medial and lateral growth rates at the proximal or distal end of the radius in foals that had received HCPTE or those used as controls [57]. There are also no studies comparing transphyseal bridging directly with HCPTE. The two procedures are sometimes used in combination, usually when the clinician decides the deformity is severe or the foal is older and has less growth potential [53].

Although there is clearly a place for more well-designed studies comparing surgical techniques for angular limb deformities, it may be hard for researchers to use subjects with naturally occurring disease. Control subjects would be difficult to obtain, because owners may not be amenable to a "wait and see" approach to a problem they perceive as detrimental to their foal's future performance or value. Without knowledge of the rate of spontaneous resolution, it is difficult to assess the true success rate of any procedure. Because there are few data comparing different surgical procedures and good evidence to support the widely used periosteal stripping is lacking, however, continued research is a must. It can aid us in making treatment recommendations using EBVM in the hopes of providing the best quality of patient care as well as a successful outcome for patients with angular limb deformity.

Second and fourth metacarpal or metatarsal fractures

Fractures of the second and fourth metacarpal or metatarsal bones (splint bones) are common injuries in horses and occur with higher frequency in the distal third of the bone [58,59]. External trauma causes some of the fractures, and such fractures can also be open or comminuted with subsequent osteitis and sequestration [60,61]. When internal fixation is necessary, a plate and screws are recommended by most texts and surgeons as the surgical treatment of choice, because, in one retrospective, 2 of 11 horses treated with screws alone returned to their intended use, whereas 6 of 11 treated with plates returned to their intended use [62].

Fractures of the distal end of the splint bone are most often associated with suspensory desmitis; up to 81% of cases reported had desmitis [58,59]. The cause of these fractures is unknown, and it has been suggested that these fractures are attributable to fatigue, internal trauma from the suspensory ligament, traction from fascial attachments, and loss of pliability of the interosseous ligaments [58–61,63].

Regardless of the cause of splint bone fractures, they are most often treated by surgical removal of the affected portion and the distal remnant if the fracture involves the distal aspect of the bone or by internal fixation if the proximal third of the bone is involved [62,63]. Closed fractures of the distal splint bones are also treated with stall rest, bandaging, and anti-inflammatory medications [58,59,63]. Evidence supporting the surgical procedures is class IV evidence, including retrospectives and an in vitro experimental study. Two of these studies question the need for surgical intervention for distal fractures based on their findings that there was no correlation between radiographic signs or location and postoperative results or that the fractures and associated lameness resolved with stall rest and that non-union fractures did not cause pain. One study discusses the need for a nonsurgically treated control population [58,59]. Both of these studies were retrospective, however, with only a moderate number of horses.

A different technique has been reviewed recently in which only the affected portion of the bone is removed and the proximal and distal portions are left [63]. This retrospective found that the surgical technique was effective for removing the fractured sections of bone, and it did not seem to be detrimental (all 17 horses returned to previous work without lameness). It does not, however, tell us that this procedure is a better choice for our patients than any of the other procedures or conservative treatment. The article does not discuss presence or degree of lameness in those cases reviewed.

A prospective study using a control group or comparing two surgical techniques might be easier to design for splint fractures. This is because, in many cases, after stall rest and healing of concurrent suspensory desmitis, horses are not lame. Owners and clinicians might be more open to participating in research in which control groups have a good chance of recovering without intervention. Because economics, cosmetic appearance, and postoperative performance are always important to horse owners, these would be appealing factors to compare between groups during future research in this area.

Dorsal cortical fractures of the third metacarpal bone

Dorsal cortical fractures, or stress fractures, of the third metacarpal bone occur most frequently in racing Thoroughbreds [64]. Treatment of these incomplete cortical fractures has ranged from nonsurgical treatment involving anti-inflammatory drugs and restricted exercise to internal fixation [64–69]. Some fractures heal with conservative treatment, whereas others may have a return of symptoms when the horse is put back into work or show no signs of radiographic healing for months [67,70].

Nonsurgical treatment recommendations have included rest periods of 7 months or more [70]. Although there are some horses that heal with conservative treatment, some fractures are refractory, and screw fixation or osteostixis is often used to treat those horses. The mechanism by which osteostixis may stimulate healing is not completely understood, but it is thought to allow osteogenic factors from the medullary cavity access to the fracture line and induction of a regional acceleratory phenomenon [65–69]. There are no studies directly comparing osteostixis with screw fixation or with untreated controls. One retrospective study reviewed the results of screw fixation combined with cortical drilling and found that horses returned to training in an average of 2.75 months and returned to racing in an average of 7.62 months [69]. In three other case series of 11, 28, and 53 horses treated with osteostixis alone (no implant), the average time to return to racing was 9.4, 6.9, and 6.8 months, respectively [65,67,68]. It is hard to compare therapies based on published evidence, but it would seem that most horses (82%–89% of horses) were reported to return to racing after either technique [65,68,69]. There is some risk involved with osteostixis for the horse during recovery or on return to racing. Drill holes create a stress riser in bone, and clustered drill holes of 2.7 or 3.5 mm in diameter reduced the breaking strength of metacarpal bones by 43.8% to 55.7% in cadaver bone [66]. Despite this, relatively few catastrophic failures are reported for horses treated with osteostixis, although some surgeons elect to apply splints or casts for recovery from this procedure [65–67]. Screws can cause pain if not removed, and if transcortical fixation is used, refracture can occur [65,69]. Osteostixis, or cortical drilling, is asserted to be the surgical treatment of choice because it does not require a second operation to remove implants [65,67–69].

Although the surgical procedures mentioned previously may speed healing of refractory dorsal cortical fractures, high-quality evidence supporting such a claim is not published. As for many of the other conditions discussed in this article, outcome has generally been reported in a case series or retrospective manner. The true incidence of horses that do not heal without some type of surgical intervention, if horses return to training and racing faster without reinjury after surgery, and which surgical technique veterinarians should choose are not clearly based on high-quality research.

Palmar digital neurectomy

Palmar digital neurectomy has been used by equine practitioners for years to allow horses with chronic heel pain to continue to compete or to be more comfortable at pasture. In many cases, it is used to treat navicular disease, but it is also used to treat other chronic conditions that cause lameness and respond to anesthesia of the palmar digital nerve [71,72]. Several different techniques have been used to destroy or transect the palmar digital nerves and desensitize the palmar foot [71–75]. Complications after any of the procedures can include painful neuromas, recurrence of lameness, sloughing of the hoof, and rupture of the deep digital flexor tendon [71,72,76].

In attempts to minimize neuroma formation, surgery has been performed using a carbon dioxide (CO_2) laser, cryotherapy units, epineural capping, insertion of the nerve in the proximal phalanx, and the guillotine technique with injection of sodium hyaluronate or doxorubicin [71,74,75,77–79]. In an experimental study on normal horses, sodium hyaluronate injection at the neurectomy site yielded no difference from injection of saline [77]. When doxorubicin was injected into the transected nerve stump, there was a high rate of incisional complications (16 of 28 cases) and the overall success rate was comparable to that of other studies [78]. Some claim that use of a CO_2 laser reduces neuroma formation [71], but the study published evaluating the use of the laser included only 10 horses, with no control or comparison group [75]. In that group of horses, there was no clinical evidence of neuroma formation, but there was also no evidence of neuroma formation in 24 horses in one study and in none of 8 horses in another study that had neurectomies performed by the guillotine technique [72,73]. Conversely, 3 of 42 horses that had a neurectomy by transection and electrocoagulation were found to have neuroma formation [72]. Dabreiner and colleagues [79] performed neurectomies in normal adult horses using the guillotine method, perineural capping, CO_2 laser transection, or CO_2 transection and coagulation (one technique per leg in each of 6 horses) and followed the horses for 1 year. The guillotine method provided the longest duration of cutaneous desensitization and significantly lower scores for nerve regeneration and neuroma formation. Although this study was performed in normal horses and had only 6 subjects (24 limbs), its use of comparison groups is better evidence that one surgical technique may be preferred to the others when the surgeon's aim is to prevent neuroma formation.

Recurrence of lameness is another complication after neurectomy and reinnervation; presence of a neuroma that goes undetected or presence of an aberrant branch of the palmar digital nerve is the reported cause [72,73,79]. Response to perineural anesthesia and lack of detectable painful neuroma on palpation or return of skin sensation are the criteria for reinnervation most often used in the literature [72–74]. It has been postulated that reinnervation of the heel pain could be explained by axons sprouting from the proximal stump anastomosing with other local nerve branches [72]. Return of skin sensation may not tell the whole story, because in one study, some horses progressed from hypoesthesia to perception of skin stimulation before response to deep pain after experimental cryotherapy of nerves [74]. Most reports of reinnervation are not accompanied by histologic evaluation, but there are descriptions of some nerve regeneration as well as nerve atrophy after neurectomy [76,79]. There is no good evidence supporting or refuting any of the theories to explain recurrence. Time that horses remain sound after a neurectomy is unclear, because follow-up time varies. In one study, 9 of 10 horses were sound at follow-up; 3 of these horses were followed for 20 months or longer, and 2 were followed for 14 months. The other 5 horses were only followed for 4 to 8 months [75]. Results of another retrospective study revealed that 15 (54%) of 28 horses were sound at 1 year [78], whereas in another study, 74% of horses were sound at one year; this rate dropped to 63% after 2 years [72]. Although it is probably performed quite frequently, there is also little published about repeated palmar digital neurectomy to address the recurrence of lameness. Most accounts explain that a small neuroma is seen in the proximal aspect of the previous surgical site [71–73,75].

With advancing diagnostics, such as ultrasound and MRI, we also now know that many horses with heel pain have more complex and varied problems than navicular bone degeneration. This is accompanied by the knowledge that the palmar digital nerve block is not specific and may desensitize the sole, lamina, coffin bone, distal interphalangeal, and other soft tissue structures as well as the heel [80]. It may be that some horses with recurrence of lameness or persistence of lameness have deep digital flexor tendon injuries, coffin joint pain, or other abnormalities that are not completely abolished by palmar digital neurectomy or that progress until the abnormalities are no longer within the area desensitized by the neurectomy. The evidence we have supporting neurectomy as a surgical therapy for horses with heel pain and which cases are optimal candidates for that treatment certainly could be bolstered by continued research. Important questions to be answered could focus on the causes of heel pain, what exactly happens to innervation of the foot after surgery, and an objective look at repeated neurectomies.

Tendonitis

Tendon injury is common among horses that race or perform at a high level but can occur in any horse. Tendon tears have a high rate of reinjury and require long periods of convalescence; attempts at treatment have been aimed at reducing healing time and reducing the odds of reinjury [81,82]. Along with rest, controlled exercise, and anti-inflammatory medications, there are several nonsurgical therapies that have been used with varying popularity and success [81,82]. Some of these include intralesional medications of various types, extracorporeal shock wave therapy, cold therapy, laser therapy, magnetic therapy, counterirritation ("firing"), and therapeutic ultrasound [81]. There is some weak evidence of efficacy for a few treatments, although there is little to none for many of them and a few are even considered injurious themselves. Surgical therapies for tendonitis include tendon splitting, desmotomy of the accessory ligament of the superficial digital flexor tendon, and tenoscopy for those tears that are intrathecal [81,83–89].

Most of the literature on surgical therapy for tendonitis examines superficial digital flexor tendon tears in racehorses. The studies are class III and IV, with a few prospective and randomized experimental studies [81–89]. The effects of tendon splitting in experimentally induced lesions are published in a randomized study on six horses. The authors used collagenase to induce tendonitis in both front legs, and splitting was performed 7 days later on one leg in each horse. Ultrasonographic lesion area was significantly less in the split tendons compared with the controls at weeks 3, 4, and 8 [83]. In another study, no benefit was seen after splitting chronic (repeated collagenase injections at 6 and 12 weeks after the first injection) experimental lesions. This publication only used four ponies in each group, and the control groups were untreated limbs and those that had been "fired" [88]. Neither of these studies is compelling evidence for or against tendon splitting, and the other available resources are mostly retrospective descriptions of the procedure and the postoperative results [90,91].

Another surgical treatment that has been widely used to treat superficial digital flexor tendonitis is transection of the accessory ligament of the superficial digital flexor tendon (superior check ligament) [84–86,89]. The evidentiary support for this procedure is class III and IV studies. Success after surgery was evaluated by reporting the percentage of horses that could complete five or more races after surgery. The percentage able to do so ranged from 52% to 71% [84–86,89]. It is hard to compare these results with those describing medically or conservatively managed cases from another study, because the populations and performance disciplines are different [82]. In one of the studies, a group treated surgically was compared with those treated nonsurgically, but trainers were allowed to choose the treatment and compliance was inconsistent [86]. In this and another publication, higher than expected rates of suspensory desmitis were seen [86,89]. This prompted in vitro evaluation of strain on the flexor tendons and the suspensory ligament after a superior check ligament desmotomy, in which it was found that there were significantly increased strains on the superficial digital flexor tendon and the suspensory ligament after desmotomy [92].

Surgical treatment of tendonitis could be better supported by evidence that clearly demonstrates the superior efficacy of one technique versus others, versus other treatments, or versus no treatment. As for technique, we should also answer the question raised by some of the retrospective and in vitro studies discussed previously; for example, "Should we perform a superior check ligament desmotomy to treat this condition if it is at the expense of the suspensory ligament?"

Summary

Surgical procedures to address equine musculoskeletal disease or injuries are used frequently by the veterinary practitioner. An evidence-based approach to veterinary medicine has recently been introduced [1–4] and can be applied to clinical decisions that equine practitioners make about these conditions. Although this article is necessarily abbreviated and is by no means a comprehensive look at this subject, the evidence currently available to answer questions directed at surgical therapy is reviewed. There are virtually no class I or II studies, which would include meta-analyses, systematic reviews, and high-quality randomized controlled clinical trials. We continue to have to rely principally on retrospective case series and expert opinion, which provide relatively weak data to guide our decision-making process. In most cases, current published research gives us information revealing the safety and outcome of performing a surgical procedure or support for the idea that the same goal can be accomplished with several methods. Most published research, however, does not tell us how those techniques compare with others or what the true efficacy is compared with a control group. At this juncture, we can use what information we have with the understanding that as the quality of research advances, we should apply stricter standards to the evidence we use to answer our clinical questions.

References

[1] Cockcroft PD, Holmes MA. Handbook of evidence-based veterinary medicine. Oxford (UK): Blackwell; 2003. p. 11–9.
[2] Geyman JP. Evidence-based medicine in primary care: an overview. In: Geyman JP, Deyo RA, Ramsey SD, editors. Evidence-based clinical practice: concepts and approaches. Boston: Butterworth-Heinemann; 2000. p. 1–11.
[3] Aragon CL, Budsberg SC. Applications of evidence-based medicine: cranial cruciate ligament injury repair in the dog. Vet Surg 2005;34:93–8.
[4] Pinsky LE, Deyo RA. Clinical guidelines: a strategy for translating evidence into practice. In: Geyman JP, Deyo RA, Ramsey SD, editors. Evidence-based clinical practice: concepts and approaches. Boston: Butterworth-Heinemann; 2000. p. 119–23.
[5] Shlipak MG. Decision analysis. In: Friedland DJ, editor. Evidence-based medicine. A framework for clinical practice. Stamford (CT): Appleton & Lange; 1998. p. 35–59.
[6] Markel MD. Fracture biomechanics. In: Nixon AJ, editor. Equine fracture repair. Philadelphia: W.B. Saunders Company; 1996. p. 10–8.
[7] Sanders-Shamis M, Bramlage LR, Gable AA. Radius fractures in the horse: a retrospective study of 47 cases. Equine Vet J 1986;18(6):432–7.
[8] Auer JA, Watkins JP. Treatment of radial fractures in adult horses: an analysis of 15 clinical cases. Equine Vet J 1987;19(2):103–10.
[9] Rodgerson DH, Wilson DA, Kramer J. Fracture repair of the distal portion of the radius by use of a condylar screw implant in an adult horse. J Am Vet Med Assoc 2001;218(12):1966–9.
[10] Watkins JP. The radius and ulna. In: Auer JA, Stick JA, editors. Equine surgery. 3rd edition. St. Louis (MO): Sauders Elsevier; 2006. p. 1267–79.
[11] Auer JA. Fractures of the radius. In: Nixon AJ, editor. Equine fracture repair. Philadelphia: W.B. Saunders Company; 1996. p. 222–30.
[12] AO-ASIF Advanced Techniques in Equine Fracture Management. April 28–May 1, 2005. Colombus (OH).
[13] Janicek JC, Wilson DA, Carson WL, et al. In vitro biomechanical comparison of the dynamic condylar screw and double broad plate fixation of distal diaphyseal osteotomized/ostectomized equine radii. In: Presented at the Proceedings 2006 ACVS Veterinary Symposium. The surgical summit. Washington, DC; 2006. p. 10.
[14] Rooney JR. Biomechanics of lameness in horses. 2nd edition. Huntington (NY): R.E. Krieger Publishing; 1977. p. 133–9.
[15] Ruggles AJ. Carpus. In: Auer JA, Stick JA, editors. Equine surgery. 3rd edition. St. Louis (MO): Sauders Elsevier; 2006. p. 1253–66.
[16] McIlwraith CW, Yovich JV, Martin GS. Arthroscopic surgery for the treatment of osteochondral chip fractures in the equine carpus. J Am Vet Med Assoc 1987;191(5):531–40.

[17] Lucas JM, Ross MW, Richardson DW. Post operative performance of racing Standardbreds treated arthroscopically for carpal chip fractures: 176 cases (1986–1993). Equine Vet J 1999; 31(1):48–52.
[18] Shimozawa K, Ueno Y, Ushiya S, et al. Survey of arthroscopic surgery for carpal chip fractures in Thoroughbred racehorses in Japan. J Vet Med Sci 2001;63(3):48–62.
[19] Kawcak CE, Norrdin RW, Frisbie DD, et al. Effects of osteochondral fragmentation and intra-articular triamcinolone acetonide treatment on subchondral bone in the equine carpus. Equine Vet J 1998;30(1):66–7.
[20] Huber MJ, Schmotzer WB, Riebold TW, et al. Fate and effect of autogenous osteochondral fragments implanted in the middle carpal joint of horses. Am J Vet Res 1992;53(9):1579–88.
[21] van Weeren PR. Osteochondrosis. In: Auer JA, Stick JA, editors. Equine surgery. 3rd edition. St. Louis (MO): Sauders Elsevier; 2006. p. 1166–78.
[22] Nixon AJ, Fortier LA, Goodrich LR, et al. Arthroscopic reattachment of osteochondritis dissecans lesions using resorbable polydioxanone pins. Equine Vet J 2004;36(5):376–83.
[23] McIlwraith CW, Foerner JJ, Davis DM. Osteochondritis dissecans of the tarsocrural joint: results of treatment with arthroscopic surgery. Equine Vet J 1991;23(3):155–62.
[24] Riley CB, Scott WM, Caron JP, et al. Osteochondritis dissecans and subchondral cystic lesions in draft horses: a retrospective study. Can Vet J 1998;39:627–33.
[25] Laws EG, Richardson DW, Ross MW, et al. Racing performance of Standardbreds after conservative and surgical treatment for tarsocrural osteochondrosis. Equine Vet J 1993; 25(3):199–202.
[26] Beard WL, Bramlage LR, Schneider RK, et al. Postoperative racing performance in Standardbreds and Thoroughbreds with osteochondrosis of the tarsocrural joint: 109 cases (1984–1990). J Am Vet Med Assoc 1994;204(10):1655–9.
[27] Howard RD, McIlwraith CW, Trotter GW. Arthroscopic surgery for subchondral cystic lesions of the medial femoral condyle in horses: 41 cases (1988–1991). J Am Vet Med Assoc 1995;206(6):842–50.
[28] Jackson WA, Stick JA, Arnoczky SP, et al. The effect of compacted cancellous bone grafting on the healing of subchondral bone defects of the medial femoral condyle in horses. Vet Surg 2000;29:8–16.
[29] Bodo G, Hangody L, Modis L, et al. Autologous osteochondral grafting (mosaic arthroplasty) for treatment of subchondral cystic lesions in the equine stifle and fetlock joints. Vet Surg 2004;33:588–96.
[30] Wallis TW, Goodrich LR, McIlwraith CW, et al. Arthroscopic injection of corticosteroids into the lining of subchondral cystic lesions of the medial femoral condyle in horses: a retrospective study of 39 cases (2001–2005). In: Presented at the Proceedings 2006 ACVS Veterinary Symposium. The surgical summit. Washington, DC; 2006. p. 27.
[31] Rechenberg BV, Auer JA. Subchondral cystic lesions. In: Auer JA, Stick JA, editors. Equine surgery. 3rd edition. St. Louis (MO): Sauders Elsevier; 2006. p. 1178–84.
[32] Rechenberg BV, McIlwraith CW, Auer JA. Cystic bone lesions in horses and humans: a comparative review. Vet Comp Orthop Traumatol 1998;11:8–18.
[33] Auer JA. Arthrodesis techniques. In: Auer JA, Stick JA, editors. Equine surgery. 3rd edition. St. Louis (MO): Saunders Elsevier; 2006. p. 1073–86.
[34] Genetzky RM, Schneider EJ, Butler HC, et al. Comparison of two surgical procedures for arthrodesis of the proximal interphalangeal joint in horses. J Am Vet Med Assoc 1981; 179(5):464–8.
[35] Schneider JE, Carnin BL, Guffy MM. Arthrodesis of the proximal interphalangeal joint in the horse: a surgical treatment for high ringbone. J Am Vet Med Assoc 1978;173(10): 1364–9.
[36] Caron JP, Fretz PB, Bailey JV, et al. Proximal interphalangeal arthrodesis in the horse. A retrospective study and modified screw technique. Vet Surg 1990;19(3):196–202.
[37] MacLellan KNM, Crawford WH, MacDonald DG. Proximal interphalangeal joint arthrodesis in 34 horses using two parallel 5.5-mm cortical bone screws. Vet Surg 2001;30:454–9.

[38] Martin GS, McIlwraith CW, Turner AS, et al. Long-term results and complications of proximal interphalangeal arthrodesis in horses. J Am Vet Med Assoc 1984;184(9):1136–40.
[39] Steenhaut M, Verschooten F, De Moor A. Arthrodesis of the pastern joint in the horse. Equine Vet J 1985;17(1):35–40.
[40] Schaer TP, Bramlage LR, Embertson RM, et al. Proximal interphalangeal arthrodesis in 22 horses. Equine Vet J 2001;33(4):360–5.
[41] James FM, Richardson DW. Minimally invasive plate fixation of lower limb injury in horses: 32 cases (1999–2003). Equine Vet J 2006;38(3):246–51.
[42] Crabill MR, Watkins JP, Schneider RK. Double-plate fixation of comminuted fractures of the second phalanx in horses: 10 cases (1985–1993). J Am Vet Med Assoc 1995;207:1458–61.
[43] Penraat JA, Allen AL, Fretz PB, et al. An evaluation of chemical arthrodesis of the proximal interphalangeal joint in the horse by using monoiodoacetate. Can J Vet Res 2000;64:212–21.
[44] Shoemaker RW, Allen AL, Richarson CE, et al. Use of intra-articular administration of ethyl alcohol for arthrodesis of the tarsometatarsal joint in healthy horses. Am J Vet Res 2006;67(5):850–7.
[45] Edwards GB. Surgical arthrodesis for the treatment of bone spavin in 20 horses. Equine Vet J 1982;14(2):117–21.
[46] Wyn-Jones G, May SA. Surgical arthrodesis for the treatment of osteoarthrosis of the proximal intertarsal, distal intertarsal and tarsometatarsal joints in 30 horses: a comparison of four different techniques. Equine Vet J 1986;18(1):59–64.
[47] Dowling BA, Dart AJ, Matthews SM. Chemical arthrodesis of the distal tarsal joints using sodium monoiodoacetate in 104 horses. Aust Vet J 2004;82(1):38–42.
[48] Adkins AR, Yovich JV, Steel CM. Surgical arthrodesis of distal tarsal joints in 17 horses clinically affected with osteoarthritis. Aust Vet J 2001;79(1):26–9.
[49] Hague BA, Guccione A. Laser-facilitated arthrodesis of the distal tarsal joints. Clin Tech Equine pract 2002;1:32–5.
[50] Scruton C, Baxter GM, Cross MW, et al. Comparison of intra-articular drilling and diode laser treatment for arthrodesis of the distal tarsal joints in normal horses. Equine Vet J 2005;37(1):81–6.
[51] Zubrod CJ, Schneider RK, Hague BA, et al. Comparison of three methods for arthrodesis of the distal intertarsal and tarsometatarsal joints in horses. Vet Surg 2005;34:372–82.
[52] Auer JA, Martens RJ, Williams EH. Periosteal transection for correction of angular limb deformities in foals. J Am Vet Med Assoc 1982;181(5):459–66.
[53] Auer JA. Angular limb deformities. In: Auer JA, Stick JA, editors. Equine surgery. 3rd edition. St. Louis (MO): Saunders Elsevier; 2006. p. 1130–49.
[54] Auer JA, Martens RJ. Periosteal transection and periosteal stripping for correction of angular limb deformities in foals. Am J Vet Res 1982;43(9):1530–4.
[55] Auer JA, Martens RJ. Angular limb deformities in foals. Proceedings of the 26th Annual Convention of the American Association of Equine Practitioners 1980;26:81–96.
[56] Read EK, Read MR, Townsend HG, et al. Effect of hemi-circumferential periosteal transection and elevation in foals with experimentally induced angular limb deformities. J Am Vet Med Assoc 2002;221(4):536–40.
[57] Slone DE, Roberts CT, Hughes FE. Restricted exercise and transphyseal bridging for correction of angular limb deformities. Presented at the 46th Annual AAEP Convention Proceedings. San Antonio (TX): 2000. p. 126–67.
[58] Bowman KF, Evans LH, Herring ME. Evaluation of surgical removal of fractured distal splint bones in the horse. Vet Surg 1982;11:116–20.
[59] Verschooten F, Gasthuys F, DeMoor A. Distal splint bone fractures in the horse: an experimental and clinical study. Equine Vet J 1984;16(6):532–6.
[60] Allen D, White NA. Management of fractures and exostosis of the metacarpals and metatarsals II and IV in 25 horses. Equine Vet J 1987;19(4):326–30.
[61] Harrison LJ, May SA, Edwards GB. Surgical treatment of open splint bone fractures in 26 horses. Vet Rec 1991;128:606–10.

[62] Peterson PR, Pascoe JR, Wheat JD. Surgical management of proximal splint bone fractures in the horse. Vet Surg 1987;(1695):367–72.
[63] Jenson PW, Gaughan EM, Lillich JD, et al. Segmental ostectomy of the second and fourth metacarpal and metatarsal bones in horses: 17 cases (1993–2002). J Am Vet Med Assoc 2004; 224(2):271–4.
[64] Norwood GL. The bucked-shin complex in Thoroughbreds. Proc Am Assoc Equine Pract 1978;24:319–36.
[65] Specht TE, Colahan PT. Osteostixis for incomplete cortical fracture of the third metacarpal bone. Results in 11 horses. Vet Surg 1990;19(1):34–40.
[66] Specht TE, Miller GJ, Colahan PT. Effects of clustered drill holes on the breaking strength of the equine third metacarpal bone. Am J Vet Res 1990;51(8):1242–6.
[67] Hanie EA, Sullins KE, White NA. Follow-up of 28 horses with third metacarpal unicortical stress fractures following treatment with osteostixis. Equine Vet J Suppl 1992;11(24):5–9.
[68] Cervantes C, Madision JB, Ackerman N, et al. Surgical treatment of dorsal cortical fractures of the third metacarpal bone in Thoroughbred racehorses: 53 cases (1985–1989). J Am Vet Med Assoc 1992;200(12):1997–2000.
[69] Dallap BL, Bramalage LR, Embertson RM. Results of screw fixation combined with cortical drilling for treatment of dorsal cortical stress fractures of the third metacarpal bone in 56 Thoroughbred racehorses. Equine Vet J 1999;31(3):252–7.
[70] Richardson DW. Dorsal cortical fractures of the equine metacarpus. Compend Contin Educ Pract Vet 1984;6:248–55.
[71] Furst AE, Lischer CJ. Foot. In: Auer JA, Stick JA, editors. Equine surgery. 3rd edition. St. Louis (MO): Saunders Elsevier; 2006. p. 1184–217.
[72] Jackman BR, Baxter GM, Doran RE, et al. Palmar digital neurectomy in horses 57 cases (1984–1990). Vet Surg 1993;24(4):285–8.
[73] Matthews S, Dart AJ, Dowling BA. Palmar digital neurectomy in 24 horses using the guillotine technique. Aust Vet J 2003;81(7):402–5.
[74] Schneider RK, Mayhew IG, Clarke GL. Effects of cryotherapy on the palmar and plantar digital nerves in the horse. Am J Vet Res 1985;46:7–12.
[75] Haugland LM, Collier MA, Panciera RJ, et al. The effect of CO_2 laser neurectomy on neuroma formation and axonal regeneration. Vet Surg 1992;21(5):351–4.
[76] Taylor TS, Vaughan JT. Effects of denervation of the digit of the horse. J Am Vet Med Assoc 1980;177(10):1033–9.
[77] Murray RC, Gaughan EM, DeBowes RM, et al. Acute effects of perineural administration of sodium hyaluronate on palmar digital neurectomy sites in horses. Am J Vet Res 1994; 55(10):1484–9.
[78] Fubini SL, Cummings JF, Todhunter RJ. The use of intraneural doxorubicin in association with palmar digital neurectomy in 28 horses. Vet Surg 1988;17(6):346–9.
[79] Dabreiner RM, White NA, Sullins KE. Comparison of current techniques for palmar digital neurectomy in horses. Proc Am Assoc Equine Pract 1997;43:231–2.
[80] Schumacher J, Steiger R, Schumacher J, et al. Effects of analgesia of the distal interphalangeal joint or palmar digital nerves on lameness caused by solar pain in horses. Vet Surg 2000; 29:54–8.
[81] Davis CS, Smith RKW. Diagnosis and management of tendon and ligament disorders. In: Auer JA, Stick JA, editors. Equine surgery. 3rd edition. St. Louis (MO): Saunders Elsevier; 2006. p. 1086–111.
[82] Dyson SJ. Medical management of superficial digital flexor tendonitis: a comparative study in 219 horses (1992–2000). Equine Vet J 2004;36(5):415–9.
[83] Henninger RW, Bramlage LR, Bailey M, et al. Effects of tendon splitting on experimentally-induced acute equine tendonitis. Vet Comp Orthop Traumatol 1992;5:1–9.
[84] Hogan PM, Bramlage LR. Transection of the accessory ligament of the superficial digital flexor tendon for the treatment of tendonitis: long term results in 61 Standardbred racehorses (1985–1992). Equine Vet J 1995;27(3):221–6.

[85] Fulton IC, MacLean AA, O'Rielly JL, et al. Superior check ligament desmotomy for treatment of superficial digital flexor tendonitis in Thoroughbred and Standardbred horses. Aust Vet J 1994;71(8):233–5.
[86] Gibson KT, Burbidge HM, Pfeiffer DU. Superficial digital flexor tendonitis in Thoroughbred race horses: outcome following non-surgical treatment and superior check desmotomy. Aust Vet J 1997;75(9):631–5.
[87] Smith MRW, Wright IM. Noninfected tenosynovitis of the digital flexor tendon sheath: a retrospective analysis of 76 cases. Equine Vet J 2006;38(2):134–41.
[88] Silver IA, Brown PM, Goodship AE. A clinical and experimental study of tendon injury, healing, and treatment in the horse. Equine Vet J 1983;1(Suppl):5–32.
[89] Hawkins JF, Ross MW. Transection of the accessory ligament of the superficial digital flexor muscle for the treatment of superficial digital flexor tendonitis in Standardbreds: 40 cases (1988–1992). J Am Vet Med Assoc 1995;206(5):674–8.
[90] Knudsen O. Percutaneous tendon splitting—method and results. Equine Vet J 1976;8(3): 101–3.
[91] Nilsson G, Bjorck G. Surgical treatment of chronic tendinitis in the horse. J Am Vet Med Assoc 1969;155(6):920–6.
[92] Alexander GR, Gibson KT, Day RE, et al. Effects of superior check desmotomy on flexor tendon and suspensory ligament strain in equine cadaver limbs. Vet Surg 2001;30:522–7.

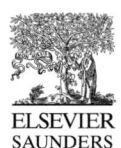

Evidence-Based Immunization in Horses

Nuria Barquero, DVM, MSc, MRCVS[a],
James R. Gilkerson, BVSc, PhD[b],
J. Richard Newton, BVSc, MSc, PhD, FRCVS[a],*

[a]Centre for Preventive Medicine, Animal Health Trust, Lanwades Park,
Kentford, Newmarket, Suffolk, United Kingdom, CB8 7UU
[b]Equine Infectious Disease Laboratory, Veterinary Pre-Clinical Centre,
Faculty of Veterinary Science, University of Melbourne, Victoria, 3010, Australia

Immunization, or vaccination, may be defined as the process of rendering a subject resistant to disease by administration of vaccines for prevention, amelioration, or treatment of infectious diseases. The twentieth century was a period of great leaps forward in veterinary science. At the forefront of these advances was the development of vaccines that enabled veterinarians to control and prevent diseases that had previously been devastating to the livestock industries. As had been proven in the field of human public health, vaccination campaigns were central in the control of these infectious diseases and, in many cases, were used to eradicate previously endemic and economically crippling diseases, such as foot and mouth disease and rinderpest. In the field of equine medicine, however, the economic impetus for development of efficacious vaccines was not as great as for the livestock industries. Thus, in many respects, it has lagged behind.

Evidence of vaccine efficacy is essential for practitioners when giving advice to clients about the relative merits of different vaccines or when trying to evaluate the economic benefits of instituting a vaccine program. Vaccine efficacy data are relatively readily available in the field of human health. When examining the evidence of efficacy of human vaccinations, there is not only the published data available from phase 2 and phase 3 trials but real-life postrelease field data. There are many governmental and nongovernmental public health agencies that record the details of vaccination programs in children as well as for particular global public health

* Corresponding author.
E-mail address: richard.newton@aht.org.uk (J.R. Newton).

initiatives, such as the smallpox eradication program. Many childhood diseases, such as measles, are notifiable in most developed countries, and such data as the total number of children vaccinated, the number of reported cases of disease, and the number of adverse reactions to vaccination are generally well reported by the public health services in many countries around the globe.

Unfortunately, in veterinary medicine in general and in equine veterinary medicine in particular, this sort of data, which is necessary to make informed decisions about vaccine use and effectiveness, is often not available. The most commonly available evidence that many veterinarians have at their disposal is the registration claim of the product, and perhaps the safety and efficacy data that were required for registration, which may or may not have been published in a peer-reviewed journal. Double-blind randomized controlled trials are uncommon. In many cases, there is a conflict between the expectations of the owner and the data at hand for the veterinarian. The owner expects that vaccination is going to prevent the disease in question, whereas the product may only claim to be an aid in the management of the disease, which can lead to dissatisfaction on behalf of the client when the disease still occurs in fully vaccinated animals. Veterinarians need to consider the epidemiology of the disease in question, the type of vaccine that they are administering to the animal, the immunologic constraints of the vaccine technology, and the available evidence of efficacy when they are evaluating which vaccine to use or whether to vaccinate at all.

The use of vaccines in controlling equine infectious diseases should be considered as only a part of a more wide-ranging strategy in disease control. In dealing with disease outbreaks, predetermined actions need to be taken, including strategies for isolation of affected animals, limiting shedding of pathogens into shared environments, heightened hygiene practices, and, possibly, adoption of vaccination in the face of an outbreak when indicated. Disease control at the herd level should be instigated through limiting the contact between infected and susceptible animals. The implementation of multiple simultaneous disease control measures, which includes the use of vaccination, may present some difficulties with respect to evaluating the true effectiveness of immunization in preventing, ameliorating, or treating infectious diseases, however.

Mechanisms of action

Immune defenses include innate and adaptive responses, but only the adaptive responses can be induced by vaccination. The immune adaptive response is mediated by antibodies or by effector cells, such as cytotoxic T lymphocytes (CTLs) and T-helper (TH) lymphocytes (CD4+). There are two subsets of TH cells: TH-1 cells, which stimulate cytotoxic and inflammatory functions, and TH-2 cells, which stimulate antibody response.

Vaccination should induce the appropriate TH response, which is influenced by the type of antigen, the type of adjuvant, and the immunization route.

Various different technologies are used in equine vaccines at the present time. In killed vaccines, the agent is completely inactivated using heat, chemicals, or irradiation; in most cases, their efficacy requires the addition of a potent adjuvant. Vaccines in this group include inactivated whole-pathogen vaccines, which are currently the most common equine vaccines; protein subunit vaccines, which incorporate inactive pathogen proteins; and recombinant subunit vaccines, which contain synthetic antigen produced using recombinant DNA technology.

In live vaccines, the pathogen is alive but expresses attenuated pathogenicity. These vaccines generally have a longer lasting duration of immunity, but they may potentially induce disease in immunocompromised animals. Vaccines in this group include modified-live vaccines, which may be attenuated through multiple cell culture passage using variants from other species or by development of temperature-sensitive mutants, and recombinant vector vaccines, which use pathogen DNA inserted in another nonpathogenic organism to express pathogenic and immunogenic peptide epitopes. Additional technologies are being investigated for use in horses but are currently not available as commercial vaccines; these include reassortant virus vaccines and DNA vaccines.

Evaluating the evidence

As with other aspects of equine veterinary medicine, it is appropriate to assess the scientific merits of immunization objectively in its intended role of disease prevention, amelioration, or treatment. This is important because vaccine production, promotion, and administration are a financially lucrative part of the equine veterinary health care business, and it should be incumbent on the veterinary profession to ensure that it is seen to use this technology for improving the health and welfare of animals in its care rather than simply as a money-making exercise. To this end, evidence-based veterinary medicine (EBVM) provides an increasingly powerful tool with which to examine the present level of proof for endorsing beneficial consequences from vaccination of horses against infection with and disease caused by a range of specific pathogens. As in all forms of EBVM, the quality or strength of the evidence varies across a spectrum according to the type of study that is presented. At the top of a theoretic pyramid of quality of evidence sits multistudy meta-analyses, followed by systematic reviews and randomized clinical trials and then by selective reviews and nonrandomized clinical trials. Behind these higher quality studies come cohort, case-control, and cross-sectional studies in that order, and the lowest quality evidence is provided by case series and reports and, finally, expert opinion.

In applying these levels of evidence for immunization against equine infectious diseases, we are not in fact aware of any notable peer-reviewed meta-analyses among this broad subject and reviews tend to be selective rather than truly systematic. Rather, much of the evidence relies on experimental challenge studies of varying quality as opposed to the randomized clinical field trials that are conducted in target human populations but remain rare for equine vaccines. Specific limitations of experimental studies may relate to insufficient sample size to detect a statistically meaningful effect from vaccination; absence of suitable masking (often referred to as blinding) of study investigators, thereby introducing unintentional observer bias; and poor generalizability to target populations through use of a healthy subset of age-restricted subjects that have been evaluated under optimal experimental conditions.

Another source of evidence relating to the effectiveness of equine vaccination in preventing infection and disease is based on field outbreak investigation. Failure of vaccination to prevent disease in the field may be related to significant antigenic and pathogenic differences between the infectious organisms included in the vaccine and those responsible for the infection, often referred to as strain variation. This is often in contrast to experimental challenge studies, in which vaccine strains and infecting viruses may be the same or closely related. Field-based cross-sectional surveys have also been used to evaluate the ability of vaccines to stimulate measurable immune responses previously demonstrated as being valid proxy measures of susceptibility to infection and disease.

Equine influenza virus

Among naive horses, equine influenza is a highly contagious respiratory disease and is characterized by pyrexia, associated depression and anorexia, a harsh dry cough, nasal discharge, and secondary bacterial respiratory infection. A novel H3N8 equine influenza A virus subtype, which first emerged in Miami, Florida in 1963, initiated a worldwide pandemic of equine respiratory disease [1–3] and was the stimulus for the development of multivalent adjuvanted influenza vaccines for horses [4–7]. This early work, based on experience from human vaccines, led to the development of the now broadly standard schedules for equine influenza vaccination. These schedules recommend that a primary course of two doses of injections be given approximately 4 to 6 weeks apart, followed by a booster vaccination 6 months after the end of the primary course and annual boosters thereafter. The same schedules are still adopted today for the product datasheet recommendations for the latest inactivated virus vaccines and are the basis for the regulatory rules for most international equine competitions.

It was recognized during several influenza outbreaks in the United Kingdom during the 1970s [8–11], and especially in the 1979 outbreak [12], that vaccinated horses generally experienced less severe disease than those that were unvaccinated. Influenza vaccination of Thoroughbred racehorses in Great Britain became mandatory under the Jockey Club Rules of Racing at the start of the flat-racing season in March 1981 and was followed soon after in Ireland and France. Since that time, British racing has not been cancelled because of equine influenza, but there have been continued seasonal peaks of infection among unvaccinated non-Thoroughbred horses associated with increased mixing at shows in the summer months. Because of the absence of systematic, consistent, and long-term surveillance data, however, it is not possible to provide conclusive evidence to support the true impact of mandatory influenza vaccination on reducing the incidence of equine influenza virus (EIV) infection and associated disease.

With the evolution of equine H3N8 influenza A viruses attributable to antigenic drift, influenza outbreaks have periodically caused periodic disruption to the training schedules of vaccinated Thoroughbreds in individual yards or training centers in the United Kingdom, despite the use of vaccination [13–16]. The adoption of more widespread vaccination has made the diagnosis of influenza infection less straightforward, however, because clinical signs are less severe, acute blood samples already possess moderate levels of serum antibody, and the quantities of live virus retrievable from the respiratory tract are greatly reduced. The development of a sensitive and rapid ELISA for the detection of influenza nucleoprotein (NP) antigen in extracts from nasopharyngeal swabs [17,18] has greatly improved the ability to diagnose influenza in previously vaccinated horses, as was demonstrated in the 1989 United Kingdom outbreak [14].

Failure of vaccine efficacy is commonly referred to as "vaccine breakdown" and is attributed to a combination of variable vaccine potency, poor response to vaccination, and antigenic drift in EIVs [19–21]. Measurement of serum antibody by the single radial hemolysis (SRH) test has been shown to be particularly sensitive for detecting influenza infection, and SRH antibody has predictive value for vaccine-induced protection [22–24]. Although cell-mediated immunity (CMI) has been suggested to be an important component of immunity to influenza, there is little evidence that it is stimulated by inactivated vaccines [25,26], although some evidence is now emerging that novel vaccine approaches based on canarypox vectors may induce meaningful CMI [27].

Small-scale controlled experimental studies using vaccinated and nonvaccinated influenza-naive Welsh Mountain Ponies provide the main evidence for the pattern of serologic responses after administration of influenza vaccines and the protective immunity that they provide. Experimental influenza viral challenge studies have repeatedly shown a strong correlation between vaccine-induced humoral antibody levels and protective immunity against infection with antigenically similar viruses ("homologous" viruses) [28–32]. Subsequent field studies have confirmed these observations in vaccinated racehorses with natural infection [24,33]. Field studies have also confirmed the need for inclusion of antigenically relevant strains in vaccines for the strong correlation between vaccine-induced antibody and immunity to remain valid [14,34], thereby corroborating findings from experimental strain variation challenge studies [35].

Several potentially important differences exist between experimental studies and the field situation, however, particularly in relation to interference with vaccine responses from maternally derived antibody (MDA) as well as the use of different types of vaccines administered in immunization schedules. Experimental studies, frequently conducted for licensing purposes on behalf of commercial companies, necessarily use the same vaccine (adjuvant and antigen strains) under optimal cold-chain conditions for all vaccinations, which are usually administered to recently weaned pony foals that have no serologic evidence of MDA. In contrast, the field situation may involve different vaccine types that are transported under suboptimal conditions and administered to horses from well-vaccinated dams. The effects of mixing vaccine types on serologic responses in experimental ponies have not been characterized, but observations from a field outbreak in Newmarket in 1995 raised the possibility that mixing of vaccine types played a part in the failure of vaccine efficacy [33]. It has also been proposed that persistence of passively acquired MDA might interfere with vaccine responses in young horses through neutralization of vaccine antigen [36–39].

It has long been recognized that young horses, especially groups of racehorses, are particularly susceptible to influenza-like infection [40], and it is harder to stimulate vaccine-induced immunity in these young horses than in older animals [5]. Failure of efficacy of vaccines is still most commonly reported in young racehorses, most likely for various reasons, including vaccine potency, the horse's immunologic response, and differences between the infecting and vaccine viruses [33]. In addition, international movement of horses has been recognized as an important factor in the spread of influenza throughout the world [16,41–43].

Although a reasonably strong body of evidence exists for EIV vaccine efficacy based on experimental vaccination and challenge studies conducted under optimal conditions in previously nonvaccinated ponies, little randomized controlled evidence exists for such vaccines being effective in field conditions. A notable exception is provided by a study describing a double-blind, randomized, placebo-controlled trial of a vaccine among 462 stabled horses at a Canadian racetrack [44]. Horses vaccinated with an inactivated aluminium phosphate–adjuvanted vaccine did not differ from those that received placebo in the severity of clinical signs in the face of a natural EIA outbreak. The results of that study showed no significant decrease in the risk of developing infectious upper respiratory tract disease between vaccinated and nonvaccinated horses, although the median duration of clinical disease was 3 days shorter in vaccinated horses [44,45].

The qualitative differences between the immune responses that follow infection or vaccination with inactivated virus suggest that improvements can be made in vaccine design. Ideally, vaccines should induce broadly reactive, local and systemic, antibody and cellular immune responses; establish memory; and consequently generate a rapid anamnestic response on field exposure to EIV. The occurrence of free and cell-associated virus is thereby reduced, and recovery is enhanced. Live-attenuated and live-vectored equine influenza vaccines that should more closely mimic natural infection are now available. A live recombinant vaccine that uses canarypox as a vector to express the haemagglutinin (HA) genes of EIVs has been available in Europe since 2003. The recombinant virus undergoes an abortive infection in mammalian cells, such that no progeny viruses are made but the expressed viral antigens are processed endogenously and presented as peptides by means of major histocompatibility complex (MHC) class I by the host cell in the same manner as occurs in natural infection but without associated infection risks. Experimental challenges with the canarypox-vectored vaccine showed that horses were protected against infection and virus shedding was markedly reduced [46]. The experiment used 15 influenza-naive Welsh Mountain Ponies randomly assigned to three groups of 5 ponies. The two vaccinated groups (one dose and two doses) had statistically significantly less severe clinical disease than the control group and did not shed as much virus. Another study used 24 ponies in an experimental challenge and also showed that the canarypox vaccine protected against development of clinical signs and viral shedding [27].

A cold-adapted, temperature-sensitive, modified-live virus equine influenza vaccine that is delivered intranasally is now licensed for use in the United States. The safety and efficacy of the vaccine have been demonstrated in experimental studies; however, the vaccine does not provide sterile immunity [47–50]. No correlation was found between the concentration of serum antibody induced by vaccination and protection against infection, although an anamnestic response was demonstrated at 7 days after infection [49]. Although there is evidence to show that primed animals develop a serologic response [50], it seems that the use of serum antibody response as a measure of live virus mucosal vaccines in naive animals is inappropriate. Although the development of reliable infectious challenge models in horses allows the experimental efficacy of all types of EIV vaccines to be consistently evaluated, the inability to measure alternative correlates of immunity for alternative vaccination strategies presents problems for the newer vaccines in extending their evaluation of effectiveness to the field situation.

Summary

The reliable experimental reproduction of EIV infection and associated disease provides strong evidence for the effectiveness of a wide range of vaccine types, including newer technologies in which good correlates of protection are not yet measurable. Although equine influenza vaccines have been available and used for several decades, convincing field-based data are extremely limited; in fact, the only truly blind randomized controlled field trial indicated that the vaccine under study was not effective.

Some care is required in interpreting experimental studies conducted under optimal conditions that use nonvaccinated control groups for comparison with vaccinated animals, because it is relatively straightforward to show apparently significant benefits from vaccination in terms of reduction of clinical signs alone. Nevertheless, it is clear from the long distance and almost global spread of equine influenza in spite of aggressive vaccination strategies that elimination of viral shedding is a more important goal, and more relevant benchmark for investigation, than is attenuation of clinical signs if future preventive strategies are to be successful.

Equine herpesviruses 1 and 4

Equine herpesvirus (EHV) 1 was first isolated from an aborted fetus at necropsy in 1932 in Kentucky [51]. Since then, EHV-1 has been recognized as a significant cause of equine fetal and neonatal losses in horse-breeding populations worldwide [52]. It was first thought that EHV-1 was responsible for outbreaks of rhinopneumonitis and abortion, but restriction endonuclease studies identified that the respiratory isolates were substantially different from the abortion isolates [53–55]. This recognition subsequently led to the differentiation of EHV-1 and EHV-4.

EHV-1 and EHV-4 are spread by the respiratory route, but EHV-1 rapidly progresses to establish a systemic infection by means of a lymphocyte-associated viremia, whereas EHV-4 remains primarily in the respiratory tract. Viremia is central to the pathogenesis of EHV-1 abortion and neurologic disease; viremia is the mechanism of transport of virus to the sites of secondary replication, such as the uterus and spinal cord [56]. Transportation to replication sites distant to the site of primary replication in the upper respiratory epithelium and EHV-1 abortigenic disease have been demonstrated to occur in mares with high levels of antibody [57,58]. Thus, the use of antibody alone as a marker for protection against EHV-1 systemic disease is of dubious value.

Recent seroepidemiologic studies in Australia have shown that a small proportion of foals are infected with EHV-1 early in life [59,60]; subsequent detection of EHV-1 and EHV-4 in nasal samples from foals less than 1 month old confirmed these findings [61]. The source of EHV-1 infection for these foals was likely to have been reactivation of a previously latent infection in the mare [60]. This silent cycle of EHV-1 infection commenced with mare-to-foal spread, with subsequent foal-to-foal spread in the preweaning and postweaning periods [60,62]. These data have implications in the design and implementation of vaccination programs, because these infected foals are lifelong latently infected carriers of EHV-1 that can become a source of infection for horses in the future. The age of first infection also is problematic, because some foals are infected before an age when they have a maximal immunologic response to the vaccine.

The immunopathogenesis and history of EHV-1 vaccination have been comprehensively reviewed [63]. An early strategy for controlling EHV-1 abortion by vaccination was based on the use of hamster attenuated-live virus in a "planned infection" program [64,65]. This attenuated virus was fully infective by the respiratory route and spread from vaccinates to in-contact susceptible horses [66]. The program was successful in reducing the incidence of abortion in mares on the breeding farms in Kentucky, where it was tested, as well as in reducing the frequency of rhinopneumonitis in racehorses [64]; however, abortions associated with planned infections, the short duration of immunity, and the period of quarantine that was required after treatment led to this method of vaccination being superseded [66]. Other attenuated vaccines have subsequently been used to control EHV-1 abortion. Another EHV-1 vaccine, first hamster attenuated, and then further attenuated in equine cells, was developed in Europe [67]. This vaccine was widely used in Europe and North America; however, questions of efficacy [68–70] and reports of abortion storms in vaccinated mares [70] led to the increased use of inactivated vaccines.

Inactivated EHV-1 vaccine and, more recently, a vaccine against EHV-1 and EHV-4 combined have been the most commonly and widely used EHV vaccines. Several trials of inactivated EHV-1 vaccine have demonstrated that the frequency of EHV-1 abortion in vaccinated mares was reduced [57,71] when using a chemically inactivated adjuvanted vaccine administered by intramuscular injection. Several subsequent studies have examined the efficacy of inactivated EHV-1 vaccines, with mixed results. One large-scale field trial in Kentucky that studied the safety and efficacy of inactivated EHV-1 vaccine (Pneumabort K) found that the incidence of EHV-1 abortion was reduced in vaccinated mares compared with unvaccinated control mares [72]. Unfortunately, such studies are problematic from an evidence-based point of view because they are not controlled or masked, and thus do not account for many potential confounding variables. There are certainly no large-scale, double-blind, randomized controlled trials, possibly because of the extraordinary cost of conducting these experiments in horses.

Different studies have found a reduction in the level of viremia in vaccinates with no reduction in the frequency of abortions [73], significantly fewer abortions in vaccinates with no sustained difference in the level or duration of viremia [74], and no evidence of protection against viremia or abortion [68]. The disparity in the data produced by these studies is partially related to the pathogenesis of EHV-1 abortion, because not all infected mares become viremic and not all viremic mares abort. The unpredictable nature of EHV-1 abortion requires that any field trial recruit large numbers of mares. This requirement has not been met by many of the studies done to date. The most significant evidence for the efficacy of an inactivated EHV-1/4 combined vaccine demonstrated that vaccinates were significantly protected against respiratory disease and also had evidence of protection against EHV-1 abortion [74]. This study, however, involved only nine pregnant mares (five vaccinates and four unvaccinated controls), and although there was a significant difference in the frequency of abortion between vaccinates and controls, one of the vaccinated mares aborted after challenge.

Despite the lack of formal efficacy data from field trials rather than experimental challenge models, inactivated EHV-1/4 vaccines are widely used in the horse industry and are widely associated with a reduction in the frequency of EHV-1 abortion. Data on the frequency of EHV-1 abortion in central Kentucky over the past 5 decades show a reduction in the frequency rate of EHV-1 abortion after the widespread commencement of vaccination with inactivated EHV-1 and, later, EHV-1/4 combined vaccines. It should be remembered, however, that during this same period, our knowledge of the pathogenesis and epidemiology of EHV-1 abortion has increased significantly and farm management practices have been adapted to reduce the impact of EHV-1 abortion storms.

EHV-1 pathogenesis studies have shown that viremia occurs in the presence of high levels of neutralizing antibody [57,58]. Because viremia is central to the pathogenesis of EHV-1 systemic disease, it has been suggested that effective EHV-1 vaccines must stimulate high levels of CTLs [75]. This has led to a recent revival in interest in attenuated EHV-1 vaccines. A temperature-sensitive EHV-1 isolate has been administered by intranasal instillation to pregnant mares, young horses, and foals [76–78]. These studies suggest that attenuated EHV-1 vaccines can be safe and efficacious; however, again, there have been only small numbers of horses tested, and some vaccinated mares aborted after challenge.

EHV-4 infection is ubiquitous in the equine population. Several serosurveys have shown that the level of EHV-4 seropositivity using a type-specific ELISA [52] approaches 100% in mares and foals [60,79,80]. EHV-4 respiratory disease is generally a mild self-limiting condition, but in performance horse stables, any loss of respiratory capacity is important; thus, EHV-4 is potentially an important pathogen. The efficacy of vaccination against EHV-4 respiratory disease has been tested [74]. Weanling foals were initially vaccinated twice, 4 weeks apart, with an EHV-1/4 combined vaccine. Two weeks after the second vaccination, these foals and a group of unvaccinated control foals were infected with EHV-4 by intranasal instillation. The vaccinated group shed less EHV-4 for a shorter duration of time than the control group and exhibited less severe clinical signs of respiratory disease, as determined by the authors' clinical scoring system.

Summary

There is some evidence that inactivated EHV-1/4 vaccines reduce the likelihood of EHV-1 abortion as well as the severity and duration of EHV-1 or EHV-4 respiratory disease after challenge infection; however, individual vaccinated animals may still experience disease. Recent studies suggest that some level of protection against EHV-1 abortion is also afforded by intranasal administration of an attenuated EHV-1 isolate. There is no available evidence that vaccination with inactivated or attenuated EHV-1 vaccines can prevent EHV-1 abortion if the challenge dose is high, however, such as might occur when management of the index case of EHV-1 abortion is inappropriate. The available studies on which vaccination recommendations are based all have problems with sample size, experimental design, and analysis, making formation of valid conclusions problematic. None of the published studies outlines the rationale behind the manufacturer's recommendations to vaccinate pregnant mares in the fifth, seventh, and ninth months of gestation. Importantly, no published studies evaluate the efficacy of EHV-1 vaccination in the prevention of EHV-1 neurologic disease, and no commercially available vaccines make any claim in this regard. There is some evidence to support claims that EHV-4 vaccination reduces the severity of EHV-4 respiratory disease as well as the duration and titer of EHV-4 shed by infected horses.

West Nile virus

West Nile fever, caused by infection with West Nile virus (WNV), takes its name from the West Nile district of Uganda, where the virus was first isolated in 1937 from the blood of a febrile woman. The virus, which is transmitted by insect vectors, has a wide geographic distribution, including Africa, the Middle East, Southwest and Central Asia, Europe, and, most recently, North America. For WNV, the principle vectors are various species of mosquito, and the main reservoir hosts are birds. The transmission cycle involves mosquitoes infecting birds and feeding on their blood. The virus is then amplified in the bloodstream of infected birds, which then infect other mosquitoes when they feed. Infected mosquitoes that feed on other animals, including human beings and horses, may infect these hosts, which usually do not become sufficiently infected to allow further transmission. It is believed that migration of infected birds between regions with suitable vectors has resulted in the emergence of the disease in areas, such as the United States, that had not previously seen WNV. Most infected migratory birds and mammals do not usually show clinical signs of infection, although the outbreaks seen in North America have resulted in large numbers of nonmigratory birds and horses demonstrating signs.

An inactivated WNV vaccine for horses has been available in North America since 2002, with a "live canarypox-vectored" vaccine launched commercially in 2004. Among the experimental evidence for WNV vaccination, the plaque reduction neutralization test (PRNT) was used to evaluate the serologic immune responses provided by intramuscular administration of two doses, given 3 weeks apart, of three different potencies of the inactivated vaccine [81]. All three groups demonstrated significant increases in serum antibody titers when tested 14 days after the second vaccine dose was administered. The medium-dose vaccine group and nonvaccinated controls were subsequently experimentally challenged 12 months after administration of the second vaccine. Nine (82%) of 11 controls compared with only 1 (5%) of 19 vaccinated horses developed viremia after challenge, thereby providing evidence of a statistically significant ($P<.0001$) protective effect from vaccination in this experimental challenge study. Several blind experimental challenge studies have been conducted on the canarypox-vectored vaccine that is licensed in United States to protect against WNV infection (Recombitek WNV). In studies, the canarypox-vectored vaccine induced detectable neutralizing antibodies among all 28 horses administered two doses intramuscularly 5 weeks apart [82]. Using a WNV-infected mosquito feeding challenge, no clinical signs of WNV were detected in any challenged animals. More than 80% of the 16 nonvaccinated controls had detectable viremia compared with none (0%) of 9 horses ($P<.001$) challenged 2 weeks and only 1 (10%) of 10 horses ($P = .001$) infected 12 months after receiving the two-dose primary vaccination. In a parallel study [83], 9 horses that received a single dose of canarypox-vectored vaccine 26 days earlier and 10 nonvaccinated animals were challenged using a WNV-infected mosquito challenge. Viremia was detected in only 1 vaccinated horse compared with 8 nonvaccinated animals ($P = .005$), and although all horses seroconverted after challenge, antibodies were detected sooner among vaccinated horses. The authors suggested that the results indicated some potential benefit from administration of a single dose of this vaccine under some field conditions. Finally, the canarypox-based vaccine was also evaluated using an experimental WNV intrathecal challenge model to assess the protective efficacy of this vaccine when neurologic clinical signs are induced [84]. In this scenario, although the challenge model was artificial, it was believed to resemble the severity of disease encountered in natural disease more closely, which had not been produced in previous mosquito-biting challenge studies. After this challenge, 8 (80%) of 10 controls developed clinical signs of encephalomyelitis, compared with only 1 vaccinated horse (10%) that exhibited a single episode of muscle fasciculation ($P = .005$). Nine controls and 1 vaccinated horse developed fever ($P = .001$). Postmortem histopathologic examination indicated that 8 controls and 1 vaccinated horse had evidence of nonsuppurative encephalitis ($P = .005$). Together, these data provide convincing experimental evidence for the efficacy of inactivated and canarypox-vectored live vaccines against WNV viremia and some evidence for the protective efficacy of live vaccination against the development of clinical signs of disease with WNV infection.

Another study described an experimental WNV-infected mosquito horse-feeding challenge study of a noncommercially available DNA vaccine (plasmid pCBWN) administered intramuscularly on one occasion [85]. In this challenge, all four (100%) vaccinated horses remained healthy and nonviremic, whereas seven (88%) of eight nonvaccinated animals developed viremia ($P = .01$) and one became febrile and developed neurologic signs 8 days after challenge, requiring euthanasia on day 9 after infection.

Although the experimental vaccine studies described previously provide controlled conditions for assessing the efficacy of vaccination using artificially induced WNV infection and clinical disease, they do not necessarily reproduce the variation in field conditions in which the vaccine is used by practitioners. Therefore, it would be valuable to assess the apparent effectiveness of field WNV vaccination in protecting against clinical disease and mortality. The annual westward spread of WNV across the United States since its first emergence in New York in 1999 and the availability of equine WNV vaccines since 2002 have provided the opportunity for several authors from different states in the United States to assess field vaccine effectiveness.

Vaccine effectiveness among 569 horses naturally exposed to WNV in North Dakota was assessed in 2002 [86]. In a final multivariable logistic regression model (n = 389), the odds of death attributable to WNV were significantly reduced (odds ratio [OR] = 0.062, 95% confidence interval [CI]: 0.007–0.58) among horses that had received vaccine administered according to the manufacturer's recommendations compared with nonvaccinated animals after controlling for horse's age and signs of incoordination, caudal paresis, or recumbency. The odds of death were also significantly reduced (OR = 0.32, 95% CI: 0.15–0.68) for horses that received one or two doses of vaccine, even though the dosing was not according to the manufacturer's recommendations. These data also indicated that a significantly lower proportion of vaccinated horses compared with nonvaccinated animals became recumbent ($P = .018$). In a similar retrospective study conducted among WNV-infected horses in Texas in 2002, investigators showed that after accounting for the clinical signs of ataxia, falling down, recumbency, and lip droop, horses that had been vaccinated at least once before the onset of disease were almost twice as likely to survive (OR = 1.8; $P = .005$) than those that had not been vaccinated in the year before the development of signs [87]. In a prospective cohort study of horses in California between December 2003 and November 2005, the occurrence of clinical disease associated with WNV infection was monitored among 37 nonvaccinated and 155 comingled vaccinated horses (87 receiving inactivated vaccine and 68 receiving canarypox recombinant vaccine). There was serologic evidence for exposure to WNV among 68% of 31 seronegative nonvaccinated horses between December 2004 and the end of the study period, confirming that WNV had been present among the cohort. Two (5%) of the 37 nonvaccinated horses compared with none of the 155 vaccinated animals developed clinical neurologic disease attributable to WNV infection, highlighting a statistically significant protective effect attributable to vaccination ($P = .036$).

Experimental challenge data for the inactivated WNV vaccine were accompanied by field-based safety information from 648 horses, including

32 pregnant mares, that demonstrated absence of local or systemic reactions in 96% of vaccinated animals and mild local reactions in the remainder [81]. Further evidence of safety among 595 pregnant mares was provided in a retrospective study showing there was no increased risk of pregnancy loss among WNV-vaccinated compared with nonvaccinated horses [88]. Under field conditions, the canarypox-vectored vaccine has been shown to provide a good anamnestic serologic response in animals that had previously only been administered the inactivated vaccine [89]. Another field-based study compared the immune responses induced by natural infection in 37 animals with those after vaccination in 187 horses [90]. For animals for which there were data available 5 to 7 months after infection or vaccination, 90% (18 of 20) of naturally infected horses had PRNT titers of 1:100 or greater 5 to 7 months after infection, whereas only 33% (28 of 84) of vaccinated horses had equivalent levels of PRNT titers 5 to 7 months after a second vaccine dose ($P<.0001$). The authors of this study concluded that revaccination every 6 months in endemic areas, in addition to good preventive methods, may be necessary to prevent WNV in some horses.

Summary

There is a growing body of experimental and field-based evidence that WNV vaccination in horses is effective in preventing viremia and the associated clinical disease and mortality that occur in a small proportion of infected animals. Field data indicate that vaccine manufacturers' recommendations should be followed but that more regular boosting, especially just before or during extended high-risk periods, may be warranted to maximize protective immunity.

Potomac horse fever (*Neorickettsia risticii*)

Potomac horse fever (PHF) is caused by infection with the small bacterial organism *Neorickettsia risticii*. This organism was formerly called *Ehrlichia risticii;* hence, the disease is frequently also referred to as equine monocytic ehrlichiosis (EME). The disease was first recognized in 1979 in areas along the Potomac River in Maryland and Virginia and has since been recognized more widely in North America and Europe. The disease is seasonal, occurring most commonly in the summer, and is characterized by fever, associated depression and inappetence, diarrhea, and demonstrable leukopenia on whole-blood examination as well as laminitis in approximately 25% of cases. Mortality may be as high as 25%, and abortion can occur in pregnant mares.

Preventive strategies are based on administration of inactivated whole-organism (bacterin) vaccines, all based on a single strain isolated from a horse in Maryland in 1984. In one experimental challenge study in 40 horses, all 13 control horses (100%) developed the disease, whereas only 6 (22%) of 27 vaccinated animals showed clinical signs ($P<.0001$) [91]. In contrast, data from a cross-sectional field study of 2587 horses on 511 farms in New York failed to demonstrate a correlation between the county's seropositive proportion and the percentage of horses vaccinated for PHF [92]. Vaccination was not associated with a reduction in prevalence or severity of clinical signs of EME, and the median date of diagnosis was not delayed compared with nonvaccinated animals [92]. A limited survey 38 (88%) of 43 PHF cases that occurred between 1994 and 1996 demonstrated a high proportion of vaccine failure [93]. The authors of this survey also demonstrated poor serologic responses among 41 horses that received one (n = 5), two (n = 20), or three (n = 16) doses of vaccine and marked heterogeneity among new *N risticii* isolates. It was thus concluded that the observed failure of vaccination against PHF [92] could be attributable to a combination of deficiency in antibody response by horses receiving even multiple doses and antigenic differences between the existing vaccine strain and new field isolates.

Summary

Although the early experimental data, probably based on homologous experimental challenge, provided statistically strong evidence in favor of a clinical benefit from vaccination for PHF, this has not been supported by subsequent data acquired from use of the vaccine in the field. Subsequent investigations have highlighted limited antibody responses and strain differences as possible reasons for poor vaccine effectiveness in the field.

Equine viral arteritis

Equine viral arteritis (EVA) is an infectious disease of horses caused by equine arteritis virus (EAV), a member of the family Arteviridae, genus *Arterivirus*. EAV was first isolated from horses during an outbreak of severe respiratory disease and abortion on a Standardbred stud farm in the town of Bucyrus, Ohio in 1953. The consequences of the infection range from subclinical infection to an influenza-like pyretic illness in adult horses, abortion in pregnant mares, and interstitial pneumonia in neonatal foals. Vaccination strategies are based on the use of formalin-inactivated and live-attenuated vaccines, with a geographic split in their use between Europe and Japan (inactivated) and North America (live attenuated). New experimental DNA and protein subunit vaccines are also being developed.

After the outbreak in the United Kingdom in 1993, a formalin-inactivated vaccine (Artervac) has been in use, predominantly in Thoroughbred stallions. Although an archive of data exists to demonstrate that the vaccine is capable of inducing long-lasting neutralizing antibody levels in animals receiving repeated booster vaccinations, no evidence is available on which to assess its efficacy in preventing establishment of the carrier state in infected stallions.

Another inactivated vaccine against EVA has been developed, and its immunogenicity and efficacy have been studied [94]. Two doses of the vaccine administered a month apart did induce antibodies, but these decreased rapidly. A further dose of vaccine given 2 months after the second dose induced an anamnestic antibody response that persisted for 6 months. Further studies have shown that vaccination with this inactivated vaccine does protect stallions from the carrier state and pregnant mares from abortion [95,96], although it apparently does not protect all animals against EAV infection, because EAV was recovered from the blood of some vaccinated horses after experimental challenge.

Early studies of EAV demonstrated that virulent virus could be attenuated by means of repeated passage through various different cell lines while, at the same time, retaining its ability to stimulate long-lasting immunity (immunogenicity) up to 2 years after vaccination [97,98]. Only the minimal side effects of short-term abnormality of sperm morphology in stallions and mild fever have been reported for the modified live virus (MLV) vaccine [99], although live virus can be recovered transiently from the blood and nasopharynx in some vaccinated animals [100,101]. The MLV vaccine protects against clinical disease and reduces virus shedding, and horses in contact with and mares covered by vaccinated stallions are not infected by EAV [102,103]. The use of MLV vaccine is not recommended in pregnant mares, however, because occasional fetal infections have been described [104].

New vaccines against EAV are under development, including a DNA vaccine that has been demonstrated to induce a long-lasting immune response [105]. Experimental challenge of recombinant subunit EAV vaccines has shown a reduction in the severity of clinical signs and virus shedding [106].

Summary

MLV and whole-virus inactivated EVA vaccines are used in geographically distinct regions of the world with little prospect that the alternative type is likely to be adopted outside their now established but limited markets because of different regulatory requirements in different countries; for example, MLV EAV vaccines are not allowed to be used in the United Kingdom. Significant data relating to efficacy exist for the MLV vaccine from experimental and field sources, particularly in preventing the carrier state in vaccinated colts. Concerns remain as to the safety of the MLV vaccine in pregnant mares late in gestation, in inducing vaccine-related clinical disease, and in the possibility of collateral transmission. In contrast, there is less clear-cut evidence to suggest efficacy of the inactivated vaccines. For these vaccines, more frequent boosting and slower onset of protection remain concerns, particularly in high-value stallions beginning their reproductive carriers. Concern also remains for both types of established EVA vaccine regarding their ready differentiation from natural infection. As such, future marker vaccines based on a range of technology, such as subunits, DNA, or viral vectors, might prove persuasive if combined with rapid onset and long-lasting immunity.

Equine encephalitides

There are three antigenically distinct alphaviruses that cause equine encephalitis, also referred to as encephalomyelitis. The three viruses are eastern equine encephalitis (EEE), western equine encephalitis (WEE), and Venezuelan equine encephalitis (VEE) viruses, thus called because of their geographic distribution in the Americas, which is where they occur as mosquito vector-borne infections. Live and inactivated virus vaccines have been developed against equine encephalitis virus infection.

The inactivated vaccines are of relatively low immunogenicity and provide only relatively short-lived protection against clinical disease. A recent prospective study showed that horses responded variably to each antigen. Some animals in the study failed to show increased titers despite recent vaccination, and others had low or undetectable antibodies 6 months after vaccination [107]. Subsequent studies have highlighted variation in responses between different commercial vaccines, including EEE antigen, which should be considered in vaccine selection [108].

Inadequate inactivation of the virus possibly caused a major epidemic or epizootic of VEE in Central America and Texas in the 1970s; subsequently, a live-attenuated VEE virus vaccine (TC-83) was developed by cell culture passage. Although inactivated vaccines continue to be used to prevent equine infections with WEE and EEE viruses, live-attenuated vaccines are only available for VEE. An experimental challenge infection of 13 vaccinated and 5 nonvaccinated control horses [109] showed complete protection among the vaccinated horses, but all the controls demonstrated signs of disease ($P < .001$), with 4 control horses dying because of the disease ($P = .002$).

Field studies have also evaluated the safety and efficacy of a live VEE vaccine [110]. In three studies, there was an overall seroconversion rate of 87% (127 of 146 vaccinated horses) observed after vaccination to the epizootic virus strain, although vaccine batch variation was believed to account for the observation of only 50% seroconversion in one population of vaccinated horses studied. Viremia was observed after vaccination in 10 of 26 horses; this was raised as a concern because of the possibility for reversion to virulence of the vaccine strain if viremia levels were high enough to allow infection of mosquitoes. No serious adverse reactions were observed, however, including no vaccine-associated abortion in 42 mares, among 100 horses vaccinated in one of the studies. The authors considered that the cessation of deaths 9 days after vaccination of 900 horses during one outbreak that had seen approximately 30 VEE-associated deaths around the time of vaccination and 12 further deaths up to the ninth day after vaccination was evidence of vaccine efficacy. The lack of nonvaccinated control animals makes this assertion difficult to corroborate definitively. Another study, however, demonstrated VEE infection after administration of live-attenuated vaccine in 10 horses [111].

More recent field observations have demonstrated that widespread vaccination with live-attenuated vaccine, in conjunction with vector control and movement restrictions, was apparently effective in quickly restricting two fatal VEE epizootics in Mexico in 1993 and 1996 [112]. The relative effectiveness of the individual measures could not be determined, however, and some cases did occur among vaccinated horses with apparently adequate levels of homologous neutralizing antibody. The occurrence of clinical cases in vaccinated horses highlights potentially significant strain variation between recent epizootic and conventional live vaccine VEE virus strains. In addition, although various studies have demonstrated cross-protective immunity conveyed from EEE and WEE against experimental and field infectious challenge with VEE [113], there also seems to be interference with VEE antibody responses with multivalent vaccination [114–118].

The safety, immunogenicity, and efficacy in horses of a new genetically engineered live-attenuated VEE vaccine candidate, V3526 [119], which had previously been shown to be the best of 14 potential candidates for a human vaccine based on animal infection models [120], have also been demonstrated. Recombinant and DNA vaccines are under investigation in rodent models and have shown promising results, although trials in horses are necessary to assess the efficacy of these new vaccines [121].

Summary

VEE is the most studied of the three alphavirus equine encephalitides that occur in the Western Hemisphere. Experimental and field challenge studies provide support for the efficacy of live-attenuated VEE virus vaccines. Care is required in the interpretation of some of this evidence, however, because of the potential confounding effects of concurrent management practices during field epizootics and evidence for cross-protective immunity from vaccinal immunity to EEE and WEE against infection with VEE virus. Antigenic differences between vaccine and field virus strains may also be important.

Strangles (*Streptococcus equi* subsp *equi*)

Streptococcus equi subsp *equi* is the causal organism of an acute and highly contagious upper respiratory disease (strangles) that mainly affects young horses. Unlike the closely related equine streptococci *S equi* subsp *zooepidemicus, S equi* subsp *equi* is not part of the normal bacterial flora of the equine pharynx. These bacteria impinge on the lingual or palatine tonsillar tissue, and hence are translocated to the lymph nodes draining the tonsillar tissue and the pharynx. Typical clinical signs of strangles include nasal discharge, fever, and abscessation of the regional lymph nodes that drain the upper respiratory tract, namely, the retropharyngeal and submandibular lymph chain. Abscessed lymph nodes rupture, if left untreated, to the external environment through the skin or into internal spaces, such as the guttural pouch. Abscess formation can occur at other sites, and this is commonly referred to as "bastard strangles." Lymph nodes of the head and neck as well as the mediastinal and mesenteric lymph nodes are sites often affected by bastard strangles. Although mortalities from strangles are not common, death can result from rupture of abscesses into the thoracic or abdominal cavity or because of respiratory distress attributable to pressure on the trachea from enlarged abscessed retropharyngeal lymph nodes (hence, the name "strangles"). Purulent discharges from the respiratory tract of affected horses or from draining abscesses are important sources of *S equi* subsp *equi* from which other horses are infected directly, by horse-to-horse contact, or indirectly by means of shared housing or feeding equipment or by contact with other fomites. In addition to obviously diseased horses, horse-to-horse spread of *S equi* subsp *equi* can occur from apparently healthy carrier horses in association with guttural pouch infection. Most infected horses recover from the disease and do not become carrier animals [122].

Commercial vaccines have been used to attempt to control strangles for many years in Australia and the United States, with limited evidence of efficacy. Bacterins of inactivated whole *Streptococcus equi* subsp *equi* or adjuvanted extracts of *S equi* subsp *equi* have been shown to be immunogenic but have had little published efficacy data to support their use [123]. A study in Australia that surveyed stud farm owners or managers to determine the incidence, risk factors, and effect of vaccination on the occurrence of strangles on horse farms found that studs at high risk from strangles (eg, they had had cases in the recent past) were more likely to vaccinate against strangles but that there was no indication that vaccination decreased the likelihood of outbreaks of strangles [124]. Vaccination with inactivated or extract vaccines has been reported to reduce the severity of clinical signs of strangles [125] and to reduce the attack rates in vaccinated animals after challenge, but adverse reactions to vaccination, such as soreness and abscessation at the injection site, have been reported [123]. The lack of efficacy of these whole-cell or extract vaccines containing high levels of M protein is likely attributable to the type of immune response stimulated after parenteral administration of an inactivated antigen.

Recent research efforts have been directed toward stimulating a local opsonizing mucosal IgA and IgG immune response [126–128]. A live-attenuated intranasal *S equi* subsp *equi* vaccine has been developed and commercially produced in the United States [129] in an attempt to stimulate the local mucosal protection observed in recovered animals. Concerns over the balance between safety as a result of sufficient attenuation and protection associated with significant immunogenicity have limited the use of this vaccine outside the United States.

Recently, a genetically attenuated vaccine has been released in the United Kingdom. Lacking the *aro A* gene required for aromatic amino acid synthesis [130], this deletion mutant has been shown to confer significant protection from challenge after intramucosal administration into the upper lip, but this protection is of short duration, thus requiring three monthly booster vaccinations [131]. Pustules at the site of administration in the lip were a commonly reported adverse reaction to vaccination in this study.

Summary

Although there are several publications that describe the safety and efficacy of a variety of S *equi* subsp *equi* vaccines, there is no definitive large-scale field trial to describe the efficacy of vaccination in the "real world." Although the new-generation vaccines, particularly the intramucosal vaccine, sound promising, further work is required to provide practitioners with the requisite evidence of efficacy in the field setting rather than in the artificial setting of the small-scale challenge trial.

Tetanus

Arguably, the most widely used equine vaccine in the world is the tetanus toxoid, but there are no publications that evaluate the efficacy of this vaccination strategy for horses under extensive field conditions. Tetanus is a sporadic infectious but not contagious disease, and as such, outbreaks of tetanus in horses are not reported. This makes evaluation of vaccine efficacy in the field difficult, because the calculation of attack rates and relative risk of vaccinated versus unvaccinated animals in the face of an outbreak is not possible. All the evidence for the use of this vaccine comes from small-scale antigenicity or challenge trials. Tetanus is an acute toxigenic disease of many species; however, the susceptibility of the different species to tetanus toxin varies considerably. Horses and human beings are highly susceptible, ruminants and pigs are intermediately susceptible, and carnivores are relatively resistant to the effects of tetanus toxin. Tetanospasmin (tetanus toxin) binds to receptors on the neuromuscular junction and is transported to the central nervous system in toxin-containing vesicles by retrograde intra-axonal flow, where it blocks transmission of inhibitory signals, resulting in spastic paralysis [132].

It is certainly true that the absence of evidence is not evidence of absence. Despite the absence of evidence from large-scale trials to demonstrate conclusively that tetanus toxoid effectively prevents tetanus, there is sufficient evidence from small-scale challenge studies and clinical data from practitioners to support the prophylactic use of tetanus toxoid in horses. A recent case series of horses with tetanus found that the most commonly reported risk factor in the affected horses was the absence of vaccination [133], and this is also consistent with other case reports in which the vaccination history was not known. Challenge trials have demonstrated adequate levels of protection against challenge with purified tetanus toxin [134], and studies have also examined the duration of immunity after multiple doses of toxoid [135,136]. At least two doses of toxoid would seem to be required to ensure that antibody levels were maintained at greater than 0.01 IU, which was the level previously determined to provide sufficient protection [137]. Many horses achieved these levels after a single dose of toxoid, but variation between individual horses was such that a single dose could not be relied on to stimulate adequate levels of antibody to provide protection for a 12-month period [136]. There is little experimental evidence to support the recommended 12-month interval between tetanus booster vaccinations, because all horses that received two tetanus toxoid vaccines 4 weeks apart had high levels of antitetanus antibodies when tested 12 months after the primary vaccine, but the duration of immunity after 12 months was not investigated [136].

It is common practice in equine medicine to use an active-passive immunization approach to protect horses at high risk of developing tetanus. This strategy has been shown to afford rapid onset of protective levels of antibody after the administration of antitoxin, with a long duration of antibody titer, particularly if the dose of toxoid was repeated [135].

Summary

The categoric nature of the evidence of protection against tetanus (immune horses survive, and nonimmune horses die) allows the practitioner to make a valid evidence-based decision to use tetanus toxoid and antitoxin, despite the absence of large-scale double-blind clinical trials. It is the view of the authors that all horses should be vaccinated routinely against tetanus, although the duration of immunity from vaccination has not been established.

References

[1] Anon. The 1963 equine influenza epizootic. J Am Vet Med Assoc 1963;143:1108.
[2] Gerber H. Equine influenza: clinical features, sequelae and epidemiology of equine influenza. In: Bryans JT, editor. Equine infectious diseases II: proceedings of the Second International Conference on Equine Infectious Diseases. New York: Karger Basel; 1970. p. 63–80.
[3] Scholtens RG, Steele JH. U.S. epizootic of equine influenza, 1963: epizootiology, public health reports. Washingtonian 1964;79:393.
[4] Bryans JT, Doll ER, Wilson JC, et al. Immunisation for equine influenza. J Am Vet Med Assoc 1966;148:413–7.

[5] Petermann HG, Fayet MT, Fontaine M, et al. Vaccination against equine influenza. In: Bryans JT, editor. Equine infectious diseases II: proceedings of the Second International Conference on Equine Infectious Diseases. New York: Karger Basel; 1970. p. 105–10.
[6] Frerichs GN, Burrows R, Frerichs CC. Serological response of horses and laboratory animals to equine influenza vaccines. In: Bryans JT, editor. Equine infectious diseases III: proceedings of the Third International Conference on Equine Infectious Diseases. New York: Karger Basel; 1973. p. 503–9.
[7] Burki F, Sibalin M. Conclusions and questions arising from a study of serology and immunology of equine influenza. In: Bryans JT, Gerber H, editors. Equine infectious diseases III: proceedings of the Third International Conference on Equine Infectious Diseases. New York: Karger Basel; 1973. p. 510–26.
[8] Powell DG, Burrows R. Field observations on influenza vaccination of Thoroughbred horses. International Symposium on Influenza Vaccines for Men and Horses. London, 1972. Symposium Series of Immunobiological Standardization 1973;20:332–7.
[9] Thomson GR, Mumford JA, Spooner PR, et al. The outbreak of equine influenza in England: January 1976. Vet Rec 1977;100:465–8.
[10] Powell DG, Burrows R, Spooner P, et al. Field observations on influenza vaccination among horses in Britain, 1971–1976. International Symposium on Influenza Immunization (II), Geneva, 1977. Dev Biol Stand 1977;39:347–52.
[11] Powell DG. A study of infectious respiratory disease among horses in Great Britain, 1971–1976. Thesis submitted for the Diploma of Fellowship of the Royal College of Veterinary Surgeons, London; 1980.
[12] Burrows R, Goodridge D, Denyer M, et al. Equine influenza infections in Great Britain, 1979. Vet Rec 1982;110:494–7.
[13] Wood JLN, Mumford JA. Epidemiology of equine influenza. Vet Rec 1992;130:126.
[14] Livesay GJ, O'Neill TO, Hannant D, et al. The outbreak of equine influenza (H3N8) in the United Kingdom in 1989: diagnostic use of an antigen capture ELISA. Vet Rec 1993;133:515–9.
[15] Newton JR, Mumford JA. Equine influenza in vaccinated horses. Vet Rec 1995;137:495–6.
[16] Powell DG, Watkins KL, Li PH, et al. Outbreak of equine influenza among horses in Hong Kong during 1992. Vet Rec 1995;136:531–6.
[17] Cook RF, Sinclair R, Mumford JA. Detection of influenza nucleoprotein antigen in nasal secretions from horses infected with A/equine influenza (H3N8) viruses. J Virol Methods 1988;20:1–12.
[18] Chomel JJ, Thouvenot D, Onno M, et al. Rapid diagnosis of influenza infection of NP antigen using an immunocapture ELISA test. J Virol Methods 1989;25:81–92.
[19] Hinshaw VS, Naeve CW, Webster RG, et al. Analysis of antigenic variation of equine 2 influenza A viruses. Bull World Health Organ 1983;61:153–8.
[20] Kawaoka Y, Bean WJ, Webster RG, et al. Origin of the A/equine/Johannesburg/86(H3N8) virus: antigenic and genetic analyses of equine-2 influenza A hemagglutinins. In: Powell DG, editor. Equine infectious diseases V: proceedings of the Fifth International Conference on Equine Infectious Diseases. Kentucky: Kentucky University Press; 1988. p. 47–50.
[21] Mumford J, Wood J. WHO/OIE meeting: consultation on newly emerging strains of equine influenza, 18–19 May 1992, Animal Health Trust, Newmarket, Suffolk, UK. Vaccine 1993;11:1172–5.
[22] Mumford JA. Progress in the control of equine influenza. In: Plowright W, Rossdale PD, Wade JF, editors. Equine infectious diseases VI: proceedings of the Sixth International Conference on Equine Infectious Diseases. Newmarket (UK): R&W Publications Ltd; 1992. p. 207–17.
[23] Morley PS, Hanson LK, Bogdan JR, et al. The relationship between single radial hemolysis, haemagglutination inhibition, and virus neutralisation assays used to detect antibodies specific for equine influenza viruses. Vet Microbiol 1995;45:81–92.

[24] Townsend HGG, Morley PS, Newton JR, et al. Measuring serum antibody as a method of predicting infection and disease in horses during outbreaks of influenza. In: Wernery U, Wade JF, Mumford JA, et al, editors. Equine Infectious Diseases VIII. Proceedings of the Eighth International Conference on Equine Infectious Diseases. Newmarket (UK): R&W Publications; 1999. p. 33–7.
[25] Hannant D. Immune effector responses to vaccination and infection with equine influenza. In: Nakajima H, Plowright W, editors. Equine infectious diseases VII: proceedings of the Seventh International Conference on Equine Infectious Diseases. Newmarket (UK): R&W Publications Ltd; 1994. p. 306.
[26] Hannant D, Jessett DM, O'Neill T, et al. Cellular immune responses stimulated by inactivated virus vaccines and infection with equine influenza virus (H3N8). In: Nakajima H, Plowright W, editors. Equine infectious diseases VII: proceedings of the Seventh International Conference on Equine Infectious Diseases. Newmarket (UK): R&W Publications Ltd; 1994. p. 169–74.
[27] Paillot R, Hannant D, Kydd JH, et al. Vaccination against equine influenza: quid novi? Vaccine 2006;24:4047–61.
[28] Mumford JA, Wood JM, Folkers C, et al. Protection against experimental infection with influenza virus A/equine/Miami/63 (H3N8) provided by inactivated whole virus vaccine containing homologous virus. Epidemiol Infect 1988;100:501–10.
[29] Mumford J, Wood J. Establishing an acceptability threshold for equine influenza vaccines. Dev Biol Stand 1993;79:137–46.
[30] Mumford JA, Jessett DM, Dunleavy U, et al. Antigenicity and immunogenicity of experimental equine influenza ISCOM vaccines. Vaccine 1994;12:857–63.
[31] Mumford JA, Jessett DM, Rollinson EA, et al. Duration of protective efficacy of equine influenza immunostimulating complex/tetanus vaccines. Vet Rec 1994;134:158–62.
[32] Mumford JA, Wilson H, Hannant D, et al. Antigenicity and immunogenicity of equine influenza vaccines containing a carbomer adjuvant. Epidemiol Infect 1994;112:421–37.
[33] Newton JR, Townsend HGG, Wood JLN, et al. Immunity to equine influenza: relationship of vaccine-induced antibody in young Thoroughbred racehorses to protection against field infection with influenza A/equine-2 viruses (H3N8). Equine Vet J 2000;32:65–74.
[34] Newton JR, Verheyen K, Wood JLN, et al. Equine influenza in the United Kingdom in 1998. Vet Rec 1999;145:449–52.
[35] Daly JM, Yates PJ, Browse G, et al. Comparison of hamster and pony challenge models for evaluation of antigenic drift on cross-protection afforded by equine influenza vaccines. Equine Vet J 2003;35:458–62.
[36] van Oirschot JT, Bruin G, de Boer-Luytze E, et al. Maternal antibodies against equine influenza virus in foals and their interference with vaccination. Zentralbl Veterinarmed 1991;38:391–6.
[37] van Maanen C, Bruin G, de Boer-Luytze E, et al. Interference of maternal antibodies with the immune response of foals after vaccination against equine influenza. Vet Q 1992;14:13–7.
[38] Holland RE, Conboy HS, Berry DB, et al. Age dependence of foal vaccination for equine influenza: new evidence from the USA. In: Wernery U, Wade JF, Mumford JA, et al, editors. Equine Infectious Diseases VIII. Proceedings of the Eighth International Conference on Equine Infectious Diseases. Newmarket (UK): R&W Publications; 1999. p. 547–8.
[39] Cullinane A, Weld J, Osborne M, et al. Field studies on equine influenza vaccination regimes in Thoroughbred foals and yearlings. Vet J 2001;161:174–85.
[40] Waldeman O, Kobe K, Pape J. The etiology of outbreaks of coughing in a racing centre (Hoppengarten) in Germany: preliminary communication. Vet Rec 1934;14:277–80.
[41] Mumford JA, Chambers TM. Equine influenza. In: Nicholson KG, Webster R, Hay A, et al, editors. Textbook of influenza. Blackwell Healthcare Communications Ltd; 1998. p. 146–62.
[42] Mumford JA. Control of influenza from an international perspective. In: Wernery U, Wade JF, Mumford JA, et al, editors. Equine Infectious Diseases VIII. Proceedings of the Eighth

International Conference on Equine Infectious Diseases. Newmarket (UK): R&W Publications; 1999. p. 11–24.

[43] Wernery R, Yates PJ, Wernery U, et al. Equine influenza outbreak in a polo club in Dubai, United Arab Emirates in 1995/96. In: Wernery U, Wade JF, Mumford JA, et al, editors. Equine Infectious Diseases VIII. Proceedings of the Eighth International Conference on Equine Infectious Diseases. Newmarket (UK): R&W Publications; 1999. p. 342–6.

[44] Morley PS, Townsend HGG, Bogdan JR, et al. Efficacy of a commercial vaccine for preventing disease caused by influenza virus infection in horses. J Am Vet Med Assoc 1999;215:61–6.

[45] Morley PS, Townsend HGG, Bogdan JR, et al. Risk factors for disease associated with influenza virus infections during three epidemics in horses. J Am Vet Med Assoc 2000; 216:545–50.

[46] Edlund Toulemonde C, Daly J, Sindle T, et al. Efficacy of a recombinant equine influenza vaccine against challenge with an American lineage H3N8 influenza virus responsible for the 2003 outbreak in the United Kingdom. Vet Rec 2005;156:367–71.

[47] Chambers TM, Holland RE, Tudor LR, et al. A new modified live equine influenza virus vaccine: phenotypic stability, restricted spread and efficacy against heterologous virus challenge. Equine Vet J 2001;33:630–6.

[48] Lunn D, Hussey S, Sebring R, et al. Safety, efficacy, and immunogenicity of a modified-live equine influenza virus vaccine in ponies after induction of exercise-induced immunosuppression. J Am Vet Med Assoc 2001;218:900–6.

[49] Townsend HGG, Penner SJ, Watts TC, et al. Efficacy of a cold-adapted, intranasal equine influenza vaccine: challenge trials. Equine Vet J 2001;33:637–43.

[50] Youngner JS, Whitaker-Dowling P, Chambers TM, et al. Derivation and characterization of a live attenuated equine influenza vaccine virus. Am J Vet Res 2001;62:1290–4.

[51] Dimock W, Edwards P. Is there a filterable virus of abortion in mares? Bulletin: Kentucky Agriculture Experiment Station 1933;333:291–301.

[52] Crabb BS, MacPherson CM, Reubel GH, et al. A type-specific serological test to distinguish antibodies to equine herpesviruses 4 and 1. Arch Virol 1995;140:245–58.

[53] Sabine M, Robertson GR, Whalley JM. Differentiation of sub-types of equine herpesvirus 1 by restriction endonuclease analysis. Aust Vet J 1981;57:148–9.

[54] Studdert MJ. Differentiation of subtypes within equine herpesvirus type 1. Aust Vet J 1980; 56:45.

[55] Studdert MJ, Simpson T, Roizman B. Differentiation of respiratory and abortigenic isolates of equine herpesvirus 1 by restriction endonucleases. Science 1981;214:562–4.

[56] Allen G, Bryans JT. Molecular epizootiology, pathogenesis and prophylaxis of equine herpesvirus-1 infections. Prog Vet Microbiol Immunol 1986;2:78–144.

[57] Bryans JT. On immunity to disease caused by equine herpesvirus 1. J Am Vet Med Assoc 1969;155:294–300.

[58] Doll ER, Wallace M, Richards MG. Thermal, hematological and serological responses of weanling horses following inoculation with equine abortion virus: its similarity to equine influenza. Cornell Vet 1954;44:181–90.

[59] Gilkerson JR, Love DN, Whalley JM. Serological evidence of equine herpesvirus 1 (EHV-1) infection in Thoroughbred foals 30-120 days of age. Australian Equine Veterinarian 1997;15:128–34.

[60] Gilkerson JR, Whalley JM, Drummer HE, et al. Epidemiology of EHV-1 and EHV-4 in the mare and foal populations on a Hunter Valley stud farm: are mares the source of EHV-1 for unweaned foals. Vet Microbiol 1999;68:27–34.

[61] Foote CE, Love DN, Gilkerson JR, et al. EHV-1 and EHV-4 infection in vaccinated mares and their foals. Vet Immunol Immunopathol 2006;111:41–6.

[62] Gilkerson JR, Love DN, Whalley JM. Incidence of equine herpesvirus 1 infection in Thoroughbred weanlings on two stud farms. Aust Vet J 2000;78:277–8.

[63] Kydd JH, Townsend HGG, Hannant D. The equine immune response to equine herpesvirus-1: the virus and its vaccines. Vet Immunol Immunopathol 2006;111:15–30.
[64] Doll ER. Immunization against viral rhinopneumonitis of horses with live virus propagated in hamsters. J Am Vet Med Assoc 1961;139:1324–30.
[65] Doll ER, Bryans JT. A planned infection program for immunizing mares against viral rhinopneumonitis. Cornell Vet 1963;53:249–62.
[66] Peacock G. Biological requirements and control of equine rhinopneumonitis virus vaccine (live virus). J Am Vet Med Assoc 1969;155:310–2.
[67] Bass E. Immunization with a modified live virus equine rhinopneumonitis vaccine and an aluminium hydroxide adsorbed equine influenza vaccine. Journal of Equine Medicine 1979;3(5):65–74.
[68] Burki F, Rossmanith W, Nowotny N, et al. Viraemia and abortions are not prevented by two commercial equine herpesvirus-1 vaccines after experimental challenge of horses. Vet Q 1990;12:80–6.
[69] Dutta SK, Shipley WD. Immunity and the level of neutralization antibodies in foals and mares vaccinated with a modified live-virus rhinopneumonitis vaccine. Am J Vet Res 1975;36:445–8.
[70] Eaglesome MD, Henry JN, McKnight JD. Equine herpesvirus 1 infection in mares vaccinated with a live-virus rhinopneumonitis vaccine attenuated in cell culture. Can Vet J 1979;20:145–7.
[71] Bryans J. Immunization of pregnant mares with an inactivated equine herpesvirus 1 vaccine. In: Bryans J, Gerber H, editors. Equine infectious diseases IV. Princeton (NJ): Veterinary Publications; 1978. p. 83–92.
[72] Bryans JT, Allen GP. Application of a chemically inactivated, adjuvanted vaccine to control abortigenic infection of mares by equine herpesvirus I. Dev Biol Stand 1982; 52:493–8.
[73] Burrows R, Goodridge D, Denyer MS. Trials of an inactivated equid herpesvirus 1 vaccine: challenge with a subtype 1 virus. Vet Rec 1984;114:369–74.
[74] Heldens JG, Kersten AJ, Weststrate MW, et al. Duration of immunity induced by an adjuvanted and inactivated equine influenza, tetanus and equine herpesvirus 1 and 4 combination vaccine. Vet Q 2001;23:210–7.
[75] Allen, G, Kydd JH, Slater JD, et al. Advances in understanding of the pathogenesis, epidemiology and immunological control of equine herpesvirus abortion. In: Wernery U, Wade JF, Mumford JA, et al. editors. Equine infectious diseases VIII. Newmarket (UK): R & W Publications; 1998. p. 129–146.
[76] Patel JR, Bateman H, Williams J, et al. Derivation and characterisation of a live equid herpes virus-1 (EHV-1) vaccine to protect against abortion and respiratory disease due to EHV-1. Vet Microbiol 2003;91:23–39.
[77] Patel JR, Didlick S, Bateman H. Efficacy of a live equine herpesvirus-1 (EHV-1) strain C147 vaccine in foals with maternally-derived antibody: protection against EHV-1 infection. Equine Vet J 2004;36:447–51.
[78] Patel JR, Foldi J, Bateman H, et al. Equid herpesvirus (EHV-1) live vaccine strain C147: efficacy against respiratory diseases following EHV types 1 and 4 challenges. Vet Microbiol 2003;92:1–17.
[79] Foote CE, Gilkerson JR, Whalley JM, et al. Seroprevalence of equine herpesvirus 1 in mares and foals on a large Hunter Valley stud farm in years pre- and postvaccination. Aust Vet J 2003;81:283–8.
[80] Gilkerson JR, Whalley JM, Drummer HE, et al. Epidemiological studies of equine herpesvirus 1 (EHV-1) in Thoroughbred foals: a review of studies conducted in the Hunter Valley of New South Wales between 1995 and 1997. Vet Microbiol 1999;68:15–25.
[81] Ng T, Hathaway D, Jennings N, et al. Equine vaccine for West Nile virus. Dev Biol (Basel) 2003;114:221–7.

[82] Minke JM, SIger L, Karaca K, et al. Recombinant canarypoxvirus vaccine carrying the prM/E genes of West Nile virus protects horses against a West Nile virus-mosquito challenge. Arch Virol Suppl 2004;18:221–30.

[83] Siger L, Bowen RA, Karaca K, et al. Assessment of the efficacy of a single dose of a recombinant vaccine against West Nile virus in response to natural challenge with West Nile virus-infected mosquitoes in horses. Am J Vet Res 2004;65:1459–62.

[84] Siger L, Bowen R, Karaca K, et al. Evaluation of the efficacy provided by a recombinant canarypox-vectored equine West Nile virus vaccine against an experimental West Nile virus intrathecal challenge in horses. Vet Ther 2006;7:249–56.

[85] Davis BS, Chang GJ, Cropp B, et al. West Nile virus recombinant DNA vaccine protects mouse and horse from virus challenge and expresses in vitro a noninfectious recombinant antigen that can be used in enzyme-linked immunosorbent assays. J Virol 2001;75:4040–7.

[86] Schuler LA, Khaitsa ML, Dyer NW, et al. Evaluation of an outbreak of West Nile virus infection in horses: 569 cases (2002). J Am Vet Med Assoc 2004;225:1084–9.

[87] Ward MP, Schuermann JA, Highfield LD, et al. Characteristics of an outbreak of West Nile virus encephalomyelitis in a previously uninfected population of horses. Vet Microbiol 2006;118:255–9.

[88] Vest DJ, Cohen ND, Berezowski CJ, et al. Evaluation of administration of West Nile virus vaccine to pregnant broodmares. J Am Vet Med Assoc 2004;225:1894–7.

[89] Grosenbaugh DA, Backus CS, Karaca K, et al. The anamnestic serologic response to vaccination with a canarypox virus-vectored recombinant West Nile virus (WNV) vaccine in horses previously vaccinated with an inactivated WNV vaccine. Vet Ther 2004;5:251–7.

[90] Davidson AH, Traub-Dargatz JL, Rodeheaver RM, et al. Immunologic responses to West Nile virus in vaccinated and clinically affected horses. J Am Vet Med Assoc 2005;226:240–5.

[91] Ristic M, Holland CJ, Goetz TE. Evaluation of a vaccine for equine monocytic ehrlichiosis. Presented at the Proceedings of a Symposium on Potomac Horse Fever. Louisville, Kentucky; 1988. p. 89.

[92] Atwill ER, Mohammed HO, Lopez JW, et al. Cross-sectional evaluation of environmental, host, and management factors associated with risk of seropositivity to Ehrlichia risticii in horses of New York State. Am J Vet Res 1996;57:278–85.

[93] Dutta SK, Vemulapalli R, Biswas B. Association of deficiency in antibody response to vaccine and heterogeneity of Ehrlichia risticii strains with Potomac horse fever vaccine failure in horses. J Clin Microbiol 1998;36:506–12.

[94] Fukunaga Y, Wada R, Matsumura T, et al. Induction of immune response and protection from equine viral arteritis (EVA) by formalin inactivated-virus vaccine for EVA in horses. Zentralbl Veterinarmed B 1990;37:135–41.

[95] Fukunaga Y, Wada R, Matsumura T, et al. An attempt to protect against persistent infection of equine viral arteritis in the reproductive tract of stallions using formalin-inactivated virus vaccine. In: Plowright W, Rossdale PD, Wade JF, editors. Equine infectious diseases VI: proceedings of the Sixth International Conference on Equine Infectious Diseases. Newmarket (UK): R&W Publications Ltd; 1991. p. 239–44.

[96] Fukunaga Y, Wada R, Kanemaru T, et al. Protection against abortion in pregnant mares vaccinated with a killed vaccine after exposure to equine arteritis virus. In: Nakajima H, Plowright W, editors. Equine infectious diseases VI: proceedings of the Sixth International Conference on Equine Infectious Diseases. Newmarket (UK): R&W Publications Ltd; 1994. p. 340.

[97] Doll ER, Bryans JT, Wilson JC, et al. Immunization against equine viral arteritis using modified live virus propagated in cell cultures of rabbit kidney. Cornell Vet 1968;48:497–524.

[98] Mcollum WH, Timoney PJ, Roberts AW, et al. Response of vaccinated and non-vaccinated mares to artificial insemination with semen from stallions persistently infected with equine arteritis virus. In: Powell DG, editor. Equine infectious diseases V: proceedings of the Fifth

International Conference on Equine Infectious Diseases. Kentucky: Kentucky University Press; 1988. p. 13–8.
[99] Timoney PJ, Umphenour NW, McCollum WH. Safety evaluation of a commercial modified live equine arteritis virus vaccine for use in stallions. In: Powell DG, editor. Equine infectious diseases V: proceedings of the Fifth International Conference on Equine Infectious Diseases. Kentucky: Kentucky University Press; 1988. p. 19–27.
[100] Fukunaga Y, Wada R, Hirasawa K, et al. Effect of the modified Bucyrus strain of equine arteritis virus experimentally inoculated into horses. Bull Equine Res Inst 1982;19:97–101.
[101] Timoney PJ, McCollum WH. Equine viral arteritis. Vet Clin North Am Equine Pract 1993; 9:295–309.
[102] McKinnon AO, Colbern GT, Collins JK, et al. Vaccination of stallions with a modified live equine arteritis virus vaccine. J Equine Vet Sci 1986;6:66–9.
[103] Timoney PJ, Klingeborn B, Lucas MH. A perspective on equine viral arteritis (infectious arteritis of horses). Rev Sci Tech 1996;15:1203–8.
[104] Moore BD, Balasuriya UB, Nurton JP, et al. Differentiation of strains of equine arteritis virus of differing virulence to horses by growth in equine endothelial cells. Am J Vet Res 2003;64:779–84.
[105] Giese M, Bahr U, Jakob NJ, et al. Stable and long-lasting immune response in horses after DNA vaccination against equine arteritis virus. Virus Genes 2002;25:159–67.
[106] Castillo-Olivares J, de Vries AA, Raamsman MJ, et al. Evaluation of a prototype sub-unit vaccine against equine arteritis virus comprising the entire ectodomain of the virus large envelope glycoprotein (G(L)): induction of virus-neutralizing antibody and assessment of protection in ponies. J Gen Virol 2001;82:2425–35.
[107] Waldridge BM, Wenzel JG, Ellis AC, et al. Serologic responses to eastern and western equine encephalomyelitis vaccination in previously vaccinated horses. Vet Ther 2003;4: 242–8.
[108] Holmes MA, Townsend HG, Kohler AK, et al. Immune responses to commercial equine vaccines against equine herpesvirus-1, equine influenza virus, eastern equine encephalomyelitis, and tetanus. Vet Immunol Immunopathol 2006;111:67–80.
[109] Spertzel RO, Kahn DE. Safety and efficacy of an attenuated Venezuelan equine encephalomyelitis vaccine for use in Equidae. J Am Vet Med Assoc 1971;159:731–8.
[110] Eddy GA, Martin DH, Reeves WC, et al. Field studies of an attenuated Venezuelan equine encephalomyelitis vaccine (strain TC-83). Infect Immun 1972;5:160–3.
[111] Walton TE, Alvarez O Jr, Buckwalter RM, et al. Experimental infection of horses with enzootic and epizootic strains of Venezuelan equine encephalomyelitis virus. J Infect Dis 1973;128:271–82.
[112] Oberste MS, Fraire M, Navarro R, et al. Association of Venezuelan equine encephalitis virus subtype IE with two equine epizootics in Mexico. Am J Trop Med Hyg 1998;59:100–7.
[113] Walton TE, Jochim MM, Barber TL, et al. Cross-protective immunity between equine encephalomyelitis viruses in equids. Am J Vet Res 1989;50:1442–6.
[114] Vanderwagen LC, Pearson JL, Franti CE, et al. A field study of persistence of antibodies in California horses vaccinated against western, eastern, and Venezuelan equine encephalomyelitis. Am J Vet Res 1975;36:1567–71.
[115] Ferguson JA, Reeves WC, Hardy JL. Antibody studies in ponies vaccinated with Venezuelan equine encephalomyelitis (strain TC-83) and other alphavirus vaccines. Am J Vet Res 1977;38:425–30.
[116] Moore RM Jr, Moulthrop JI, Sather GE, et al. Venezuelan equine encephalitis vaccination survey in Arizona and New Mexico, 1972. Public Health Rep 1977;92:357–60.
[117] Baker EF Jr, Sasso DR, Maness K, et al. Venezuelan equine encephalomyelitis vaccine (strain TC-83): a field study. Am J Vet Res 1978;39:1627–31.
[118] Ferguson JA, Reeves WC, Milby MM, et al. Study of homologous and heterologous antibody response in California horses vaccinated with attenuated Venezuelan equine encephalomyelitis vaccine (strain TC-83). Am J Vet Res 1978;39:371–6.

[119] Fine DL, Roberts BA, Teehee ML, et al. Venezuelan equine encephalitis virus vaccine candidate (V3526) safety, immunogenicity and efficacy in horses. Vaccine 2007;25:1868–76.
[120] Pratt WD, Davis NL, Johnston RE, et al. Genetically engineered, live attenuated vaccines for Venezuelan equine encephalitis: testing in animal models. Vaccine 2003;21:3854–62.
[121] Minke JM, Audonnet JC, Fischer L. Equine viral vaccines: the past, present and future. Vet Res 2004;35:425–43.
[122] Sweeney CR, Timoney JF, Newton JR, et al. Streptococcus equi infections in horses: guidelines for treatment, control, and prevention of strangles. J Vet Intern Med 2005;19: 123–34.
[123] Hoffman AM, Staempfli HR, Prescott JF, et al. Field evaluation of a commercial M-protein vaccine against Streptococcus equi infection in foals. Am J Vet Res 1991;52:589–92.
[124] Jorm LR. Strangles in horse studs; incidence, risk factors and effect of vaccination. Aust Vet J 1990;67:436–9.
[125] Bryant S, Brown KK, Lewis S, et al. Protection against strangles with an enzymatic *Streptococcus equi* extract. Vet Med 1985;80:58–70.
[126] Galan JE, Timoney JF. Immune complexes in purpura hemorrhagica of the horse contain IgA and M antigen of Streptococcus equi. J Immunol 1985;135:3134–7.
[127] Galan JE, Timoney JF. Mucosal nasopharyngeal immune responses of horses to protein antigens of Streptococcus equi. Infect Immun 1985;47:623–8.
[128] Sheoran AS, Sponseller BT, Holmes MA, et al. Serum and mucosal antibody isotype responses to M-like protein (SeM) of Streptococcus equi in convalescent and vaccinated horses. Vet Immunol Immunopathol 1997;59:239–51.
[129] Walker JA, Timoney JF. Construction of a stable non-mucoid deletion mutant of the Streptococcus equi Pinnacle vaccine strain. Vet Microbiol 2002;89:311–21.
[130] Kelly C, Bugg M, Robinson C, et al. Sequence variation of the SeM gene of Streptococcus equi allows discrimination of the source of strangles outbreaks. J Clin Microbiol 2006;44: 480–6.
[131] Jacobs AA, Goovaerts D, Nuijten PJ, et al. Investigations towards an efficacious and safe strangles vaccine: submucosal vaccination with a live attenuated Streptococcus equi. Vet Rec 2000;147:563–7.
[132] Quinn PJ, Markey BK, Carter ME, et al. Veterinary microbiology and microbial disease. Ames (IA): Blackwell Science Ltd; 2002.
[133] van Galen G, Delguste C, Sandersen C, et al. Tetanus in horses: a review of 31 cases. In: Handbook of presentations and free communications, BEVA Congress, Birmingham, UK, 13–16 September 2006. p. 203–4.
[134] Lohrer J, Radvila P. [Active tetanus prevention in the horse and the duration of immunity]. Schweiz Arch Tierheilkd 1970;112:307–14.
[135] Liefman CE. Combined active-passive immunisation of horses against tetanus. Aust Vet J 1980;56:119–22.
[136] Liefman CE. Active immunisation of horses against tetanus including the booster dose and its application. Aust Vet J 1981;57:57–60.
[137] Tasman A, Huygen FJA. Immunization against tetanus of patients given injections of anti-tetanus serum. Bull World Health Organ 1954;26:397.

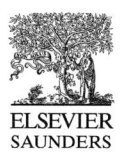

Evidence-Based Parasitology in Horses
Christine A. Uhlinger, VMD, MPH

Brandywine Equine Clinic, 350 Highland Road, Apex, NC 27502–5462, USA

There is a large body of literature on internal parasites in horses. Over the past 60 years, several scientific investigations have elucidated life cycles, described pathophysiologic responses to parasitic infection, evaluated effects of specific anthelmintics on parasite burden and fecal egg count, and assessed the putative "success" of various anthelmintic treatment regimens.

It is also true, however, that although much evidence has been gathered, the answers to some basic questions have not been answered. The emergence of parasites resistant to most available anthelmintics has raised new and troubling issues that have thrown some traditionally accepted tenets of parasite control into question. Thus, this article focuses on what has been established concerning the interaction of equine parasites and their hosts, highlighting those issues for which convincing data are still lacking.

Intestinal parasitism causes disease, doesn't it?

It is a widely accepted tenet of equine management that horses are at significant risk of disease unless parasite control measures are instituted. Centuries of clinical experience suggested that gastrointestinal distress, identified as "colic" and "ill thrift," was caused by "worms." Thus, for most modern horse owners, the rationale for the administration of anthelmintics is the prevention of colic. Within the past century, numerous scientific publications have described the pathophysiologic responses to parasitism and the relation of these responses to the clinical picture of weight loss, poor condition, gastrointestinal dysfunction, and the broad category of conditions grouped under the term *colic*.

Large strongyles

The association of large strongyle infection with lesions in the ileocolic arteries as well as in horses with severe and often fatal colic has been long

E-mail address: cau@bellsouth.net

established. The primary damage is done by the larval forms, which cause mucosal and subserosal damage to the gut before inflicting their well-known effect on the ileocolic arteries [1–4].

Although concern over large strongyle colic has decreased with the development of modern anthelmintics (most of which are effective in the prevention of significant large strongyle disease), this parasite is still present in equine populations. It is important to note that large strongyle colic still occurs, even in horses treated with apparently adequate anthelmintic programs [5]. In one review of 58 horses with recurrent colic, 4 had thromboembolic disease or verminous arteritis [6].

Small strongyles

Initially, there was more debate concerning the role of small strongyles as the cause for colic. Small strongyles are the predominant group of worms present in wild and domestic horses [7]. These species confine their migration to the submucosa of the large colon and cecum [8,9], where they may encyst in large numbers. It has been established that small strongyles may be pathogenic at times of penetration into and emergence from the large intestinal mucosa. Cyathostomes can undergo arrested larval development within the large intestinal mucosa for more than 2 years. When in the hypobiotic stage, small strongyles are difficult to treat with anthelmintics. The clinical manifestation occurs in the prepatent stage of infection. It has been documented that the clinical manifestation of small strongyle disease may be brought about by the administration of anthelmintics [10].

There is good evidence that small strongyle infection may result in poor condition, weight loss, failure to gain weight, and diarrhea [10–13]. The diarrhea is caused by an inflammatory enteropathy characterized by diarrhea and may be accompanied by edema and fever. These horses may exhibit a neutrophilia, decreases in total protein and albumin, and increases in β-globulin. Fecal egg counts are often negative [10,11], although adult and L4 larvae may be found in the feces. The effects on infection on young horses are more profound than the effects on older animals, and most reports of clinical cyathostomiasis have been in animals younger than 5 years of age [10,13].

There has been work on the development of diagnostic techniques for the prepatent stages of cyathostome infection [14] using serum IgG(T) responses to larval antigen complexes. If this test can be perfected, it would be a powerful tool in establishing the level of parasitism in an individual horse, in determining the role of cyathostome infection in gastrointestinal disease, and in evaluating anthelmintic programs. Currently, however, there are no accepted parameters to measure the subclinical impact of cyathostome infection in well-managed horses.

The association of small strongyle colic in adult horses is indirect at best, however. One study reported that an unusually high incidence of colic decreased after the horses were treated with anthelmintic regimens specifically designed to control small strongyles [15]. Another study found an increased incidence of colic in horses that had not been treated with ivermectin or moxidectin but treated with product that might be expected to control large strongyles [16].

Tapeworms

As was the case with small strongyles, the association between *Anoplocephala perfoliata* infection and significant clinical disease was long a topic of debate. Although heavy infections were associated with unthriftiness [17], their role in the cause of colic was long suspected but unproven. Recent work has strengthened the role of *A perfoliata* in the cause of some types of colic, however. This work indicated an association between levels of an antigen-specific equine IgG and IgG(T) and the intensity of infection with *A perfoliata* [18]. Subsequent studies with the assay demonstrated an association between tapeworm infection and the risk of ileal impaction colic and spasmodic colic [19,20]. A dose-response relation between infection intensity and risk of disease was also shown. Another study [21] demonstrated that the risk of ileal impaction was higher in horses that had not been treated with an anthelmintic effective against tapeworms than in those that had received treatment with products effective against these parasites.

When to treat

There is little controversy on the need to treat animals showing signs suggestive of parasitic disease or young animals, which are more susceptible to the effects of parasitic infection. Further, in view of this somewhat overwhelming body of work documenting the potential adverse effects of parasites on the adult horse, questioning the need for preventative strategies in this population seems heretical. The traditional view is that horses at pasture in nonarid regions are inevitably at risk of disease from parasites. Thus, it has been recommended that they should routinely be put on parasite control programs in the absence of the results of blood tests or fecal examinations, which are regarded as nonspecific at best and unreliable at worst [22]. Many veterinarians adhere to this approach, which is justified more or less reasonably under the "better safe than sorry" principle of practice.

It is also true, however, that many, if not most, well-managed horses, particularly well-nourished adult horses, tolerate parasitic burdens without apparent ill effects. There has been a recent report in the literature of the good health of research animals that have not been treated with anthelmintics for prolonged periods of up to 26 years [23]. It has also been observed that adult horses may be parasitized by millions of cyathostomes in the absence of recognizable clinical disease [24]. Indeed, it seems that horses acquire a resistance to cyathostome infection with age [25]. Host resistance seems to confer protection against disease rather than infection; thus, animals unlikely to express signs of disease continue to shed parasitic ova [26,27].

In sum, with the exception of the few studies cited previously, there is little support in the literature for the role of parasitism as a major risk factor for colic. It may be that the conditions in herds investigated in these studies are not generalizable to the larger equine population. Still, a meta-analysis evaluating risk factors in colic has failed to find an association with anthelmintic history or fecal egg count in horses that did and did not experience colic [28]. These types of observations suggest a need for re-evaluation of high-intensity anthelmintic regimens in herds of apparently healthy adult animals.

Anthelmintics kill worms, don't they?

Most of the available published literature on equine anthelmintics consists of reports of the effect of various products on reductions in parasite burdens or fecal egg counts. Of the two, studies using reductions in fecal egg counts are more common. Combination studies have shown that products that decrease fecal egg count also result in the elimination at least some proportion of the worm burden [28–32]. It has been noted that evaluations based on fecal egg count indicate more activity by anthelmintics than assessments based on the actual removal of worms, however [33].

The inability of usual doses of many anthelmintics to kill hypobiotic cyathostome larvae has been well documented. Of the currently available anthelmintics, only moxidectin and fenbendazole (at high doses) have been shown to be effective against the encysted larval stages of the parasites [10].

Unfortunately, the selection pressure caused by frequent administration of anthelmintics has resulted in the development of resistance of small strongyle parasites to the effects of benzimidazoles (BZDs) and pyrantel salts. BZD-resistant small strongyles have been identified worldwide. More recently, there have been reports of populations of cyathostomes resistant to pyrantel salts [34–36]. In addition, many researchers consider the development of ivermectin or moxidectin resistance as inevitable [24]. This concern about anthelmintic resistance is one of the factors fueling re-evaluation of current methods of parasite control in the horse.

Effective parasite control programs rely on the administration of anthelmintics to all herd members at frequent intervals, right?

The well-accepted goal of preventative parasite control programs is to minimize parasitic damage by reducing the number of infective larvae in the environment. The intent of this approach is to reduce the number of infective larval stages by the removal of adult egg-producing parasites from the host.

It has been frequently stated in the literature that the best treatment interval is ideally selected with an eye to parasite prepatent periods, life cycles, climatic and environmental variables, and management and health concerns of individual farms. In practice, most owners and veterinarians pick one interval and stick with it. According to some surveys, treatment every 8 to 12 weeks using anthelmintics of two or three classes is the most common regimen in use [37]. There is no reason to believe that this treatment interval, or indeed any specific treatment interval, is appropriate in all animals or herds, however. This interval may be insufficient in herds showing signs of animals with parasitic disease [15] or in herds of young susceptible animals grazing contaminated pastures. Equally, an 8- to 12-week interval may be unnecessarily short in herds of healthy adult horses or in animals with limited turn out [38,39]. Given the local seasonal transmission patterns of parasites in most climates and management systems that keep horses off pasture at certain times of the year, it is unlikely that the same treatment interval is appropriate year round in any group of animals. The reliance on a set treatment interval is probably primarily chosen because such a treatment schedule is easy to remember and implement.

The repeated administration of anthelmintics at short intervals has been associated with the development of anthelmintic resistance. As anthelmintic choices dwindle, there is an increasing interest in alternate methods of parasite control and a re-evaluation of the idea that the goal of parasite control is to eradicate parasitic infection totally. Strategic treatments based on an understanding of strongyle epidemiology have been suggested [22]. This program administers larvicidal treatment to animals joining the herd and to all herd members when larval burdens are high and transmission is low (often, during winter in the temperate regions of the United States). Animals with fecal egg counts higher than an "acceptable" level (stated as 100 or 300 eggs per gram [epg]) are then to be treated at times of high transmission. This approach depends on an intimate knowledge of transmission patterns in various climates, however, and there is reason to suspect that these vary regionally and even yearly [26,38,40].

Most recently, there has been a growing interest in "targeted" or "selected" treatments, in which treatment is limited to animals demonstrating signs of parasitic disease and animals that shed an unusually high number of parasitic ova in the feces. This strategy developed out of the observation that horses may be relatively consistent in the number of eggs they shed [41,42]; horses with high (or low) fecal egg counts at one assessment are likely to have high (or low) fecal egg counts at subsequent assessments. Therefore, efforts to minimize the contamination of pasture with parasitic ova while minimizing the use of anthelmintics rely on treating the horses most likely to be shedding high numbers of parasitic ova. It has been suggested that mature horses with consistently low fecal egg counts need not be treated [39,43]. This strategy has been used with apparent success in maintaining low fecal egg counts in a herd infected with BZD- and pyrantel-resistant small strongyles [21]. Although these strategies are likely to minimize the contamination of grazing areas with parasitic larvae, there is no assurance that this promotes the well-being of the individual herd members. Indeed, it may well be that some horses with low fecal egg counts would benefit from antiparasitic treatment. Therefore, the effect of these targeted programs on the health of the horses is no more certain that the effect of treatment at some set interval.

Different strategies for control have been suggested in a report describing the use of anthelmintics in Denmark, where these drugs are only available by prescription and their use for routine preventative treatment is not permitted [44]. Most veterinarians surveyed used fecal egg counts for diagnosis and surveillance. Treatment decisions were based on cutoff values from 20 to 500 epg. Treatment without prior fecal examinations was most common for young horses and when there was clinical suspicion of parasitic disease. The authors of this study noted that control strategies based on surveillance make huge demands on the accuracy and reliability of the test. Further, they note that the use of the fecal egg test has the potential to overlook serious infections, because fecal egg counts lack sensitivity and specificity [45].

If herd or individual animal fecal egg counts are kept low, all is well, right?

In targeted programs, the cutoff point for selecting animals for anthelmintic treatment has variously been stated as 100 or less epg [21] or 100 or less epg for foals and 300 or less epg for adult horses [22]. The outcome measures for defining the success of these anthelmintic programs is often given as 100 or less epg or 200 or less epg.

It is important to be aware of the fact that all these cutoff points are chosen arbitrarily, based on best guesses in regard to acceptable levels of parasitic burdens in the individual or in the environment. The levels selected for herd management are based on assumptions concerning the effect of a given level of fecal shedding on pasture larval counts, which may or may not be accurate. In an individual animal, there is no reliable correlation between fecal egg count and parasitic burden; indeed, the most serious manifestations of strongyle disease may occur in the absences of ova in the feces. Further, as previously mentioned, animals that have acquired resistance to parasitic disease continue to shed parasitic markers. This essentially leaves veterinarians without a reliable marker of subclinical parasitic disease. Until assays that allow an estimate of actual cyathostome burden exist, the reliance on fecal egg count is likely to continue.

The real measure of the success of parasite control programs is the well-being of the herd members. Although fecal egg counts are widely used for surveillance and management, it must be acknowledged that the fecal egg counts are a poor proxy for the health and well-being of the animals.

So where are we now?

Despite the large body of scientific work into the pathophysiology of parasitic infections and the effect of anthelmintics, basic questions concerning parasite control have not been answered. Do adult horses need regular treatment at a set interval? If so, what are the variables that control that interval? What are the best strategies for minimizing the effects of parasitism while maintaining the efficacy of ivermectin or moxidectin? Until there is a more or less reliable measure of the level of parasitism in individual horses, these questions are likely to go largely unanswered. Furthermore, even if veterinarians identify new parasite control strategies, are they likely to be able to get horse owners to implement them?

In the United States over the past 20 years, the administration and selection of anthelmintics have largely passed out of the hands of veterinarians and into the hands of the horse-owning public. The selection of anthelmintics by the owners is largely driven by marketing and is not affected by cost or concerns about anthelmintic resistance [37]. The selection of the treatment interval is largely driven by fundamentally unsupported belief in the necessity for an 8- to 12-week treatment interval. As anthelmintic choices dwindle, there is a compelling need for the participation of the veterinarian in the design of appropriate anthelmintic treatments and prevention strategies. Whether the horse-owning public can be weaned away from their belief in the need for "cookbook" anthelmintic schedules remains to be seen.

References

[1] Klei TR. Morphologic and clinicopathologic changes following Strongylus vulgaris infections of immune and nonimmune ponies. Am J Vet Res 1982;43:1300–7.

[2] Klei TR. Antibody responses of young ponies to initial and challenge infections of Strongylus vulgaris. Vet Parasitol 1983;3:187–98.

[3] Wynne E. Antigenic analysis of tissues and excretory and secretory products from Strongylus vulgaris. Can J Comp Med 1980;45:259–65.

[4] Lyons ET, Drudge JH, Tolliver SC. Ivermectin: activity against larval Strongylus vulgaris and adult Trichostrongylus axei in experimental infections in ponies. Am J Vet Res 1982; 43(8):1449–50.

[5] DeLay J, Peregrine AS, Parsons DA. Verminous arteritis in a 3-month-old Thoroughbred foal. Can Vet J 2001;42(4):289–91.

[6] Hillyer MH, Mair TS. Recurrent colic in the mature horse: a retrospective review of 58 cases. Equine Vet J 1997;29(6):421–4.

[7] Young KE, Garza V, Snowden K, et al. Parasite diversity and anthelmintic resistance in two herds of horses. Vet Parasitol 1999;85(2–3):205–14.

[8] Ogbourne CP. Epidemiological studies on horses infected with nematodes of the family Trichonematidae (Witenberg, 1925). Int J Parasitol 1975;5(6):667–72.

[9] Ogbourne CP. The prevalence, relative abundance, and site distribution of nematodes of the subfamily Cyathostominae in horses killed in Britain. J Helminthol 1976;50: 203–14.

[10] Lyons ET, Drudge JH, Tolliver. Larval cyathostomiasis. Vet Clin North Am Equine Pract 2000;16(3):501–13.

[11] Smets K, Shaw DJ, Deprez P, et al. Diagnosis of larval cyathostominosis in horses in Belgium. Vet Rec 1999;144(24):665–8.
[12] Steinbach T, Bauer C, Sasse H, et al. Small strongyle infection: consequences of larvicidal treatment of horses with fenbendazole and moxidectin. Vet Parasitol 2006;139(1–3): 115–31, [Epub 2006 May 3].
[13] Love S, Murphy D, Mellor D. Pathogenicity of cyathostome infection. Vet Parasitol 1999; 85(2–3):113–21.
[14] Dowdall SM, Proudman CJ, Klei TR, et al. Characterisation of IgG(T) serum antibody responses to two larval antigen complexes in horses naturally- or experimentally-infected with cyathostomins. Int J Parasitol 2004;34(1):101–8.
[15] Uhlinger C. Effects of three anthelmintic schedules on the incidence of colic in horses. Equine Vet J 1990;22(4):251–4.
[16] Hillyer MH, Taylor FG, French NP. A cross-sectional study of colic in horses on Thoroughbred training premises in the British Isles in 1997. Equine Vet J 2001;33(4):380–5.
[17] Proudman CJ, Edwards GB. Are tapeworms associated with equine colic? A case control study. Equine Vet J 1993;25(3):224–6.
[18] Proudman CJ, Trees AJ. Correlation of antigen specific IgG and IgG(T) responses with Anoplocephala perfoliata infection intensity in the horse. Parasite Immunol 1996;18(10):499–506.
[19] Proudman CJ, Holdstock NB. Investigation of an outbreak of tapeworm-associated colic in a training yard. Equine Vet J Suppl 2000 Jun;(32):37–41.
[20] Proudman CJ, French NP, Trees AJ. Tapeworm infection is a significant risk factor for spasmodic colic and ileal impaction colic in the horse. Equine Vet J 1998;30(3):194–9.
[21] Little D, Blikslager AT. Factors associated with development of ileal impaction in horses with surgical colic: 78 cases (1986–2000). Equine Vet J 2002;34(5):464–8.
[22] Herd RP, Coles GC. Slowing the spread of anthelmintic resistant nematodes of horses in the United Kingdom. Vet Rec 1995;136(19):481–5.
[23] Mendell C. Researchers complete 40-year parasite study. The Horse. September 26, 2006, Article #7754. Available at: http://www.thehorse.com/ViewArticle.aspx?ID=7754&; kw=Lyons. Accessed April 27, 2007.
[24] Love S. Treatment and prevention of intestinal parasite-associated disease. Vet Clin North Am Equine Pract 2003;19(3):791–806.
[25] Klei TR, Chapman MR. Immunity in equine cyathostome infections. Vet Parasitol 1999; 85(2–3):123–33, [discussion: 133–6, 215–25].
[26] Reinemeyer CR. Small strongyles. Recent advances. Vet Clin North Am Equine Pract 1986;2(2):281–312.
[27] Goncalves S, Julliand V, Leblond A. Risk factors associated with colic in horses. Vet Res 2002;33(6):641–52.
[28] Tolliver SC, Lyons ET, Drudge JH, et al. Critical tests of thiabendazole, oxibendazole, and oxfendazole for drug resistance of population-B equine small strongyles (1989 and 1990). Am J Vet Res 1993;54(6):908–13.
[29] Lyons ET, Tolliver SC, Drudge JH. Critical tests in equids with fenbendazole alone or combined with piperazine: particular reference to activity on benzimidazole-resistant small strongyles. Vet Parasitol 1983;12(1):91–8.
[30] Drudge JH, Lyons ET. Methods in the evaluation of antiparasitic drugs in the horse. Am J Vet Res 1977;38(10):1581–6.
[31] Drudge JH, Lyons ET, Tolliver SC, et al. Critical tests and clinical trials on oxibendazole in horses with special reference to removal of Parascaris equorum. Am J Vet Res 1979;40(6): 758–61.
[32] Drudge JH, Lyons ET, Tolliver SC. Benzimidazole resistance of equine strongyles—critical tests of six compounds against population B. Am J Vet Res 1979;40(4):590–4.
[33] Lyons E. Population-S benzimidazole- and tetrahydropyrimidine-resistant small strongyles in a pony herd in Kentucky (1977–1999): effects of anthelmintic treatment on the parasites as determined in critical tests. Parasitol Res 2003;91(5):407–11.

[34] Brazik EL, Luquire JT, Little D. Pyrantel pamoate resistance in horses receiving daily administration of pyrantel tartrate. J Am Vet Med Assoc 2006;228(1):101–3.
[35] Tarigo-Martinie JL, Wyatt AR, Kaplan RM. Prevalence and clinical implications of anthelmintic resistance in cyathostomes of horses. J Am Vet Med Assoc 2001;218(12):1957–60.
[36] Kaplan RM, Klei TR, Lyons ET, et al. Prevalence of anthelmintic resistant cyathostomes on horse farms. J Am Vet Med Assoc 2004;225(6):903–10.
[37] Lloyd S, Smith J, Connan RM, et al. Parasite control methods used by horse owners: factors predisposing to the development of anthelmintic resistance in nematodes. Vet Rec 2000; 146(17):487–92.
[38] Reinemeyer CR. Current concerns about control programs in temperate climates. Vet Parasitol 1999;85(2–3):163–9, [discussion 169–72, 215–25].
[39] Eysker M, van Doorn DC, Lems SN, et al. [Frequent deworming in horses; it usually does not do any good, but it often harms]. Tijdschr Diergeneeskd 2006;131(14–15):524–30, [in Dutch].
[40] Nielsen MK, Kaplan RM, Thamsborg SM, et al. Climatic influences on development and survival of free-living stages of equine strongyles: implications for worm control strategies and managing anthelmintic resistance. Vet J 2006 [Epub ahead of print].
[41] Nielsen MK, Haaning N, Olsen SN. Strongyle egg shedding consistency in horses on farms using selective therapy in Denmark. Vet Parasitol 2006;135(3–4):333–5, [Epub 2005 Oct 13].
[42] Dopfer D, Kerssens CM, Meijer YG, et al. Shedding consistency of strongyle-type eggs in Dutch boarding horses. Vet Parasitol 2004;124(3–4):249–58.
[43] Gomez HH, Georgi JR. Equine helminth infections: control by selective chemotherapy. Equine Vet J 1991;23(3):198–200.
[44] Nielsen MK, Monrad J, Olsen SN. Prescription-only anthelmintics—a questionnaire survey of strategies for surveillance and control of equine strongyles in Denmark. Vet Parasitol 2006;135(1):47–55, [Epub 2005 Nov 23].
[45] Coles CC, Jackson F, Pomroy WE, et al. The detection of anthelmintic resistance in nematodes of veterinary importance [review]. Vet Parasitol 2006;136(3–4):167–85, [Epub 2006 Jan 19].

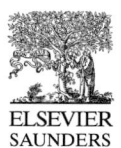

Evidence-Based Equine Dentistry: Preventive Medicine

James L. Carmalt, MA, VetMB, MVetSc, MRCVS*

Scone Veterinary Hospital, 106 Liverpool Street, Scone, NSW 2337, Australia

Equine dentistry is one of the most common tasks performed by large animal practitioners [1]. Dental publications exist from circa 600 BC. By the time of Aristotle (330 BC), ageing horses by their teeth and the effects of periodontal disease had been noted and treatments described. Knowledge progressed slowly, and it was not until Markham (1610–1723) that the technique to remove sharp overgrowths on the lateral edges of the upper cheek teeth to prevent soft tissue damage was reported. Despite this incredible history, equine dentistry sadly remains an art and not a science.

An evidence-based approach to equine dentistry is poorly used because of the perceived importance of the intervention by veterinarians and owners. Consequently, a critical evaluation of what is being achieved by so-called "occlusal equilibration" or other routine procedures is often not performed. The benefits of interventional dentistry (ie, oral extraction, repulsion in cases of diseased teeth) are obvious and preclude the need for randomized controlled trials, whereas the importance of routine dental floating (also known as occlusal equilibration) has not been fully determined.

The purpose of this article is to review the veterinary literature to evaluate the evidence supporting the role of equine dentistry in weight loss or gain and as a cause of poor performance. Several modern equine texts cite dental disease as a possible cause of oral pain, colic, gastrointestinal impaction, weight loss, and poor performance [2–7]. It has also been stated that horses focus on the pain rather than on performance when experiencing oral discomfort, which supposedly leads to a failure to respond to bit cues by evading the action of the bit or by ignoring it completely. The research behind these accepted statements is completely lacking. The literature does not conclusively define oral pain in the horse, nor does it confirm that poor

---

* Western College of Veterinary Medicine, University of Saskatchewan, 52 Campus Drive, Saskatoon, SK, S7N5B4, Canada.
  E-mail address: carmalt_vet@hotmail.com

dentition affects performance or weight loss or is a factor in the pathogenesis of colic. In addition to this, a recent prospective, matched, case-controlled study examining dietary and other management factors associated with colic in horses did not find a statistical association between horses floated at least once yearly and control horses [8].

Occlusal equilibration (floating, rasping, or filing) is the most common equine dental procedure performed [9], the goal of which has been stated as "... to maintain the symmetry and balance of the arcades and to allow a free elliptical chewing motion" [10]. This single goal has subsequently been refined to focus on four separate but integrated goals: (1) to relieve discomfort associated with oral soft tissue injuries caused by sharp enamel points, (2) to improve mastication and digestion of feedstuffs, (3) to alleviate stresses on abnormally worn teeth, and (4) to prevent discomfort associated with the bit, [11] all of which should hopefully improve mastication, maintain proper alignment, and increase the longevity of the dental arcade. Nowhere in this definition does it state that occlusal equilibration improves performance or weight gain.

Occlusal equilibration and weight loss

Consider a 15-year-old horse that is presented to a veterinary practice in poor body condition. The history is one of insidious weight loss over the past 6 months. Most readers have automatically formulated a differential diagnosis list and treatment plan during the preceding two sentences. The author would suggest that most veterinarians would have parasites and dental disease at the top of the list, with deworming and a dental float as a treatment plan.

The literature would suggest that dental malocclusions alone play a limited role in weight loss. Staggeringly, despite a 2600-year history of dental publications, publication of the results of the first clinical trial only occurred in 1995. Trials in 1995 [12] and 2001 [13] examined the role of dentition in equine nutrition using clinical trials. The former study pronounced a benefit of dental floating on feed digestibility, whereas the latter did not. Careful examination of the former study reveals the use of historical controls and small numbers of animals in the study, which questions the validity of the conclusions reached.

Numerous studies have been published subsequently. These suggest that although occlusal equilibration increases the rostrocaudal mobility (RCM) of the mandible, it does not improve feed digestibility, fecal particle size, or weight gain in the pregnant mare. Cheek tooth occlusal angle and molar occlusion percentage also have no discernable effect on the same outcome variables [14–17]. In the first of these studies, the authors found that it was the feed group and not the treatment group (floated or controls) that had a significant effect on weight gain. There was also no statistical interaction between feed and treatment group. This information suggests that it is the feed and not the occlusal equilibration that accounts for the weight gain. This is significant, because in clinical cases of weight loss where occlusal equilibration has been performed, it is common veterinary practice to alter the nutrition in favor of a higher quality feed. Credit for improvement may go to the procedure when, in fact, the nutritional changes are responsible.

Studies showing a lack of effect of routine dental procedures [13,15] have been subjected to a certain amount of criticism. One of the major critiques has been that normal horses were used for the study, and thus do not represent the population as a whole. Although the first portion of the argument is certainly true, current legislation rightly precludes the use of cachectic animals in a clinical trial. With respect to a trial conducted in 2004, investigators knew categorically that the horses had never had their teeth floated. Horses ranging in age from 3 to 18 years that had a variety of dental malocclusions commonly cited as needing correction (and potentially the cause of weight loss) [15]. If these normal horses—horses that had never had dental procedures but had a variety of dental abnormalities—were not to show benefit from treatment, perhaps the definition of a clinically significant malocclusion or "normal" should be adjusted.

It is important to note that the aforementioned reports have focused on dental malocclusions, namely because this is the main focus of occlusal equilibration and the portion of equine dentistry that is most easily understood. Nevertheless, this is likely to prove a shortsighted view of the oral cavity; it is soft tissue pathologic conditions (and the prevention thereof) that should be under scrutiny. The interaction between dental malocclusions and periodontal disease is complex, however, and not fully understood in most cases.

One dental malocclusion consistently leading to the development of periodontal disease is a valve diastema. Congenital or acquired in nature, diastemata are abnormal gaps between teeth and refer (in the horse) almost exclusively to the cheek teeth. Subcategorization of the pathologic findings into open or closed/valved is based on the architecture of the boundary walls of the space [18]. The open diastema allows cycling of feed material through the space with little to no concurrent bacterial putrefaction and periodontal disease. Conversely, the valve diastema prevents egress of feed material and leads to periodontal disease, which itself has been described as "one of the most painful conditions in the horse's mouth" and "one which is difficult to treat" [19]. In select cases, treatment of the diastema (a dental malocclusion) may to lead to resolution of periodontal disease and, in early cases, to cessation of clinical signs and weight gain.

Occlusal equilibration and performance

There is a strong anecdotal history of the link between equine performance and dentition. "Performance" is a difficult word to define fully in respect to the horse. It may mean feed conversion ratios in feedlot animals, speed in the racehorse (eg, Thoroughbred, trotter/pacer, barrel horse), or judged score in the show and dressage horse. Making claims as to the effectiveness of a dental procedure with respect to performance is difficult and should be tightly defined to avoid exaggeration.

The detrimental effect of "wolf teeth" (rudimentary first premolars) on performance is the focus of heated debate among veterinarians involved in equine dentistry. Even among ourselves, veterinarians can come to no common understanding with regard to the importance of this tooth. Some may state that "no wolf tooth has ever done a horse any good," and others may claim that they have "never seen a wolf tooth cause a problem with respect to performance." As a result of their personal perspective, some clinicians routinely remove wolf teeth of all horses going into training, whereas others reserve the right to wait until a problem develops and then remove the offending tooth. Once again, however, there are no clinical data to substantiate either of these views.

Occlusal equilibration increases the RCM of the mandible, and authors have suggested that the amount of RCM may be correlated with height or weight (because heavy-breed horses have a greater range of motion than do light-breed horses). They have theorized further that RCM of the mandible is an important aspect of performance, especially in those equine disciplines that require extreme poll flexion, such as dressage [14].

Sharp lateral cingulae and other perceived dental abnormalities on the upper cheek teeth have been linked statistically to the presence of buccal ulceration in the horse [15]. Theoretically, soft tissue pathologic conditions may have a negative effect on performance. A recent blind, randomized, controlled clinical trial examining the effect of occlusal equilibration on dressage horse performance failed to find a correlation between treatment group (occlusal equilibration and placebo treatment) and performance or between increased RCM and improved performance [20]. Some criticisms of this study are that the judged scores are wholly subjective (as is the nature of the dressage discipline) and that there was only a short time between pre- and posttreatment testing, possibly negating the positive benefits of the procedure if such benefits were to require time to be recognized. The horses in this study had not had occlusal equilibration performed in more than a year, they did have dental abnormalities, and any immediate relief should have been apparent.

The major problem, insofar as conducting good studies on the necessity for and the benefits of commonly advocated dental procedures is concerned, is that performance horses (however defined) are kept and trained within their chosen discipline to win. For this reason, randomized, controlled, performance-related clinical trials are difficult to perform in equine dentistry. Owners or trainers are unwilling to accept or become enrolled in a clinical trial, especially if they perceive a performance-limiting condition in their horse. This is especially true when winning comes with financial gain or prestige.

As a result, many upper level performance horses may have their teeth "done" at least every 6 months and more frequently in some cases. The "benefit" in these cases may be to the rider and not to the horse, even possibly resulting in subconscious adjustments of bit-induced cues by the former.

Summary

In spite of the difficulties posed in evaluating the effect of occlusal equilibration on performance and weight loss or gain, the current resurgence of interest in equine dentistry is driving the need for knowledge. Routine occlusal equilibration is commonly performed. The treatment interval and abnormalities that constitute "malocclusions of significance" are still not known. There is obviously a level of malocclusion that is clinically silent. It is certainly possible that these malocclusions will continue to develop and may lead to further problems. Currently, however, it is not fully understood what is normal. Nor is it understood whether it is pain or a mechanical impediment to jaw motion (or a combination of the two) that purportedly leads certain malocclusions to affect feed digestibility or performance. This leaves the most basic question unanswered: when should occlusal equilibration be performed and on what basis?

It is of paramount importance that the equine veterinarian approach dental problems in the horse with an open mind. Equine dentistry can generate a significant portion of practice income. Although that, in itself, makes dentistry attractive, veterinarians also have an ethical responsibility to justify not only the procedure, but also the extent and frequency by which they are performed. The author believes that a complete oral examination (comprising sedation and the use of a full-mouth speculum, mirror, and some method of illumination) every 6 to 12 months is acceptable to identify dental malocclusions or other dental pathologic conditions that may become clinically significant in time. In the author's opinion, blanket statements as to the need for biannual occlusal equilibration are not acceptable and can certainly not be supported by any evidence.

The field of equine dentistry would benefit from multifaceted research. There is a lack of basic biomechanical research with respect to dentition and the temporomandibular joint. Tightly controlled studies investigating the effect of occlusal equilibration on performance across different disciplines and the true effect of wolf teeth on performance in the horse need to be done. It is incredible in that in the field of clinical equine dentistry, so much is performed in the face of so little published research.

References

[1] Traub-Dargatz JL, Salman MD, Ross JL. Medical problems of adult horses as ranked by equine practitioners. J Am Vet Med Assoc 1991;198:1745–7.
[2] Jones SL. Oral diseases. In: Reed SM, Bayly WM, Sellon DC, editors. Equine internal medicine. 2nd edition. Philadelphia: Saunders; 2004. p. 848.
[3] Dart AJ, Dowling BA, Hodgson DR. Large intestine. In: Auer JA, Stick JA, editors. Equine surgery. 2nd edition. Philadelphia: W.B. Saunders Company; 1999. p. 266.

[4] White NA, Lopes MAF. Large colon impaction. In: Current therapy in equine medicine. 5th edition. Philadelphia: Saunders; 2003. p. 131.
[5] Hanson RR. Diseases of the large colon that can result in colic. In: Mair T, Divers T, Ducharme N, editors. Manual of equine gastroenterology. Philadelphia: Saunders; 2002. p. 279.
[6] Knottenbelt DC. The systemic effects of dental disease. In: Baker GJ, Easley J, editors. Equine dentistry. Philadelphia: WB Saunders; 1999. p. 127–38.
[7] Knottenbelt DC. Poor performance: what role do alimentary tract functions have to play? In: Lindner A, editor. The elite dressage and three-day-event horse. 2nd Conference on equine Sports Medicine and Science, Arbeitsgruppe Pferde; 2002. p. 61–7.
[8] Cohen ND, Gibbs PG, Woods AM. Dietary and other management factors associated with colic in horses. J Am Vet Med Assoc 1999;215:53–60.
[9] Scrutchfield WL. Dental prophylaxis. In: Baker GJ, Easley J, editors. Equine dentistry. Philadelphia: WB Saunders; 1999. p. 185–205.
[10] Fischer D, Easley J. Floating: making equine dentistry a practice profit center. Large Animal Veterinarian 1994 Nov-Dec;16–22.
[11] Easley J. Corrective dental procedures. In: Baker GJ, Easley J, editors. Equine dentistry. 2nd edition. Philadelphia: Elsevier Limited; 2005. p. 221–47.
[12] Gatta D, Krusic L, Casini L, et al. Influence of corrected teeth on digestibility of two types of diets in pregnant mares. In: Proceedings 14th Symposium Equine Nutrition and Physiology Society 1995;326–31.
[13] Ralston SL, Foster DL, Divers T, et al. Effect of dental correction on feed digestibility in horses. Equine Vet J 2001;33(4):390–3.
[14] Carmalt JL, Townsend HGG, Allen AL. A preliminary study to examine the effect of dental correction on rostro-caudal mobility of the equine mandible. J Am Vet Med Assoc 2003;223: 666–9.
[15] Carmalt JL, Townsend HGG, et al. The effect of dental correction on weight gain, body condition score, feed digestibility and fecal particle size in the pregnant mare. J Am Vet Med Assoc 2004;225:1889–93.
[16] Carmalt JL, Townsend HGG, Cymbaluk NJ. The effect of premolar and molar occlusal angle on feed digestibility, water balance and fecal particle size in horses. J Am Vet Med Assoc 2005;227:110–3.
[17] Carmalt JL, Allen AL. The effect of rostro-caudal mobility of the mandible on feed digestibility and fecal particle size in the horse. J Am Vet Med Assoc 2006;229(8):1275–8.
[18] Carmalt JL. Understanding the equine diastema. Equine Vet Educ 2003;15(1):34–5.
[19] Dixon PM, Tremaine WH, Pickles K, et al. Equine dental disease (part 2): a long-term study of 400 cases: disorders of development and eruption and variations in position of cheek teeth. Equine Vet J 1999;31:519–28.
[20] Carmalt JL, Carmalt KP, Barber SM, et al. The effect of occlusal equilibration on sport horse performance (dressage). J Vet Dent 2006;23(4):226–30.

Index

Note: Page numbers of article titles are in **boldface** type.

A

Age, effects on glucose and insulin metabolism, 369

Airway(s)
 lower, respiratory conditions of, 215–223
 upper, diseases of, evidence-based respiratory medicine for, 223–224

Analgesia/analgesics, for colic, 244–245

Angular limb deformities, evidence-based surgery for, 468–469

Animal fecal egg counts, 514

Anthelmintic(s)
 in effective parasite control programs, 512–514
 worms killed by, 512

Antibiotic(s), infusion of, postbreeding, in broodmares, 387–390

Antioxidant(s), for PPID, 355–356

Arteritis, viral, evidence-based immunizations for, 495–497

Arthrodesis, in evidence-based surgery, 467–468

Arytenoidectomy, for laryngeal hyperplasia, 234

B

Bandage(s), incisional, incisional complications associated with, 279–280

Bee pollen, as nutritional supplement, 376–377

Bias, publication, drug use and, 208

Biomechanical effects of shoeing and farriery techniques, evidence-based assessment of, **425–442**. See also *Shoeing, biomechanical effects of.*

Biomechanical terminology, 426–428

Bone(s), third metacarpal, dorsal cortical fractures of, evidence-based surgery for, 470–471

Broodmare practice, procedures in, **385–402**
 postbreeding antibiotic infusion, 387–390
 progesterone supplementation in early pregnancy, 390–392
 retained placenta, 393–398
 thyroid supplementation, 385–387

C

Catecholamine-resistance vasodilatory shock, vasopressin and norepinephrine for, 306–307

Celiotomy
 exploratory. See *Exploratory celiotomy.*
 repeat
  incisional complications associated with, 280
  postoperative ileus and, 283

Cervical vertebral compressive myelopathy (CVCM)
 clinical signs of, 319–320
 evidence-based approach to, **317–328**
 imaging of, 320–327
 neurologic examination in, 319–320
 pathogenesis of, 317–319
 pathologic findings in, 317–319

Chip fractures, evidence-based surgery for, 464–465

Cisapride, for ileus, 246–247

Colic
 analgesia for, 244–245
 epidemiology of, 255–258
 evidence-based gastrointestinal surgery for, **267–292**. See also *Gastrointestinal surgery, evidence-based.*
 risk factors for, 255–258
 treatment of, 258–261

Colloid solutions, crystalloids vs., in resuscitation of hypovolemic patients, 300–305

Colon, large, renospenic entrapment of, 247–249

Conflict of interest, drug use and, 208

Conformation, shoeing and, injuries related to, 437–438

Corticotropin stimulation test, in PPID diagnosis, 348

Critical care, evidence-based medicine in, **293–316**
colloid solutions vs. crystalloids, in resuscitation of hypovolemic patients, 300–305
dobutamine in, 308–310
EGDT in, 294, 295–300
norepinephrine in, 310–312
phenylephrine in, 310
vasopressin, in septic patients, 305–308

Crystalloid(s), colloid solutions vs., in resuscitation of hypovolemic patients, 300–305

Cushing's syndrome
described, 336–337
evidence-based literature on, **336–357**
historical background of, 336–337
incidence of, 336

CVCM. See *Cervical vertebral compressive myelopathy (CVCM)*.

Cyproheptadine, for PPID, 353

D

Dentistry, equine, evidence-based, **519–524**. See also *Equine dentistry, evidence-based*.

Dexamethasone suppression test, low-dose, in antemortem diagnosis of PPID, 343–344

Dexamethasone suppression test/ corticotropin stimulation test, 348

Dexamethasone suppression test/ thyrotropin-releasing hormone stimulation test, 345–346

DIP joint. See *Distal interphalangeal (DIP) joint*.

Distal interphalangeal (DIP) joint, shoeing effects on, 432

Diurnal variation, effects on glucose and insulin metabolism, 369

Dobutamine, in evidence-based medicine in critical care, 308–310

Domperidone, pituitary gland effects of, in PPID diagnosis, 351–352

Dopaminergic inhibition, loss of, pituitary gland effects of, 338–340

Dorsal cortical fractures, of third metacarpal bone, evidence-based surgery for, 470–471

Drug(s)
absorption of, 205–206
appropriateness of, 207–208
conflict of interest and publication bias, 208
described, 201–203
efficacy of, 209–210
systemic effective concentration of, 205–206
treatment effects of
accurate diagnosis in, 206–207
if disease does not exist, 206

Drug use. See also *Drug(s)*.
evidence-based
herbs, 208–209
in equine medicine and surgery, **201–213**
clinical examples of, 210–211

E

Early goal-directed therapy (EGDT), 294, 295–300

Echinacea, as nutritional supplement, 377

EGDT. See *Early goal-directed therapy (EGDT)*.

EIPH. See *Exercise-induced pulmonary hemorrhage (EIPH)*.

Encephalitides, equine, evidence-based immunizations for, 497–498

Epiglottic entrapment, upper respiratory surgery for, 239–240

Equine dentistry, evidence-based, **519–524**
occlusal equilibration and performance in, 521–523
occlusal equilibration and weight loss in, 520–521

Equine encephalitides, evidence-based immunizations for, 497–498

Equine gastric ulcer syndrome
evidence-based medicine for, 253–255
risk factors for, 252–253

Equine herpesviruses 1 and 4, evidence-based immunizations for, 488–491

Equine influenza virus, evidence-based immunizations for, 485–488

Equine viral arteritis (EVA), evidence-based immunizations for, 495–497

EVA. See *Equine viral arteritis (EVA)*.

Evidence-based approach, to clinical questions in neurology, **317–328**

Evidence-based assessment, of biomechanical effects of shoeing and farriery techniques, **425–442**. See also *Shoeing, biomechanical effects of*.

Evidence-based drug use, in equine medicine and surgery, **201–213**. See also *Drug(s); Drug use, evidence-based, in equine medicine and surgery*.

Evidence-based equine dentistry, **519–524**. See also *Equine dentistry, evidence-based*.

Evidence-based gastrointestinal medicine, **243–266**. See also *Gastrointestinal medicine, evidence-based*.

Evidence-based gastrointestinal surgery, **267–292**. See also *Gastrointestinal surgery, evidence-based*.

Evidence-based immunizations, **481–508**. See also *Immunization(s), evidence-based*.

Evidence-based medicine, in critical care, **293–316**. See also *Critical care, evidence-based medicine in*.

Evidence-based musculoskeletal surgery, **461–479**. See also *Musculoskeletal surgery, evidence-based*.

Evidence-based nutrition, **365–384**. See also *Nutrition, evidence-based*.

Evidence-based parasitology, **509–517**. See also *Intestinal disease, parasitic*.

Evidence-based pharmacology, 203

Evidence-based respiratory medicine, **215–227**. See also *Respiratory medicine, evidence-based*.

Exercise, effects on glucose and insulin metabolism, 369

Exercise-induced pulmonary hemorrhage (EIPH), evidence-based respiratory medicine for, 221–223

Exploratory celiotomy, complications after, 272–280
   incisional, 273–275
      bandages and, 279–280
      repeat celiotomy and, 280
      risk factors for, 275–280
      suture materials and patterns and, 276–279

F

Farriery techniques. See also *Shoeing*.
   biomechanical effects of, evidence-based assessment of, **425–442**

Fecal egg counts, 514

Fever(s), Potomac horse, evidence-based immunizations for, 494–495

Flaxseed, as nutritional supplement, 377

Fluid therapy, for gastrointestinal disease, 249–251

Foot, biomechanics of, in lame horses, 436–437

Fracture(s)
   chip, evidence-based surgery for, 464–465
   dorsal cortical, of third metacarpal bone, evidence-based surgery for, 470–471
   long bone, evidence-based surgery for, 463–464
   metacarpal, second and fourth, evidence-based surgery for, 469–470
   metatarsal, second and fourth, evidence-based surgery for, 469–470

G

Garlic, as nutritional supplement, 377

Gastric ulcer syndrome
   evidence-based medicine for, 253–255
   risk factors for, 252–253

Gastric ulcers, nutritional prevention of, 375–376

Gastrointestinal medicine, evidence-based, **243–266**
   analgesia for colic, 244–245
   fluid therapy in, 249–251
   for colic, 258–261
   for equine gastric ulcer syndrome, 252–255
   for ileus, 246–247

Gastrointestinal medicine (*continued*)
  for renospenic entrapment of large colon, 247–249
  for salmonellosis, 251–252

Gastrointestinal surgery, evidence-based, **267–292**
  complications of, 284–285
  exploratory celiotomy, complications after, 272–280. See also *Exploratory celiotomy, complications after*.
  large intestinal surgery, survival after, 272
  long-term survival after, 284–285
  postoperative ileus, 280–283
  small intestinal surgery, short-term survival after, 270–272
  survivors of, 268–270

Gender, as factor in PPID, 340–341

Genetic traits, effects on glucose and insulin metabolism, 369

Geriatric horses, feeding of, 378–380

Ginger, as nutritional supplement, 377–378

Ginseng, as nutritional supplement, 378

Glucose, metabolism of, evaluation of, 366–370

Glucose-intolerant horses, feeding of, 370–371

Glycemic index, in evaluation of glucose and insulin metabolism, 366–367

Guttoral pouches, evidence-based respiratory medicine for, 223–224

H

Hemiplegia, laryngeal, 231–235. See also *Laryngeal hyperplasia*.

Hemorrhage, pulmonary, exercise-induced, evidence-based respiratory medicine for, 221–223

Herb(s), in evidence-based practice, in equine medicine and surgery, 208–209

Herbal supplements, 376–378
  bee pollen, 376–377
  echinacea, 377
  flaxseed, 377
  garlic, 377
  ginger, 377–378
  ginseng, 378
  propolis, 376–377
  valerian, 378

Herpesvirus(es)
  1, evidence-based immunizations for, 488–491
  4, evidence-based immunizations for, 488–491

Hoof balance, biomechanics and, 429

Hormone(s), thyrotropin-releasing, in PPID diagnosis, 344–345

Hyperinsulinemia, 348–349

Hypotension, refractory, in septic patients, vasopressin for, 305–312

Hypothyroidism
  diagnosis of, 333–334
  primary, existence of, 329–330
  secondary, 334–335
    management of, 335

Hypovolemic patients, resuscitation of, colloid solutions vs. crystalloids in, 300–305

I

Ileus
  postoperative, 280–283
    repeat celiotomy and, 283
  prokinetic agents for, 246–247

Immunization(s), evidence-based, **481–508**
  evaluation of, 483–484
  for equine encephalitides, 497–498
  for equine herpesviruses 1 and 4, 488–491
  for equine influenza virus, 485–488
  for equine viral arteritis, 495–497
  for Potomac horse fever, 494–495
  for strangles, 498–500
  for tetanus, 500–501
  for West Nile virus, 491–494
  mechanisms of action of, 482–483

Incisional bandages, incisional complications associated with, 279–280

Influenza virus, evidence-based immunizations for, 485–488

Insulin, metabolism of, evaluation of, 366–370

Insulin resistance, demonstration of, 349–350

Insulin sensitivity, measurement of, in PPID diagnosis, 348–349

Insulinresistant horses, feeding of, 370–371

Intestinal disease, parasitic, 509–511
  strongyles
    large, 509–510
    small, 510–511

tapeworms, 511
treatment of, timing of, 511–512

Intestinal parasitism, disease due to, 509–511

L

Lame horses, foot biomechanics of, 436–437

Large colon, renospenic entrapment of, 247–249

Large intestinal surgery, survival after, 272

Laryngeal hyperplasia, 231–235
arytenoidectomy for, 234
laryngeal reinnervation for, 233
prosthetic laryngoplasty for, 231–233

Laryngeal reinnervation, for laryngeal hyperplasia, 233

Laryngoplasty, prosthetic, for laryngeal hyperplasia, 231–233

Lidocaine, for ileus, 246

Literature, evidence-based, on thyroid dysfunction, **329–336**. See also *Thyroid dysfunction, evidence-based literature on.*

Long bone fractures, evidence-based surgery for, 463–464

M

Metacarpal bones, third, dorsal cortical fractures of, evidence-based surgery for, 470–471

Metacarpal fractures, second and fourth, evidence-based surgery for, 469–470

Metacarpophalangeal joint, shoeing effects on, 433–434

Metatarsal fractures, second and fourth, evidence-based surgery for, 469–470

Metoclopramide, for ileus, 246

Musculoskeletal surgery, evidence-based, **461–479**
arthrodesis, 467–468
for angular limb deformities, 468–469
for chip fractures, 464–465
for dorsal cortical fractures of third metacarpal bone, 470–471
for long bone fractures, 463–464
for osteochondrosis, 465–467
for second and fourth metacarpal or metatarsal fractures, 469–470

for tendonitis, 473–474
palmar digital neurectomy, 471–473

N

Neorickettsia risticii, evidence-based immunizations for, 494–495

Neurectomy, palmar digital, 471–473

Neurology, clinical questions in, evidence-based approach to, **317–328**

Noise, respiratory, upper respiratory surgery for, 235

Norepinephrine
in evidence-based medicine in critical care, 310–312
vasopressin with, for catecholamine-resistance vasodilatory shock, 306–307

Nutrition, evidence-based, **365–384**
evaluation of glucose and insulin metabolism
age in, 369
clinical implications in, 368
diurnal variation in, 369
exercise in, 369
genetic traits in, 369
glycemic index in, 366–367
obesity in, 369
quality of evidence in, 368
ration adaptation in, 367–368
stress in, 369
for geriatric horses, 378–380
for glucose-intolerant horses, 370–371
for insulin-resistant horses, 370–371
for young horses, 371–375
herbal supplements in, 376–378. See also *Herbal supplements.*
in gastric ulcer prevention, 375–376

O

Obesity, effects on glucose and insulin metabolism, 369

Occlusal equilibration
performance and, 521–523
weight loss and, 520–521

Oteochondrosis, evidence-based surgery for, 465–467

P

Palate(s), soft, dorsal placement of, upper respiratory surgery for, 235–239

Palmar digital neurectomy, 471–473

Parasite control programs, anthelmintics in, 512–514

Parasitism, intestinal, disease due to, 509–511

Parasitology, evidence-based, **509–517**. See also *Intestinal disease, parasitic.*

Pergolide, for PPID, 353–354

Pharmacology, evidence-based, 203

Phenylephrine, in evidence-based medicine in critical care, 310

PIP joint. See Proximal interphalangeal (PIP) joint.

Pituitary gland
　domperidone effects on, in PPID diagnosis, 351–352
　imaging of, in PPID diagnosis, 352
　loss of dopaminergic inhibition effects on, 338–340

Pituitary pars intermedia dysfunction (PPID)
　cause of, 337–338
　diagnosis of
　　antemortem, low-dose dexamethasone suppression test in, 343–344
　　clinical, corroborating of, 342
　　corticotropin stimulation test in, 348
　　domperidone effects on pituitary gland in, 351–352
　　from single blood samples, proopiomelanocortin peptide assays in, 350–351
　　imaging of pituitary gland in, 352
　　insulin sensitivity in, 348–349
　　plasma cortisol concentration determination in, 342
　　plasma insulin concentration measurement in, 348–349
　　resting plasma corticotropin concentration measurement in, 346–348
　　thyrotropin-releasing hormone in, 344–345
　　timing of, 352
　gender predilection for, 340–341
　management of, 352–355
　　antioxidants in, 355–356
　　cyproheptadine in, 353
　　pergolide in, 353–354
　　response to, evaluation of, 356–357
　　trilostane in, 354–355
　seasonality of, 340–341

Placenta, retained, in broodmares, treatment of, 393–398

Plasma corticotropin concentration, resting, measurement of, in PPID diagnosis, 346–348

Plasma cortisol concentration, determination of, in PPID diagnosis, 342

Plasma insulin concentration, measurement of, in PPID diagnosis, 348–349

Postbreeding antibiotic infusion, in broodmares, 387–390

Potion mixing, 201–203

Potomac horse fever, evidence-based immunizations for, 494–495

PPID. See *Pituitary pars intermedia dysfunction (PPID).*

Pregnancy, early, in broodmares, progesterone supplementation in, 390–392

Progesterone supplementation, in broodmares, in early pregnancy, 390–392

Prokinetic agents, for ileus, 246–247

Proopiomelanocortin peptide assays, from single blood samples, in PPID diagnosis, 350–351

Propolis, as nutritional supplement, 376–377

Prosthetic laryngoplasty, for laryngeal hyperplasia, 231–233

Proximal interphalangeal (PIP) joint, shoeing effects on, 432–433

Publication bias, drug use and, 208

Pulmonary hemorrhage, exercise-induced, evidence-based respiratory medicine for, 221–223

R

Ration adaptation, in evaluation of glucose and insulin metabolism, 367–368

Recurrent airway obstruction (RAO), evidence-based respiratory medicine for, 215–221

Refractory hypotension, in septic patients, vasopression for, 305–312

Renospenic entrapment of large colon, 247–249

Repeat celiotomy
    incisional complications associated with, 280
    postoperative ileus and, 283

Respiratory medicine, evidence-based, **215–227**
    for EIPH, 221–223
    for guttoral pouches, 223–224
    for lower airway conditions, 215–223
    for upper airway diseases, 223–224

Respiratory noise, upper respiratory surgery for, 235

Resting plasma corticotropin concentration, measurement of, in PPID diagnosis, 346–348

Resuscitation, of hypovolemic patients, colloid solutions vs. crystalloids in, 300–305

S

Salmonellosis, diagnosis of, 251–252

Seasonality, of PPID, 340–341

Sepsis
    mortality due to, tissue oxygenation in reduction of, EGDT in, 295–300
    refractory hypotension and, vasopressin for, 305–312

Septic shock, vasopressin in patients with, 307–308

Shock
    catecholamine-resistance vasodilatory, vasopressin and norepinephrine for, 306–307
    septic, vasopressin in patients with, 307–308

Shoe(s), applying of, effects of, 428–429

Shoeing
    biomechanical effects of
        artificial manipulations, 431–436
        change in frontal plane, 436
        change in ground contact, 429–430
        change in heel or toe height, 431–432
        change in toe position or length, 435–436
        changes in sagittal plane, 430–431
        DIP joint–related, 432
        evidence-based assessment of, **425–442**
        metacarpophalangeal joint–related, 433–434
        PIP joint–related, 432–433
        stance characteristics, 432
        tendon strains–related, 434–435
    conformation and, injuries related to, 437–438

Small intestinal surgery, short-term survival after, 270–272

Soft palate, dorsal placement of, upper respiratory surgery for, 235–239

Strain(s), tendon, shoeing effects on, 434–435

Strangles, evidence-based immunizations for, 498–500

Streptococcus equi, subsp. *equi,* evidence-based immunizations for, 498–500

Stress, effects on glucose and insulin metabolism, 369

Strongyle(s)
    large, intestinal disease due to, 509–510
    small, intestinal disease due to, 510–511

Suture materials and patterns, incisional complications associated with, 276–279

T

Tendon strains, shoeing effects on, 434–435

Tendonitis, evidence-based surgery for, 473–474

Tetanus, evidence-based immunizations for, 500–501

Third metacarpal bone, dorsal cortical fractures of, evidence-based surgery for, 470–471

Thyroid dysfunction
    described, 330–333
    evidence-based literature on, **329–336**
        hypothyroidism, 329–335
        hypothyroidism in, primary, 329–330
        thyroid tumors, 335–336

Thyroid supplementation, in broodmares, 385–387

Thyroid tumors, 335–336

Thyrotropin-releasing hormone, in PPID diagnosis, 344–345

Trilostane, for PPID, 354–355

Tumor(s), thyroid, 335–336

U

Ulcer(s), gastric, nutritional prevention of, 375–376

Upper airway diseases, evidence-based respiratory medicine for, 223–224

Upper respiratory surgery, **229–242.** See also specific indication, e.g., *Laryngeal hyperplasia.*
for dorsal placement of soft palate, 235–239
for epiglottic entrapment, 239–240
for laryngeal hemiplegia, 231–235
for respiratory noise, 235

V

Vaccination(s). See *Immunization(s).*

Valerian, as nutritional supplement, 378

Vasopressin
for refractory hypotension in septic patients, 305–312
in patients with septic shock, 307–308
norepinephrine with, for catecholamine-resistance vasodilatory shock, 306–307

Viral arteritis, evidence-based immunizations for, 495–497

Vitex agnus castus extract, for PPID, 355

W

Weight loss, occlusal equilibration and, 520–521

West Nile virus, evidence-based immunizations for, 491–494

Worm(s), anthelmintics for killing, 512

Y

Young horses, feeding of, 371–375

Moving?

Make sure your subscription moves with you!

To notify us of your new address, find your **Clinics Account Number** (located on your mailing label above your name), and contact customer service at:

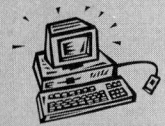

E-mail: elspcs@elsevier.com

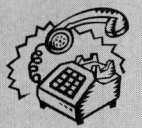

800-654-2452 (subscribers in the U.S. & Canada)
407-345-4000 (subscribers outside of the U.S. & Canada)

Fax number: 407-363-9661

Elsevier Periodicals Customer Service
6277 Sea Harbor Drive
Orlando, FL 32887-4800

*To ensure uninterrupted delivery of your subscription, please notify us at least 4 weeks in advance of move.